Epidemiologic Analysis

EPIDEMIOLOGIC ANALYSIS

A Case-Oriented Approach

STEVE SELVIN

University of California, Berkeley

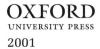

OXFORD
UNIVERSITY PRESS
2001

OXFORD
UNIVERSITY PRESS

Oxford   New York
Athens   Auckland   Bangkok   Bogotá   Buenos Aires   Calcutta
Cape Town   Chennai   Dar es Salaam   Delhi   Florence   Hong Kong   Istanbul
Karachi   Kuala Lumpur   Madrid   Melbourne   Mexico City   Mumbai
Nairobi   Paris   São Paulo   Shanghai   Singapore   Taipei   Tokyo   Toronto   Warsaw

and associated companies in

Berlin   Ibadan

Published by Oxford University Press, Inc.,
198 Madison Avenue, New York, New York, 10016
http://www.oup-usa.org

Library of Congress Cataloging-in-Publication Data
Selvin, S.
Epidemiologic analysis: a case-oriented approach / Steve Selvin.
p. cm.   Includes bibliographical references and index.
ISBN 0-19-514618-2—ISBN 0-19-514489-9 (pbk.)
1. Epidemiology—Statistical methods.   I. Title.
RA652.2.M3 S445 2001   614.4'07'2—dc21   00-053039

9 8 7 6 5 4 3 2 1

Printed in the United States of America
on acid-free paper

for Nancy and Liz

Preface

My intent in these pages is to describe a path through the forest of biostatistical/ statistical procedures to efficient and effective analytic methods. No one method automatically yields the right answer, but a variety of methods creates a well-equipped tool kit, which is essential for dealing with the increasing complexity of modern data. Our choices among the varied tools are dictated by the kind of data we collect and the questions we ask. In practice, the application of statistical methods is very much an art form; its effectiveness depends largely on the tools, knowledge, and skills of the user.

We will explore 19 case studies, each illustrating important approaches to analyzing an actual research problem. These cases are based on real data from published sources, spotlighting a number of areas found in medical and epidemiologic research. They range from Mendel's classic sweet pea experiments to current studies of the risk of AIDS and the association of birth defects with exposure to electromagnetic field radiation. A few data sets were drawn from readily available survey data (for example, the Surveillance, Epidemiology, and End Results database) and routinely collected public data (for example, California state vital records). As might be expected, these casebook examples involve a number of different sampling patterns and kinds of data (for example, case/control, prospective and cross-sectional samples as well as observational, experimental and clinical data). All data sets are obtainable from an Internet website.*

The statistical techniques also span a broad range of analytic strategies. These techniques, like the data, range from classic (for example, *t*-tests and

*http://socrates.berkeley.edu/~biostat/Courses/Spring/Ph29632/

regression models) to modern methods (for example, randomization tests, bootstrap estimation, and general additive models). Most case studies include both model-free (nonparametric) and model-based (parametric) approaches applied to the same data set. Such approaches as logistic regression, Poisson regression, matched data analysis, log-linear models, survival analysis, multivariate methods, and nonparametric regression are illustrated and explored, with a focus on describing, interpreting, and presenting results.

Graphic methods and computer-intensive analytic tools are particularly emphasized in a number of case studies. Graphic displays of both the data and the analytic results enhance the understanding of the statistical approach, frequently providing key insights of their own into the topics under study. For example, the analysis of vitamin use and the risk of a birth defect (a three-way table) is enriched with four plots illustrating the geometry of contingency table analysis. To quote Will Rogers, "You must never tell a thing. You must illustrate it. We learn through the eye and not the noggin." In short, the more than 100 plots, charts, figures, and graphs display the geometry of the data analyses. Computer-intensive methods such as bootstrap estimation and randomization tests, illustrated in several analyses, are conceptually simple and widely applicable but do not enjoy the popularity they deserve. These techniques harness the power of a modern computer to produce estimated variances, estimated distributions, and confidence intervals based on only minimal assumptions. These estimated quantities are necessities in understanding the issues that frequently arise in statistically analyzing a data set.

Each case analysis is designed to produce realistic answers to concrete research questions. I have maintained a sharp focus on real-world issues, illustrated by applied examples, to give a wide audience access to valuable statistical tools. Theoretical concepts are usually replaced by intuitive explanations and casebook examples. Readers interested in pursuing any topic in more depth will find references to the relevant textbooks and journal articles. Each of these 19 studies begins with a statement of the problem followed by a concise description of the relevant data and an explanation of their computer-file structure. Then, a bit of background is presented, leading to a detailed account of the data analysis. Each analysis starts with a few simple descriptive statistics and plots before turning to the increasingly specific and sophisticated analytic methods. The overall purpose is to provide useful answers to the proposed questions based on statistical analysis, illustrating effective statistical practice in general.

The analyses in this text are one person's opinion as to how the data should be explored, but there is abundant room for other ideas and approaches. Based on the data and the description given in the first two pages of each case study, readers are encouraged to try alternative analytic strategies, draw their own conclusions, and compare the results to those formally presented. An appendix explains some of the technical details used in the case analyses for readers who wish to delve into the more mathematical side of data analysis. With a bit of algebra, some of the mysteries of the statistical procedures are unveiled, leading to a better understanding of the statistical process. For example, expressions for calculating the variance of many statistical summaries are widely used in elementary tasks but are less widely explained. The appendix contains some explanations. The technical material in this text is generally at the advanced beginner or intermediate level. These 19 case studies are the basis of a biostatistics/epidemiology course taught at the University of California, Berkeley, to graduate students with a background of two or three semesters of biostatistics.

One last note: Clearly, the data analysis was executed with modern computer hardware and software. The analyses and plots are direct applications of the S-Plus system (Version 3.4 Release 1 for Sun SPARC, SunOS 5.3 : 1996). The same techniques, however, can certainly be found in other popular statistical analysis systems (for example, SAS, Stata, and Statistica). The use of another analytic system should present no special problems to those who wish to duplicate the presented results or use the data to explore their own approaches.

Contents

Appendix

Epidemiologic Analysis

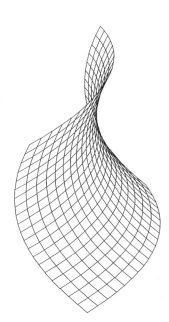

CHAPTER 1

Measurement of Trend (a 2 by *c* Table)

OBJECTIVE

To compare the frequency of infants with a single congenital malformation to that of infants with multiple congenital malformations, focusing on evaluating changes over time.

DATA

Extensive data on infants with major congenital malformations are routinely collected as part of a state surveillance system called the California Birth Defects Monitoring Program. Records of infants identified as having a single major malformation or more than one major malformation were obtained from this program. A selection of these infants was made from the years 1983 to 1991 in two Bay Area counties (San Francisco and Santa Clara). A total of 9119 sampled infants were tabulated by the number of birth defects (rows: more than one major birth defect and only one major birth defect) and the year of birth (columns: year of birth—1983, 1984, . . . , 1991), forming a 2 by 9 table. Since no population at risk is recorded, it should be kept in mind that these data cannot be used to compute rates of birth defects (estimate risk) but were collected to study the trends in the frequency of multiple defects over time.

METHODS

Chi-square and regression techniques are used to assess the overall association between the occurrence of multiple birth defects and the year of birth.
In addition, a summary chi-square statistic is partitioned into compartments
reflecting linear and nonlinear trends over time. A parallel logistic regression
model is also used to evaluate the pattern of change during the nine years.

Data type: surveillance
Reference: public data, California Birth Defects Monitoring Program

The variables are:

1. Year of birth: year as recorded
2. Number of congenital defects: coded 1 for infants with more than one major
   defect and 0 for infants with only one major defect

The tabulated data file of 9119 infants is:

```
file name = multiple.1.data

    year    one+    one
    1983    369     460
    1984    434     434
    1985    506     487
    1986    521     518
    1987    526     488
    1988    605     481
    1989    649     477
    1990    733     395
    1991    688     348
```

DISCUSSION

Observations, such as birth defects, classified by a binary variable and a
c-level categorical variable, such as year of occurrence, produce a table of
counts with two rows and c columns. Such a 2 by c table can be treated like
any contingency table. Chi-square tests for independence apply, a number of
measures of association indicate the dependence of one categorical variable
on the other, and extensive theory justifies these and other analytic approaches. Additionally, when the variable with c levels consists of an ordered
sequence of meaningful numeric values, a 2 by c table takes on an additional
dimension. Issues of trend become relevant. In a similar context, a 2 by c
table occasionally provides a description of a dose–response relationship. In
either case, it is important to describe and analyze changes reflected by the
binary variable over differing levels of the numeric but categorical variable.

Table 1.1. Number of Infants with More Than One and Only One Congenital
Defect Born Between 1983 and 1991 in San Francisco and
Santa Clara Counties, California

Defects/Years	1983	1984	1985	1986	1987	1988	1989	1990	1991	Total
more than one	369	434	506	521	526	605	649	733	688	5031
only one	460	434	487	518	488	481	477	395	348	4088
total	829	868	993	1039	1014	1086	1126	1128	1036	9119
proportion ($\hat{p}_i$)	0.445	0.500	0.510	0.501	0.519	0.557	0.576	0.650	0.664	0.552

The number of infants born with one congenital defect or more than one during the years 1983 to 1991 are naturally displayed in a 2 by 9 table (Table 1.1). A strategic first question to address is whether any relationship whatsoever exists between the proportion of infants with multiple birth defects and the year of birth. The analysis starts with this question because if no relationship exists, then the counts in the table are unrelated to each categorical variable, making a table unnecessary.

When the two categorical variables (defects and years) in Table 1.1 are statistically independent, the number of counts in each cell depends separately on the row and column marginal frequencies. Such independence allows the calculation of an expected frequency for each of the 18 cells in the defects by year table. For example, in terms of probabilities,

P (a birth with more than one defect in 1988)
$$= P \text{ (more than one defect)} \times P \text{ (born in 1988)}.$$

Then

$$P \text{ (a birth with more than one defect in 1988)} = \frac{5031}{9119} \times \frac{1086}{9119} = 0.0657.$$

The expected number of infants born in 1988 with multiple defects is $9119(0.0657) = 599.2$ if the probability of more than one defect (among all infants with at least one birth defect) is unrelated to the year of birth. In other words, each cell frequency is completely determined by two marginal probabilities. For 1988, the observed number of multiple defects is 605.

From another perspective, independence requires that

$$P \text{ (more than one defect | year of birth)} = P \text{ (more than one defect)}$$

and P (more than one defect) is estimated by $5031/9119 = 0.552$ (ignoring year of birth). The expected number of infants with multiple defects born in

1988 is again $1086(0.552) = 599.2$. In general, the estimated cell frequencies are identical regardless of which definition of independence is considered. The 18 expected frequencies of infants with more than one defect and infants with only one defect for all nine years are given in Table 1.2 based on the conjecture of independence and the observed marginal probabilities.

The estimated cell frequencies in Table 1.2 are exactly independent (absolutely no association between the occurrence of a birth defect and year of birth) and have marginal frequencies identical to those in the original table. A consequence of independence is that the nine ratios of the row frequencies are identical for all columns and the ratio of any two column frequencies is the same for both rows. Also note that, as expected, independence dictates that the proportion of infants with more than one major birth defect is the same for all years (last row—0.552).

A summary comparison of the 18 expected values (denoted e_i—Table 1.2) and the 18 observed values (denoted o_i—Table 1.1) is readily achieved using Pearson's classic chi-square test statistic (a.5), where

$$X^2 = \sum \left[\frac{(o_i - e_i)^2}{e_i} \right] = \frac{(369 - 457.4)^2}{457.4} + \cdots + \frac{(348 - 464.4)^2}{464.4} = 169.376.$$

The test statistic X^2 has an approximate chi-square distribution with $c - 1 = 9 - 1 = 8$ degrees of freedom when the number of birth defects and the year of birth are statistically independent.[1] The significance probability or p-value is $P(X^2 \geq 169.376 \mid \text{no association}) < 0.001$, indicating that the conjecture of independence is not plausible.

The next question is: *since an association likely exists, what sort of association is it?* To begin to sort out the relationship between two categorical variables, a table of residual values is usually helpful. A residual value measures the relative correspondence between each observed and expected value. One definition (there are several) of a residual value is

$$\text{residual}_i = \frac{o_i - e_i}{\sqrt{e_i}}$$

Table 1.2. Expected Number of Infants with More Than One and Only One Major Congenital Defect Born Between 1983 and 1991 (Assuming Independence)

Defects/Years	1983	1984	1985	1986	1987	1988	1989	1990	1991	Total
more than one	457.4	478.9	547.8	573.2	559.4	599.2	621.2	622.3	571.6	5031
one	371.6	389.1	445.2	465.8	454.6	486.8	504.8	505.7	464.4	4088
total	829	868	993	1039	1014	1086	1126	1128	1036	9119
proportion ($\bar{p}$)	0.552	0.552	0.552	0.552	0.552	0.552	0.552	0.552	0.552	0.552

for the ith observation. The chi-square statistic is a sum of these squared residual values or

$$X^2 = \sum(\text{residual}_i)^2 = \sum \left[\frac{(o_i - e_i)^2}{e_i} \right].$$

Large absolute values of these contributions to the chi-square statistic (say, greater than 2) show where the lack of independence is most extreme. For the birth defects data, Table 1.3 contains the residual values calculated from the 18 observed and expected frequencies (Tables 1.1 and 1.2).

Inspection of the residual values shows that the smallest and largest values are associated with the most extreme years. In addition, an increasing pattern from low to high in the first row is apparent, indicating substantial and systematic changes in the frequency of multiple defects over the nine year period. An increasing frequency of multiple defects suggests that a good way to start a more formal description of this pattern is to postulate a linear relationship between the proportion of multiple defects and the year of birth (a.14).

The proportion of infants with more than one defect among all newborns with at least one birth defect calculated for each year is a natural description of data from the 2 by c table (denoted $\hat{p}_i$). A plot displaying these nine proportions (Table 1.1—last row) is given in Figure 1.1 (dotted line). The consistent increase over the nine years is clearly visible and appears at least approximately linear. In symbols, a straight line is represented as

$$\text{expected proportion in the } i\text{th year} = p_i = a + b\,(x_i - 1982)$$

where x_i represents the year of birth. To estimate a straight line summarizing trend, ordinary least squares estimation directly applies.

A 2 by c table, like all two-way tables, is a compact representation of pairs of observations (x_i, y_i). The data tabulated in Table 1.1 are 9119 pairs of observations (one observation for each recorded infant), where each pair is made up of a year and a binary variable indicating one or more than one defect

Table 1.3. Residual Values* from the 2 by c Table of Birth Defects Frequencies

Defects/Years	1983	1984	1985	1986	1987	1988	1989	1990	1991
more than one	−4.13	−2.05	−1.79	−2.18	−1.41	0.24	1.11	4.44	4.87
one		4.58	2.28	1.98	2.42	1.57	−0.27	−1.24	−4.92	−5.40

*The sum of these 18 squared residual values equals $X^2 = 169.376$.

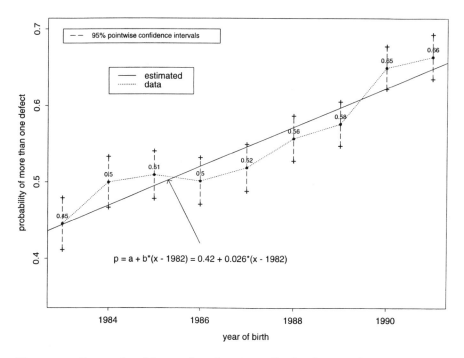

Figure 1.1. Proportion (observed and estimated) of infants with more than one major birth defect by the year of birth (1983–1991).

(a.14). To calculate the least squares estimated line, three sums based on all 9119 observations are necessary. They are

$$S_{xx} = \sum (x_i - \bar{x})^2$$

$$S_{yy} = \sum (y_i - \bar{y})^2$$

$$S_{xy} = \sum (x_i - \bar{x})(y_i - \bar{y}) \quad i = 1, 2, 3, \ldots, 9119$$

where x_i = year of birth and $y_i = \{0, \text{ or } 1\}$. Specifically,

$$S_{xx} = 58{,}000.320$$

$$S_{yy} = 2255.371$$

$$S_{xy} = 1481.174.$$

Shortcut expressions for these calculations are available[1] but are not necessary for a computer implementation.

The estimated slope of the line describing the proportion of infants with multiple defects (the $\hat{p}_i$-values) is $\hat{b} = S_{xy}/S_{xx} = 1481.174/58{,}000.320 = 0.026$, and the estimated intercept is $\hat{a}' = \bar{y} - \hat{b}\bar{x} = -50.197$ (usual theory[1]). These two estimates produce the least squares estimated line

$$\tilde{p}_i = \hat{a} + \hat{b}(x_i - 1982) = 0.418 + 0.026(x_i - 1982).$$

The year of birth generates estimates of the proportion of malformed infants with more than one birth defect (denoted $\tilde{p}_i$) based on a straight line, succinctly describing the nine year trend in the probability of multiple congenital malformations. The estimated straight line is displayed in Figure 1.1 (solid line), and the estimated values for each year are given in Table 1.4 ($\tilde{p}_i$—column 3). The year of birth is scaled by subtracting 1982 (sometimes called *centering*) so that the intercept is a meaningful value (i.e., when $x_0 = 1982$, then $\tilde{p}_0 = \hat{a} = 0.418$). Standardized deviations from the estimated straight line (represented by z_i—last column in Table 1.4) are

$$z_i = \frac{\hat{p}_i - \tilde{p}_i}{S_{\hat{p}_i}} = \frac{\hat{p}_i - \tilde{p}_i}{\sqrt{\hat{p}_i(1 - \hat{p}_i)/n_i}}$$

reflecting the correspondence between the data-generated proportions ($\hat{p}_i$) and the proportions generated by the estimated line ($\tilde{p}_i$). Thus, the nine z_i-values measure the degree of nonlinearity. Furthermore, each z_i-value has an approximate standard normal distribution when the trend in the p_i-values is linear. A summary measure of the lack of linearity then becomes the sum of the squared z_i-values or $X_{fit}^2 = \sum z_i^2 = 16.359$ (a.5). This summary has an approximate chi-square distribution with $c - 2 = 9 - 2 = 7$ degrees of freedom when the underlying annual proportion of multiple birth defects among all major defects is linearly related to the year of birth. The associated p-value is $P(X_{fit}^2 \geq 16.359 \mid \hat{p}_i \text{ randomly differs from } \tilde{p}_i) = 0.02$, indicating a statistically significant nonlinear component. When large numbers of observations are involved, however, small deviations that are unlikely by chance may

Table 1.4. Summary Results from the Least Squares Estimated Model
Applied to the Birth Defects Data

Year	$\hat{p}_i$	$\tilde{p}_i$	$\hat{p}_i - \tilde{p}_i$	$S_{\hat{p}_i}$	z_i
1983	0.445	0.444	0.001	0.017	0.063
1984	0.500	0.470	0.030	0.017	1.791
1985	0.510	0.495	0.014	0.016	0.907
1986	0.501	0.521	−0.019	0.016	−1.244
1987	0.519	0.546	−0.028	0.016	−1.758
1988	0.557	0.572	−0.015	0.015	−0.982
1989	0.576	0.597	−0.021	0.015	−1.442
1990	0.650	0.623	0.027	0.014	1.886
1991	0.664	0.649	0.015	0.015	1.055

not be particularly meaningful from the overall perspective of summarizing the observed trend by a straight line.

Another view of the role of linearity (or nonlinearity) in describing a series of proportions derived from a 2 by c table comes from a partitioning of the summary chi-square statistic. That is, the chi-square test statistic X^2 is divided into two pieces (a.14), one measuring the degree of linear trend (denoted X_L^2) and the other measuring the degree of nonlinearity (denoted X_{NL}^2). In symbols,

$$X^2 = X_L^2 + X_{NL}^2.$$

For the birth defects data, the overall summary chi-square statistic $X^2 = 169.376$ partitions into $X_L^2 = 153.350$ and $X_{NL}^2 = 16.026$. A measure of linear trend scaled to be between 0 and 1 then becomes $\hat{c} = X_L^2/X^2$ ($0 \leq \hat{c} \leq 1$). Specifically, $\hat{c} = 153.350/169.376 = 0.905$. In this sense, a straight line "explains" slightly more than 90% of the variation in the observed proportions.

The linear chi-square statistic X_L^2 is directly related to the least squares estimated slope $\hat{b}$. In fact,

$$z = \frac{\hat{b}}{S_{\hat{b}}} \quad \text{and} \quad z^2 = X_L^2$$

where $S_{\hat{b}}^2$ is the estimated variance of $\hat{b}$ given by $S_{yy}/(nS_{xx})$. Therefore,

$$S_{\hat{b}}^2 = \frac{S_{yy}}{nS_{xx}} = \frac{2255.371}{9119(58{,}000.320)} = 0.00000426$$

and

$$X_L^2 = z^2 = \left[\frac{0.026}{\sqrt{0.00000426}}\right]^2 = (12.383)^2 = 153.350.$$

Under the condition that the year of birth has absolutely no linear influence ($b = 0$) on the probability of a multiple defect (a.14), the value of the test statistic X_L^2 has an approximate chi-square distribution with one degree of freedom. The value X_L^2 reflects the differences between the $\tilde{p}_i$-estimates based on a straight line with slope $\hat{b}$ and a constant proportion ($\bar{p} = 5031/9119 = 0.552$—a horizontal line).

In addition, the chi-square statistic measuring nonlinearity is directly calculated by subtraction where $X_{NL}^2 = X^2 - X_L^2$. The test statistic X_{NL}^2 has a chi-square distribution when the observed proportions $\hat{p}_i$ differ from a straight line only because of chance variation. The value X_{NL}^2 is not very different from the previous measure of lack of linearity. Specifically, $X_{NL}^2 = X^2 - X_L^2 = 169.376 - 153.350 = 16.026$ and $X_{fit}^2 = 16.359$. As before, the chi-square statistic X_{NL}^2 summarizes the differences between the proportions $\hat{p}_i$ observed for each year of birth and the estimated $\tilde{p}_i$-values based on an estimated straight line (again columns 2 and 3 in Table 1.4).

Another seemingly different approach to assessing the linearity of a series of proportions is the comparison of two mean values. Instead of comparing the proportions of birth defects among columns, the mean values summarizing the distributions of the c-level categorical variable are compared between the two rows. These two mean values are the mean year of occurrence of the multiple defects and the mean year of occurrence of the single defects; specifically, $\bar{x}_1 = 1987.505$ (row 1—multiple defects) based on $m_1 = 5031$ observations and $\bar{x}_2 = 1986.848$ (row 2—single defects) based on $m_2 = 4088$ observations (Table 1.1). A large difference implies that the two distributions of multiple defects differ systematically over the time period 1983 to 1991; conversely, mean values that hardly differ imply that no association exists with year of birth.

A t-like test statistic measuring the difference between these two mean values is

$$z = \frac{(\bar{x}_1 - \bar{x}_2) - 0}{S_{\bar{x}_1 - \bar{x}_2}} = \frac{1987.505 - 1986.848}{0.053} = \frac{0.657}{0.053} = 12.383$$

where

$$S_{\bar{x}_1 - \bar{x}_2}^2 = \frac{S_{xx}}{n}\left[\frac{1}{m_1} + \frac{1}{m_2}\right] = \frac{58{,}000.32}{9119}\left[\frac{1}{5031} + \frac{1}{4088}\right] = 0.00282$$

and, as usual, z^2 has an approximate chi-square distribution with one degree of freedom when no difference exists between the two mean values (a.14). For the birth defects data, $z^2 = (12.383)^2 = 153.350$. The birth defects example shows what is true in general: $z^2 = X_L^2$. Therefore, the "t-test" between mean values is no more than an alternative form of the previous chi-square test based on the estimated slope.

Another form of the linear chi-square statistic X_L^2 is related to the correlation within the $n = 9119$ pairs of observations. A correlation coefficient is estimated by applying the usual expression $r_{xy} = S_{xy}/\sqrt{S_{xx}S_{yy}}$, and using the birth defects data gives $r_{xy} = 1481.174/\sqrt{(58{,}000.320)(2255.371)} = 0.130$. Then $X_L^2 = nr_{xy}^2 = 9119(0.130)^2 = 153.350$ (a.14).

The summary quantities $\hat{b}$, $\bar{x}_1 - \bar{x}_2$, and r_{xy} are expected to be zero or close to zero when no linear association exists between a binary variable and the c-level numeric variable in a 2 by c table. All three statistics address the same question: *is there evidence that the slope of a straight line summarizing the data differs systemically from zero?* Thus, from an analytic point of view, no persuasive reason exists to choose one description over the other, since each can be transformed to have the same test statistic (X_L^2) and, therefore, yield identical statistical results.

Logistic Model Approach

A linear logistic model is yet another way to describe and analyze the probabilities associated with a binary outcome and certainly applies to a binary outcome summarized in a 2 by c table. A logistic model relating year of birth (again, denoted x_i) and the risk of more than one major birth defect, in terms of log-odds, is

$$\text{log-odds}_i = \log\left(\frac{p_i}{1 - p_i}\right) = A + B\,(x_i - 1982)$$

or, in terms of logistic probabilities

$$p_i = \frac{1}{1 + e^{-\text{logs-odds}_i}} = \frac{1}{1 + e^{-[A + B(x_i - 1982)]}}$$

where $p_i = P$ (a birth with more than one defect | year of birth = x_i) (a.17). The logistic model parameters A and B are estimated either from the 9119 pairs of observations or from the nine proportions ($\hat{p}_i$—Table 1.1). In either case, the estimates are $\hat{A} = -0.333$ and $\hat{B} = 0.104$. The estimated log-odds are displayed in Figure 1.2 (solid line) based on the expression log-odds = $-0.333 + 0.104(x_i - 1982)$. Figure 1.2 also displays the observed log-odds values calculated directly from the data (dotted line). The estimated parameters yield model-generated annual probabilities of a multiple birth defect where

$$\tilde{p}_i' = \frac{1}{1 + e^{-[-0.333 + 0.104(x_i - 1982)]}} \qquad x_i = 1983, 1984, 1985, \ldots, 1991.$$

These 9 estimated probabilities are not very different from the least squares estimates based on a straight line ($\tilde{p}_i$ and $\hat{p}'$—Tables 1.4 and 1.5). An analysis based on the observed proportions (linear) and an analysis of the log-odds (logistic) generally give similar results when the values of $\hat{p}_i$ are in the neighborhood of 0.5 (say, $0.3 \leq \hat{p}_i \leq 0.7$). The reason for the similarity relates to the fact that the log-odds associated with a probability close to 0.5 is approximately a linear function of that probability (i.e., $-2.072 + 4.145p \approx \log[p/(1 - p)] = \text{log-odds}$).

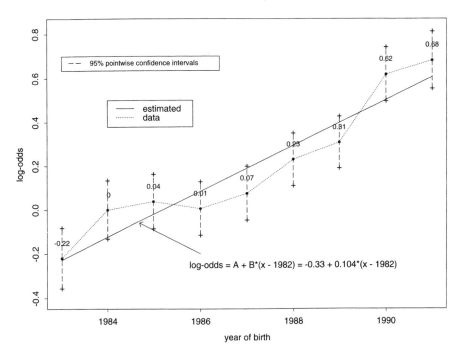

Figure 1.2. Log-odds (observed and logistic model estimated) associated with the risk of more than one major birth defect by the year of birth.

CONCLUSIONS

The process of estimating the slope (either $\hat{b}$ or $\hat{B}$) of a regression line from a 2 by c table and assessing its statistical importance is sometimes referred to as a *"test for trend"* but, more precisely, it is a test for linear trend—a linear trend based on proportions ($\hat{b}$) or a linear trend based on log-odds values ($\hat{B}$). A classic paper on strengthening the chi-square analysis of contingency

Table 1.5. Summary of the Results from the Logistic Model Analysis Applied to the Birth Defects Data

Year	$\hat{p}_i$	$\tilde{p}_i'$	$\hat{p}_i - \tilde{p}_i'$	$S_{\hat{p}_i}$	z_i
1983	0.445	0.443	0.002	0.017	0.113
1984	0.500	0.469	0.031	0.017	1.824
1985	0.510	0.495	0.014	0.016	0.913
1986	0.501	0.521	−0.020	0.016	−1.271
1987	0.519	0.547	−0.029	0.016	−1.808
1988	0.557	0.573	−0.016	0.015	−1.043
1989	0.576	0.598	−0.022	0.015	−1.477
1990	0.650	0.623	0.027	0.014	1.894
1991	0.664	0.647	0.017	0.015	1.158

table data by W. Cochran provides the original description of the test for linear trend.[1]

Several different analyses of the California birth defects surveillance data contained in a 2 by 9 table show a clear increase, almost linear, in the risk of multiple major birth defects among children with at least one major congenital anomaly over the period 1983 to 1991. A straight line summary "explains" about 90% of the variance in the proportions of multiple birth defects. A number of statistical tests indicate that random variation is an extremely implausible explanation for this observation (p-value < 0.001). A logistic regression model approach produces almost identical conclusions.

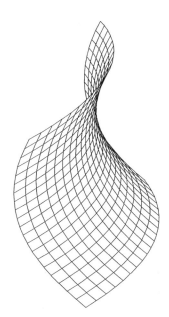

CHAPTER 2

Odds Ratio
and Relative Risk

PART I: ODDS RATIO

OBJECTIVE

To describe the relationship between exposure to maternal cigarette smoking during pregnancy and the risk of a low birth weight infant among four race/ethnicity groups.

DATA

A series of nonobese women delivering live-born infants at the University of California, San Francisco Moffitt Hospital between the years 1980 and 1990 provided data on their smoking histories and race/ethnicity (white, African-American, Hispanic, and Asian). The birth weight of each mother's infant was also recorded and classified as low birth weight (<2500 grams) or "normal" birth weight (≥2500 grams). For mothers with more than one delivery during the study period, a delivery was selected at random. After births with major congenital malformations, multiple births, and observations with missing data were removed, a total of 8859 mothers–infant pairs were available for study.

METHODS

A variety of model-free statistical measures are employed to evaluate the birth weight–smoking association, including odds ratios, Woolf's test for homogeneity, and the Mantel-Haenszel summary odds ratio. In addition, regression techniques were applied, essentially repeating the model-free analysis in the context of a logistic model.

Data type: cross-sectional (hospital records)
Reference: *Obstetrics and Gynecology*, 1995, 86(2): 163–9

The variables are:

1. Birth weight: coded 1 for infants weighing less than 2500 grams and 0 otherwise
2. Smoking: coded 1 if the mother reported smoking and 0 otherwise
3. Race/ethnicity: coded 1 for white, 2 for African-American, 3 for Hispanic, and coded 4 for Asian

The tabulated data file of 8859 mother–infant pairs is:

```
file name = lowbwt.2.data

x1      x2      x3      count
 0       0       1      3520
 1       0       1       169
 0       1       1       832
 1       1       1        98
 0       0       2       686
 1       0       2        55
 0       1       2       227
 1       1       2        54
 0       0       3       926
 1       0       3        61
 0       1       3        85
 1       1       3        11
 0       0       4      1936
 1       0       4        90
 0       1       4       102
 1       1       4         7

    x1 = birth weight,
   x2 = smoking exposure,
   x3 = race/ethnicity and
   count = cell frequency.
```

DISCUSSION

At the heart of many epidemiologic data sets is a 2 by 2 table or a series of 2 by 2 tables. Typically, a 2 by 2 table contains the counts of the joint occurrences of the four possible combinations of two binary variables (denoted a_i, b_i, c_i, and d_i forming the ith table). The notation for two binary variables, represented as "disease" and "exposure," producing four counts, is:

$table_i$	Disease	No Disease	Total
exposed	a_i	b_i	$a_i + b_i$
unexposed	c_i	d_i	$c_i + d_i$
total	$a_i + c_i$	$b_i + d_i$	n_i

where n_i represents the total number of observations ($n_i = a_i + b_i + c_i + d_i$) for a specific table, that is, the ith table in a series of $i = 1, 2, 3, . . . , k$ tables. For the smoking and low birth weight data, there are four race-specific 2 by 2 tables (Table 2.1).

There are two distinct ways to describe the association between smoking and low birth weight—one model-free and one model-based. In addition to selecting an analytic approach, a measure of association needs to be chosen. Among several useful measures of association, the most popular is the odds ratio (a.11). The odds ratio estimated from a 2 by 2 table (again, the ith table) is

$$\hat{or}_i = \frac{a_i/b_i}{c_i/d_i} = \frac{a_i/c_i}{b_i/d_i} = \frac{a_id_i}{b_ic_i}.$$

Four estimated odds ratios are given in Table 2.2 measuring the association between smoking and low birth weight for each race/ethnicity group.

Table 2.1. Data on Mother–Infant Pairs Classified by Smoking, Birth Weight, and Race/Ethnicity

White	<2500 g	≥2500 g	Total
smokers	98	832	930
nonsmokers	169	3520	3689
total	267	4352	4619
African-American	<2500 g	≥2500 g	Total
smokers	54	227	281
nonsmokers	55	686	741
total	109	913	1022
Hispanic	<2500 g	≥2500 g	Total
smokers	11	85	96
nonsmokers	61	926	987
total	72	1011	1083
Asian	<2500 g	≥2500 g	Total
smokers	7	102	109
nonsmokers	90	1936	2026
total	97	2038	2135

Table 2.2. Odds Ratios for Each Race/Ethnicity Group and Their
Approximate 95% Confidence Intervals

Race/Ethnicity	n_i	$\hat{or}_i$	Lower Bound	Upper Bound
white	4619	2.453	1.892	3.182
African-American	1022	2.967	1.980	4.446
Hispanic	1083	1.965	0.996	3.875
Asian	2135	1.476	0.667	3.267

A direct analysis of an estimated odds ratio is not very tractable. The fact that the complex distribution associated with an estimated odds ratio is not symmetric and that the odds ratio is fundamentally a multiplicative measure of association complicates statistical analysis. The situation is considerably simplified by transforming the odds ratio. An empirically successful transformation results from taking the logarithm of the odds ratio (using log ($\hat{or}_i$) instead of $\hat{or}_i$). The distribution of the transformed value is close to symmetric, and the log-odds ratio becomes an additive measure of association. The distribution of the log-odds ratio is then accurately approximated by a normal distribution, which is almost always the basis for analysis rather than the complicated distribution of the odds ratio itself. A log-odds ratio of zero ($or = 1$) implies no association, and both positive and negative values reflect the degree of association. Furthermore, log (or) and $-$log (or) are equal but opposite measures of association (additive scale). For the birth weight data, the estimated log-odds ratios are given in Table 2.3. The estimated variance associated with the logarithm of an estimated odds ratio [a.11] is calculated from the expression

$$\text{estimated variance log-odds ratio} = S^2_{\log(\hat{or}_i)} = \frac{1}{a_i} + \frac{1}{b_i} + \frac{1}{c_i} + \frac{1}{d_i}$$

and the race-specific values for the low birth weight data are given in Table 2.3. Two natural questions arise from Table 2.2 or 2.3: *do these four measures of association systematically differ among the race/ethnicity groups?* and *if the measures differ only because of random variation, what is their common value?*

Table 2.3. Logarithm of the Odds Ratios and Their Estimated Variances
for Each Race/Ethnicity Group

Race/Ethnicity	n_i	$\log(\hat{or}_i)$	$S^2_{\log(\hat{or}_i)}$	w_i
white	4619	0.897	0.018	56.795
African-American	1022	1.088	0.043	23.494
Hispanic	1083	0.675	0.120	8.323
Asian	2135	0.390	0.164	6.087

The first question is directly addressed by evaluating the amount of variation among the observed log-odds ratios. The degree of variability is measured relative to the mean log-odds ratio. An estimated mean log-odds ratio is achieved by a weighted average of the individual estimated values (a.12). That is, for k observed 2 by 2 tables

$$\text{mean log-odds ratio} = \overline{\log{(or)}} = \frac{\sum w_i \log{(\hat{or}_i)}}{\sum w_i} \quad i = 1, 2, 3, \ldots, k$$

where k log-odds ratios are combined and the weights are the reciprocal of the variances (denoted w_i—Table 2.3). Using weights $w_i = 1/S^2_{\log{(\hat{or}_i)}}$ emphasizes log-odds ratios estimated with high precision (small variances) and deemphasizes the less precise values (large variances). Weighting a series of estimates by their reciprocal variances produces a single summary estimate. This kind of weighted average is used in several of the following analyses (a.12). In fact, weighted averages are a fundamental statistical tool in epidemiologic analysis in general. From Table 2.3, the weighted average

$$\overline{\log{(or)}} = [56.795(0.897) + 23.494(1.088) + 8.323(0.675)$$
$$+ 6.087(0.390)]/94.699 = 0.892$$

is the estimated mean log-odds ratio. The somewhat awkward mean log-odds ratio is an effective measure of association and is easily interpreted when the averaged quantities estimate the same underlying value. Like the individual log-odds ratios, it too has an approximately normal distribution and is an additive measure of association.

Comparison of each observed value with the estimated common mean value measures the variation among the k individual log-odds ratios, and evaluation follows a typical chi-square pattern (a.5). Quantities with approximate standard normal distributions are created and squared; then the sum has an approximate chi-square distribution when the variation among the estimated log-odds ratios is strictly random. Specifically,

$$z_i = \frac{\log{(\hat{or}_i)} - \overline{\log{(or)}}}{S_{\log{(\hat{or}_i)}}}$$

has an approximate standard normal distribution. Therefore, the sum of squared values

$$X^2_W = \sum z_i^2 = \sum \left[\frac{\log{(\hat{or}_i)} - \overline{\log{(or)}}}{S_{\log{(\hat{or}_i)}}} \right]^2 = \sum w_i \left[\log{(\hat{or}_i)} - \overline{\log{(or)}} \right]^2$$

has an approximate chi-square distribution with $k - 1$ degrees of freedom when the estimates log $(\hat{or}_i)$ differ only because of chance variation $(i = 1, 2, 3, \ldots, k$ and k is the number of log-odds ratios compared). This test statistic is frequently referred to as *Woolf's chi-square test for homogeneity*[2] (a.5).

For the low birth weight data, Woolf's test statistic is

$$X_W^2 = 56.795(0.897 - 0.892)^2 + \cdots + 6.087(0.390 - 0.892)^2 = 2.828$$

and has an approximate chi-square distribution with three degrees of freedom when the underlying race-specific odds ratios are homogeneous (i.e., $or_1 = or_2 = or_3 = or_4 = or$). The probability of more extreme variation among the four estimated log-odds ratios by chance alone is p-value $= P(X_W^2 \geq 2.828$ | homogeneous) $= 0.42$. This result provides no persuasive evidence that the four odds ratios differ systematically among the four race/ethnicity groups.

Since no substantial evidence exists to the contrary, one usually proceeds as if the underlying odds ratios were homogeneous. Therefore, the next step is to estimate the common odds ratio. If one assumes that the four estimated odds ratios differ only because of random variation, three estimates of the common odds ratio are:

1. Woolf's estimate[2]: $\hat{or}_w = e^{\overline{\log (or)}} = e^{0.892} = 2.441$ (a.5),
2. Mantel-Haenszel estimate[3]: $\hat{or}_{MH} = (\sum a_i d_i / n_i)/(\sum b_i c_i / n_i) = 2.448$ (a.6), and
3. Maximum likelihood estimate[4]: $\hat{or}_{mlk} = 2.423$ (discussion to follow).

No important differences exist among the three estimates, which is typical for most sets of 2 by 2 tables, especially when the observed counts are large in all cells of all tables.

The estimated variance [a.12] of Woolf's weighted average estimate $\overline{\log (or)}$ is

$$S_{\overline{\log(or)}}^2 = \frac{1}{\sum w_i}$$

where the weights w_i are again the reciprocal of the estimated variances of each estimate log $(\hat{or}_i)$, given in Table 2.3. The smoking–birth weight data yield an estimate of $\overline{\log (or)} = 0.892$ with associated estimated variance of $S_{\overline{\log(or)}}^2 = 1/94.699 = 0.011$.

Because estimated summary values tend to have approximate normal distributions (particularly estimates that combine values sampled from symmetric distributions), accurate tests of significance can be conducted and approximate confidence intervals constructed. The estimated common odds ratio $\overline{\log (or)}$ is no exception. To compare the observed log-odds ratio to

$\log (or) = \log (1) = 0$ (i.e., no association between smoking and the risk of a low birth weight infant—$or = 1$), then

$$z = \frac{\overline{\log (or)} - \log (1)}{S_{\overline{\log (or)}}} = \frac{\overline{\log (or)} - 0}{\sqrt{1/\sum w_i}} = \frac{0.892 - 0}{\sqrt{0.011}} = 8.683$$

is a value from a standard normal distribution when no association exists. The corresponding p-value is $P (Z \geq 8.683 \mid$ no association$) < 0.001$, showing clear evidence of an association.

In addition, an approximate 95% confidence interval based on the estimate $\overline{\log (or)} = 0.892$ is

$$\text{lower bound} = \log (\hat{or}) - 1.960 \, S_{\log (\hat{or})} = 0.892 - 1.960\sqrt{0.011} = 0.691,$$

$$\text{lower bound} = \log (\hat{or}) + 1.960 \, S_{\log (\hat{or})} = 0.892 + 1.960\sqrt{0.011} = 1.093,$$

giving a confidence interval of (0.691, 1.093). Because $\hat{or}_w = e^{\overline{\log (or)}} = 2.441$, an approximate 95% confidence interval for the underlying summary odds ratio estimated by $\hat{or}_w = 2.441$ is

$$(e^{\text{lower bound}}, e^{\text{upper bound}}) = (e^{0.691}, e^{1.093}) = (1.996, 2.986).$$

In words, the 95% confidence interval indicates that the "true" common odds ratio is unlikely to be less than 1.996 or greater than 2.986.

A Natural Summary

The relationship between smoking exposure and low birth weight is naturally summarized by two conditional probabilities:

$$p_1 = P \text{ (low birth weight infant} \mid \text{smoking mother)}$$

and

$$p_2 = P \text{ (low birth weight infant} \mid \text{nonsmoking mother)}.$$

These two probabilities are estimated for each race/ethnicity group by the observed proportions of low birth weight infants delivered by mothers who smoke and mothers who do not smoke (denoted $\hat{p}_1$ and $\hat{p}_2$, respectively—Table 2.4).

Parallel to the odds ratio analysis, these proportions also show a strong influence of maternal smoking on the risk of a low birth weight infant. In all

Table 2.4. Observed Proportions and the Corresponding Log-Odds Associated with Low Birth Weight Infants by Smoking Status and Race/Ethnicity

Race/Ethnicity	Smokers		Non-Smokers	
	$\hat{p}_1$	Log-odds$_1$	$\hat{p}_2$	Log-odds$_2$
white	0.105	−2.139	0.046	−3.036
African-American	0.192	−1.436	0.074	−2.524
Hispanic	0.115	−2.045	0.062	−2.720
Asian	0.064	−2.679	0.044	−3.069

Note that log-odds = log $[\hat{p}/(1 - \hat{p})]$.

four race/ethnicity groups the proportion of low birth weight infants is higher among smokers ($\hat{p}_1 > \hat{p}_2$). Figure 2.1 clearly displays these substantial and consistent differences between smokers and nonsmokers for each race/ethnicity group (distance between the dotted lines).

Like the comparison of the observed proportions, the differences between the log-odds values also measure the risk associated with smoking. Figure 2.2 displays the risk of a low birth weight infant among smoking and non-smoking mothers in terms of estimated log-odds (again, distance between the

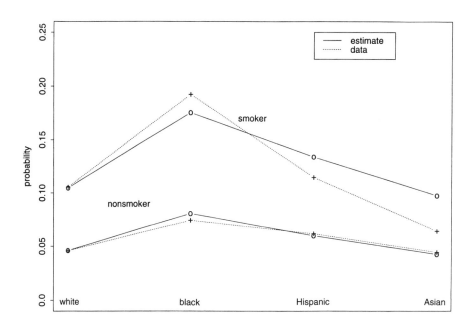

Figure 2.1. Proportion (observed and linear model estimated) of low birth weight infants by race/ethnicity.

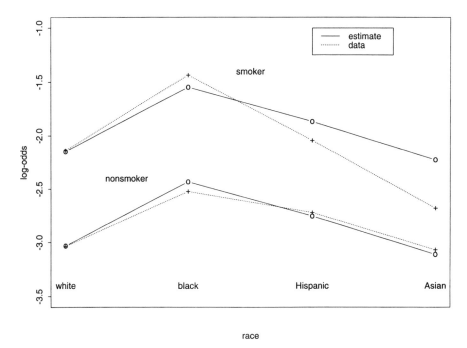

Figure 2.2. Log-odds (observed and logistic model estimated) associated with a low birth weight infant by race/ethnicity.

dotted lines). The link between comparing two proportions p_1 and p_2 and the odds ratio is the difference in log-odds values. An estimated odds ratio is the exponentiated difference between two estimated log-odds values or

$$\hat{or} = e^{\text{difference in log odds}} = e^{(\text{log-odds}_1) - (\text{log-odds}_2)}.$$

For example, $\hat{or}_{\text{white}} = e^{-2.139 - (-3.036)} = e^{0.897} = 2.453 = (98/832)/(169/3520)$ (Table 2.1).

Geometrically, the distance between log-odds for the smokers and non-smokers directly indicates the risk of a low birth weight infant associated with smoking exposure. These four distances (Figure 2.2) are approximately equal for the four race/ethnicity groups, making the "lines" representing risk close to parallel on a log-odds scale. Thus, the plotted log-odds values reveal, from a geometric point of view, approximate homogeneity of the odds ratios among the race/ethnicity groups (Table 2.2). A more general link between an odds ratio and the probability of a low birth weight infant is provided by the linear logistic model (a.17) where homogeneity is again an issue.

Logistic Model Approach

The relationship between a probability (denoted p_{ij}), such as the probability of a low birth weight infant, and several risk factors, such as maternal smoking and race/ethnicity, frequently can be effectively modeled by a logistic function where

$$p_{ij} = \frac{1}{1 + e^{-(\text{log-odds}_{ij})}}$$

making the log-odds a linear function. Specifically, the risk of a low birth weight infant associated with smoking (x_i) and race/ethnicity (y_j) in terms of the log-odds is described as a linear function (a.17) where

$$\text{log-odds}_{ij} = a + bx_i + c_1 y_{1j} + c_2 y_{2j} + c_3 y_{3j} \qquad i = 0, 1 \quad \text{and} \quad j = 0, 1, 2, 3.$$

The variable x_i represents a binary indicator that equals 0 for nonsmokers and 1 for smokers. The three y_j-components are also indicator variables, called *dummy variables*, and make up a design variable representing the four race/ethnicity groups. The detailed additive model representing the log-odds in each of the eight smoking/race categories is as follows:

Race/Ethnicity	y_{1j}	y_{2j}	y_{3j}	Nonsmokers—log-odds$_{0j}$	Smokers—log-odds$_{1j}$
white	0	0	0	a	$a + b$
African-American	1	0	0	$a + c_1$	$a + b + c_1$
Hispanic	0	1	0	$a + c_2$	$a + b + c_2$
Asian	0	0	1	$a + c_3$	$a + b + c_3$

The parameter b measures the independent influence of smoking on the risk of a low birth weight infant. The parameters c_1, c_2, and c_3 measure the independent influences of race/ethnicity on risk. Independence in this context means that the model is constructed so that the coefficients associated with one variable are not influenced by levels of the other variable. For example, the risk of a low birth weight infant associated with smoking (b) is the same for the four race/ethnicity category (c_j). The postulated logistic model dictates this independent impact of smoking since

[log-odds (smokers)] − [log-odds (nonsmokers)]
$$= [a + b(1) + c_j] - [a + b(0) + c_j] = b$$

within all four race/ethnicity groups. Geometrically, the "lines" representing smoking versus nonsmoking risk in terms of log-odds are exactly parallel (Figure 2.2—solid line). That is, the logistic model structure requires the log-odds (smoking versus nonsmoking) to differ by a constant distance b for each race/ethnicity category (perfect homogeneity or perfect independence). A similar argument applies to the independence of the race/ethnicity influences. Independence (homogeneity) is a property of the model and may or may not be a property of the data.

Since an additive (no interaction) model postulates the same relationship between smoking and the risk of a low birth weight infant for all four race/ethnicity groups, an important question arises about the usefulness of the model in representing the data. In other words, the fit of the model is a function of the homogeneity of the relationship between smoking and low birth weight. Two choices exist; the underlying risk relationship is the same within the four race/ethnicity groups, and the observed differences occurred only because of random variation (*fit* = good, when b is assumed constant) or important differences, in addition to random variation, exist among one or more of the four groups (*fit* = poor, when b is assumed constant). Geometrically, the issue of homogeneity becomes a question of the similarity of the distances between two observed "lines" (Figure 2.2—dotted lines) on a log-odds scale.

Like most statistical models, the goodness-of-fit of a logistic model is reflected by the size of the *residual deviance* (or, more technically, -2 times the log-likelihood value). Specifically, the residual deviance is 3.042 (Table 2.5). This test statistic has an approximate chi-square distribution with three degrees of freedom, and the interpretation is the same as the previous Woolf's chi-square value ($X_W^2 = 2.828$). Like X_W^2, the residual deviance shows no persuasive evidence that the association (p-value = 0.42) between smoking and the risk of a low birth weight infant differs among the four race/ethnicity groups. Both chi-square statistics equally assess homogeneity and rarely give very different answers.

Again, behaving as if the risk of smoking is the same in all four race/ethnicity groups (b = constant), the focus becomes the estimated coefficients from the additive logistic model (Table 2.5), particularly the coefficient reflecting the risk associated with smoking ($\hat{b} = 0.885$).

Table 2.5. Coefficients Estimated from the Linear Logistic Model from the Low Birth Weight Data

	Coefficients	Estimate	Std. Error
intercept	a	-3.032	—
smoking	b	0.885	0.101
African-American	c_1	0.598	0.121
Hispanic	c_2	0.279	0.139
Asian	c_3	-0.080	0.124

residual deviance = 3.042 with degrees of freedom = 3

The model coefficients provide estimates of the eight log-odds values which then produce estimates of the corresponding probabilities of a low and a "normal" birth weight infant for the four race/ethnicity groups and the two maternal smoking exposure categories. These 16 model estimated probabilities are given in Table 2.6 (denoted $\tilde{p}_{ij}$). Figure 2.1 displays the eight probabilities of a low birth weight infant estimated from the logistic model and the eight observed proportions calculated directly from the data.

For example, the model-estimated probability than an Asian mother who smokes will have a low birth weight infant is

$$\text{estimated log-odds} = \hat{a} + \hat{b} + \hat{c}_3 = -3.032 + 0.885 - 0.080 = -2.227$$

giving

$$\tilde{p}_{13} = P \text{ (low birth weight } | \text{ Asian, smoking mother)} = \frac{1}{1 + e^{-(-2.227)}} = 0.097.$$

Since $\tilde{p}_{13} = 0.097$, then among the 109 Asian smokers, $109(0.097) = 10.61$ low birth weight infants are expected compared to the 7 observed and $109(1 - 0.097) = 109(0.903) = 98.39$ "normal" birth weight infants are expected compared to the 102 observed. Similarly, the other 14 expected values based on the logistic model are estimated (Table 2.6) and compared to the observed values (Table 2.1 or 2.6) to assess the accuracy of the logistic model. The classic Pearson chi-square goodness-of-fit statistic summarizes the differences, producing a third evaluation of the correspondence between the model and the data (homogeneity?) where

$$X^2 = \sum \left[\frac{(o_i - e_i)^2}{e_i} \right] = 2.866 \quad i = 1, 2, 3, \ldots, 16.$$

The Pearson chi-square test statistic ($X^2 = 2.866$) indicating the goodness-of-fit of the estimated additive model hardly differs from the previous two assessments of homogeneity (Woolf's and residual deviance measures). Table 2.6 contains the details of the chi-square calculation, specifically displaying the 16 observed cell frequencies (o_i) and the 16 estimated cell frequencies (e_i) based on the logistic model.

As usual, to assess the impact of smoking on the risk of a low birth weight infant as reflected by the single estimated coefficient $\hat{b} = 0.885$, the quantity

$$z = \frac{\hat{b} - 0}{S_{\hat{b}}}$$

Table 2.6. Observed and Expected Cell Frequencies for the 16 Birth Weight, Smoking, and Race/Ethnicity Categories

Weight	Race/Ethnicity	Exposure	Total	$\bar{p}_{ij}{}^{*}$	o_i	e_i
<2500 g	white	smoker	930	0.105	98	97.3
≥2500 g	white	smoker	930	0.895	832	832.7
<2500 g	white	nonsmoker	3689	0.046	169	169.7
≥2500 g	white	nonsmoker	3689	0.954	3520	3519.3
<2500 g	African-American	smoker	281	0.175	54	49.2
≥2500 g	African-American	smoker	281	0.825	227	231.8
<2500 g	African-American	nonsmoker	741	0.081	55	59.8
≥2500 g	African-American	nonsmoker	741	0.919	686	681.2
<2500 g	Hispanic	smoker	96	0.134	11	12.8
≥2500 g	Hispanic	smoker	96	0.866	85	83.2
<2500 g	Hispanic	nonsmoker	987	0.060	61	59.2
≥2500 g	Hispanic	nonsmoker	987	0.940	926	927.8
<2500 g	Asian	smoker	109	0.097	7	10.6
≥2500 g	Asian	smoker	109	0.903	102	98.4
<2500 g	Asian	nonsmoker	2026	0.043	90	87.1
≥2500 g	Asian	nonsmoker	2026	0.957	1936	1938.9

*Estimated from the logistic model (e.g., Asian smokers—$\bar{p}_{13}$ = 0.097).

is appropriate and has an approximate standard normal distribution (mean = 0 and variance = 1) when no association exists ($b = 0$). The estimated logistic regression coefficient associated with smoking ($\hat{b} = 0.885$) measures risk in terms of the log-odds, and the test statistic $z = 8.756$ yields a p-value = $P\,(Z \geq 8.756 \mid b = 0) < 0.001$. Once again, a formal assessment shows clear evidence of an association between smoking and the risk of a low birth weight infant. Not unexpectedly, similar results were observed using Woolf's estimate $\overline{\log\,(or)} = 0.892$, where $z = 8.683$.

As before, assuming that the estimate $\hat{b} = 0.885$ accurately estimates the common differences in log-odds between smokers and nonsmokers within each race/ethnicity group, the common odds ratio is estimated by $\hat{or}_{mlk} = e^{\text{difference in log-odds}} = e^{\hat{b}} = e^{0.885} = 2.423$. Since the coefficients of the logistic model are estimated by maximum likelihood techniques, the estimated summary odds ratio 2.423 is also a maximum likelihood estimate. The standard error of $\hat{b}$ is produced as part of the estimation procedure ($S_{\hat{b}} = 0.101$—Table 2.5). To repeat, the differences among the three estimates (Woolf's, Mantel-Haenszel, and maximum likelihood estimates) are small, which is generally the case when estimating a common odds ratio from a series of 2 by 2 tables.

Confounding

Informally, the term *confounding* refers to the influence one risk factor or a set of risk factors has on the relationship between the outcome variable and a specific risk factor. The confounding influence of the four race/ethnicity groups on the relationship between low birth weight and smoking is assessed by comparing two odds ratios. An odds ratio calculated ignoring any possible influence of race/ethnicity is compared to a second odds ratio calculated accounting for any influence. The difference measures confounding.

The odds ratio reflecting the influence of smoking on the risk of a low birth weight infant ignoring race/ethnicity is

$$\hat{or} = \frac{\sum a_i / \sum b_i}{\sum c_i / \sum d_i} = \frac{170/1246}{375/7068} = 2.572 \quad i = 1, 2, 3, 4.$$

The estimate $\hat{or} = 2.572$ is the odds ratio calculated from the single 2 by 2 table ignoring race/ethnicity (created by adding the four race-specific tables). Specifically, the table ignoring race/ethnicity is

Combined	<2500 g	≥2500 g	Total
smokers	170	1246	1416
nonsmokers	375	7068	7443
total	545	8314	8859

The second odds ratio, assuming that the association between smoking and low birth weight is the same for all four race/ethnicity groups (homogeneity or no interaction), is any one of the previously estimated common odds ratios. All three estimates account for the influence of race/ethnicity. For example, the logistic model generated estimate is 2.423 ($\hat{or}_{mlk} = 2.423$). The difference, 2.572 versus 2.423, measures the confounding influence of race/ethnicity.

Although the two estimated odds ratios are subject to sampling variation, a statistical test to evaluate the observed difference is usually not performed. Confounding is a property of the sampled observations and primarily becomes an issue of how the data should be analyzed. That is, confounding addresses the question of whether the odds ratio should be reported including or excluding the influence of race/ethnicity. The likelihood that the observed differences arose by chance is much less of an issue.

An unequivocal assessment of a confounding influence is complicated by the fact that the degree of confounding depends on how it is measured. If confounding is measured by comparing two proportions, or comparing two odds ratios or comparing any two measures of association, then the degree of confounding influence will differ. As in many situations that arise in statistical analysis, the magnitude of the confounding effect associated with a risk factor or set of risk factors depends on the way the confounding influence is measured. Therefore, the degree of confounding is, at least to some extent, a function of the choice of the measure of association.

PART II: RELATIVE RISK

OBJECTIVE

To describe the association between the risk of a coronary event and a binary classification of behavior type (labeled *type A* and *type B*) while accounting for the influence of differences in body weight.

DATA

As part of the Western Collaborative Group Study (WCGS), a cohort of 3154 men at high risk of a coronary heart disease (CHD) event were observed over a nine to ten year period. These study participants were middle-aged men (ages 39 to 49) selected from among employees of 10 California companies. Three specific variables were abstracted from the data acquired during this study: the presence/absent of a coronary event, the participant's body weight at the beginning of the study, and an assessment of behavior type, called *type A* or *type B behavior*. In general terms, type A behavior is characterized by a sense of time urgency, aggressiveness, and ambition. A type A individual is typically thought of as having a competitive personality. A type B individual is essentially the opposite, with a relaxed, noncompetitive, less hurried personality. A total of 1589 type A and 1565 type B individuals were identified using extensive interview techniques. The occurrence of a CHD event was determined by an independent medical referee who was unaware of each patient's behavior type. Such CHD events occurred in 257 study participants during the follow-up period, producing an annual crude incidence of CHD of about 1.1 cases per 100 study subjects. Only 7.5% of all possible person-years were lost to follow-up. To study the relationship between behavior and CHD while accounting for the possible influences of body weight, the data were classified into a series of 2 by 2 tables (CHD by behavior type) for five body weight categories.

METHODS

Model-free estimates are used to assess the behavior–CHD association, particularly relative risk and summary relative risk measures. Also, the same issues are addressed with regression techniques employing a Poisson regression model.

Data type: prospective
Reference: *American Journal of Cardiology*, 1976, 37: 903–10

The variables are:

1. Coronary disease: coded 1 if a coronary event was observed and 0 otherwise
2. Behavior type: coded 1 if type A and 0 if type B
3. Body weight classification: <150 lb = 1, 150 to 160 lb = 2, 160 to 170 lb = 3, 170 to 180 lb = 4, and >180 lb = 5

The tabulated data file of the 3154 WCGS men is:

```
file name = chd.2.data

chd       a/b       wt       count
 1         0         1          10
 0         0         1         305
 1         1         1          22
 0         1         1         253
```

1	0	2	10
0	0	2	270
1	1	2	21
0	1	2	235
1	0	3	21
0	0	3	297
1	1	3	29
0	1	3	297
1	0	4	19
0	0	4	253
1	1	4	47
0	1	4	248
1	0	5	19
0	0	5	361
1	1	5	59
0	1	5	378

chd = coronary event,
a/b = A-type or B-type behavior,
wt = body weight category
count = cell frequencies

DISCUSSION

Relative risk, like an odds ratio, measures association. For the ith observed 2 by 2 table in a series of tables ($i = 1, 2, 3, \ldots, k$), the relative risk (denoted rr_i) is estimated by the ratio

$$\text{estimated relative risk} = \hat{rr}_i = \frac{a_i/(a_i + b_i)}{c_i/(c_i + d_i)} = \frac{\hat{P}_i}{\hat{p}_i}$$

using the same notation defined in Part I. This estimate measures association by contrasting two conditional probabilities. The numerator is an estimate of the probability of disease among those who were exposed to a risk factor (denoted P_i), and the denominator is an estimate of the probability of disease among those who were not exposed to the risk factor (denoted p_i). In terms of the WCGS data, for the ith weight category,

$$\text{relative risk} = rr_i = \frac{P_i}{p_i} = \frac{P \,(\text{CHD} \mid \text{type A behavior})}{P \,(\text{CHD} \mid \text{type B behavior})}.$$

The quantity $\hat{rr}_i = \hat{P}_i/\hat{p}_i$ is an estimate of the relative risk in the sampled population.[5]

Estimation and interpretation of a relative risk ratio follows the same pattern described in conjunction with an odds ratio (Part I). The fundamental difference concerns the way the data are collected. To estimate a meaningful relative risk, the data must be collected so that the probability of disease among the exposed and unexposed individuals estimates the probabilities in the populations sampled. This condition is fulfilled by many prospective studies. For example, the numbers of type A and type B individuals in the WCGS cohort are representative of the frequency in the sampled population. In other words, the proportion of coronary events among type A and type B individuals estimates the population conditional probabilities.

The weight variable divided into five categories (<150 lb, 150 to 160 lb, 160 to 170 lb, 170 to 180 lb, and >180 lb) produces five weight-specific 2 by 2 tables (Table 2.7). The relative risk measure calculated from each of these tables reflects the behavior–CHD association in each table (Table 2.8), where the type A and type B individuals compared have essentially the same weight distributions.

As with all estimates, assessing the impact of random variation is a necessary part of describing an association measured by an observed relative risk ratio. This assessment begins by taking the logarithm of the relative risk esti-

Table 2.7. Frequency of Coronary Heart Disease (CHD) Events Classified by Type A and Type B Behavior for Five Weight Categories

<150 lb	CHD	No CHD	Total
type A	22	253	275
type B	10	305	315
total	32	558	590
150 to 160 lb	CHD	No CHD	Total
type A	21	235	256
type B	10	270	280
total	31	505	536
160 to 170 lb	CHD	No CHD	Total
type A	29	297	326
type B	21	297	318
total	50	594	644
170 to 180 lb	CHD	No CHD	Total
type A	47	248	295
type B	19	253	272
total	66	501	567
>180 lb	CHD	No CHD	Total
type A	59	378	437
type B	19	361	380
total	78	639	817

Table 2.8. The Relative Risks, the Logarithm of the Relative Risks and Their Estimated Variances for the Western Collaboration Group Study Data

Weight (lb)	n_i	$\hat{rr}_i$	$\log(\hat{rr}_i)$	$S^2_{\log(\hat{rr}_i)}$	w_i
<150	590	2.520	0.924	0.139	7.213
150–160	536	2.297	0.832	0.140	7.136
160–170	644	1.347	0.298	0.076	13.177
170–180	567	2.281	0.825	0.067	14.961
>180	817	2.700	0.993	0.065	15.465

mate or $\log(\hat{rr}_i)$. Taking the logarithm of the risk ratio produces a distribution associated with the transformed value that is more symmetric, allowing the normal distribution to be employed as an accurate approximation. Similar to most statistical measures evaluated using a normal distribution, an estimate of the variance of $\log(rr_i)$ is needed. Let $P_i = P$ (disease | exposed) and let $p_i = P$ (disease | not exposed) in the ith table. Then the variance of $\log(\hat{rr}_i)$ is approximately (a.9)

$$\text{variance } [\log(\hat{rr}_i)] = \frac{1 - P_i}{N_i P_i} + \frac{1 - p_i}{n_i p_i}$$

where $N_i = a_i + b_i$ and $n_i = c_i + d_i$. A natural estimate of this variance is

$$S^2_{\log(\hat{rr}_i)} = \frac{1 - \hat{P}_i}{a_i} + \frac{1 - \hat{p}_i}{c_i}$$

where again $\hat{P}_i = a_i/(a_i + b_i)$ and $\hat{p}_i = c_i/(c_i + d_i)$. The estimated relative risk and the logarithm of the estimated relative risk calculated from each of the five weight-specific 2 by 2 tables are given in Table 2.8.

Confidence intervals are constructed in the same fashion as those for an odds ratio. Using the logarithm of the estimated relative risk, an approximate 95% confidence interval is

$$\log(\hat{rr}_i) \pm 1.960\, S_{\log(\hat{rr}_i)}$$

and an approximate 95% confidence interval for the quantity estimated by $\hat{rr}_i$ is

$$e^{\log(\hat{rr}_i) \pm 1.960\, S_{\log(\hat{rr}_i)}} = \hat{rr}_i^{\pm 1.960\, S_{\log(\hat{rr}_i)}}$$

yielding the five confidence intervals in Table 2.9.

Figure 2.3 displays these five relative risk measures and their approximate 95% confidence intervals. Two properties of the behavior–CHD data

Table 2.9. Log-Relative Risk and Relative Risk Along with Their Respective
Approximate 95% Confidence Limits for the Five Weight Categories

Weight (lb)	n_i	$\log(\hat{r}r_i)$	Lower	Upper	$\hat{r}r_i$	Lower	Upper
<150	590	0.924	0.194	1.654	2.520	1.215	5.228
150–160	536	0.832	0.098	1.565	2.297	1.103	4.784
160–170	644	0.298	−0.242	0.838	1.347	0.785	2.311
170–180	567	0.825	0.318	1.331	2.281	1.374	3.786
>180	817	0.993	0.490	1.492	2.700	1.640	4.445

clearly emerge from the plot of these five estimated risk ratios. The relative
risk for each weight category probably differs from 1.0 ($rr = 1$ implies no association) since the value 1.0 is excluded from four of the confidence intervals
and almost excluded from the fifth. Also, little evidence exists to indicate
that the underlying relative risk differs systematically among weight categories since the estimated values are approximately equal (about 2.4, except
perhaps for individuals weighing 160–170 lb) and the five confidence intervals generally overlap. The lack of remarkable differences among the five risk
measures motivates the calculation of a single summary relative risk based
on combining information from the five weight-specific tables to estimate the
underlying common association between behavior type and CHD.

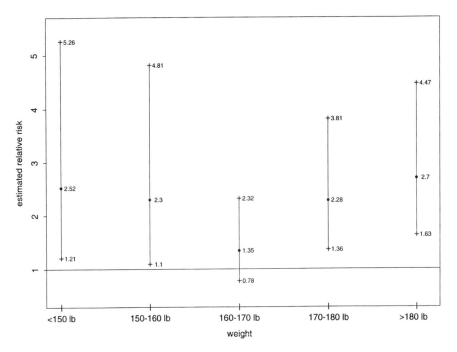

Figure 2.3. Estimated relative risk of coronary heart disease for five weight groups
with 95% confidence intervals.

Behaving as if the relative risk is homogeneous among the five weight categories ($rr_1 = rr_2 = rr_3 = rr_4 = rr_5 = rr$) and following the pattern described for the odds ratio, a weighted average provides a single summary relative risk. In symbols, a weighted average of k values of log-relative risk (a.12) is

$$\text{mean log-relative risk} = \overline{\log{(rr)}} = \frac{\sum w_i \log{(\hat{rr}_i)}}{\sum w_i} \quad i = 1, 2, 3, \ldots, k$$

based on the k individual log-relative risk estimates. Again, the weights w_i are the reciprocal values of the estimated variances (i.e., $w_i = 1/S^2_{\log{(\hat{rr}_i)}}$—Table 2.8). For the CHD data, the weighted average is

$$\overline{\log{(rr)}} = [7.213(0.924) + \cdots + 15.465(0.993)]/57.951 = 0.763.$$

The estimated summary relative risk is then $\hat{rr} = e^{0.763} = 2.145$.

As before, an estimate of the variance of this weighted average is $S^2_{\overline{\log{(rr)}}} = 1/\sum w_i = 1/57.951 = 0.017$ (a.12). An approximate 95% confidence interval for the underlying log-relative risk based on the estimate $\overline{\log{(r)}} = 0.763$ is

$$\text{lower bound} = \overline{\log{(rr)}} - 1.960 \, S_{\overline{\log{(rr)}}} = 0.763 - 1.960\sqrt{0.017} = 0.506$$

$$\text{upper bound} = \overline{\log{(rr)}} + 1.960 \, S_{\overline{\log{(rr)}}} = 0.763 + 1.960\sqrt{0.017} = 1.021$$

and the approximate 95% confidence interval for the underlying common relative risk is

$$(e^{\text{lower bound}}, e^{\text{upper bound}}) = (e^{0.506}, e^{1.021}) = (1.658, 2.775).$$

Like all confidence intervals, the bounds provide the likely range of the values of the true underlying common relative risk (rr).

Poisson Model Approach

Most measures of association can be estimated, assessed, and interpreted in the context of a linear model. The logistic model is the natural representation of the risk factor relationships when the measure of association chosen is the odds ratio. The parallel model for the relative risk postulates that the logarithm of the probability of disease is a linear function of the risk factors. Specifically, for the ith behavior type and the jth weight category, a Poisson model is

$$\text{log-probability of CHD} = \log{(p_{ij})} = a + bx_i + c_1y_{1j} + c_2y_{2j} + c_3y_{3j} + c_4y_{4j}$$

where x_i is a binary variable representing behavior type ($x_i = 0$ for type B and $x_i = 1$ for type A individuals). The design variable components y_1, y_2, y_3, and

y_4 in conjunction with the coefficients c_1, c_2, c_3, and c_4 reflect the independent impact of the five body weight categories ($j = 0, 1, 2, 3, 4$). Totally analogous to the smoking–birth weight logistic model, the behavior type–CHD Poisson model represents 10 log-probabilities as follows:

Weight (lb)	y_{1j}	y_{2j}	y_{3j}	y_{4j}	type B—log (p_j)*	type A—log (P_j)*
<150	0	0	0	0	a	$a + b$
150–160	1	0	0	0	$a + c_1$	$a + b + c_1$
160–170	0	1	0	0	$a + c_2$	$a + b + c_2$
170–180	0	0	1	0	$a + c_3$	$a + b + c_3$
>180	0	0	0	1	$a + c_4$	$a + b + c_4$

*Note the notation: $p_{0j} = p_j$ and $p_{1j} = P_j$.

The usefulness of this additive Poisson model depends on two fundamental requirements. First, it requires the relative risks underlying each weight category to be identical (homogeneous); therefore, the observed differences in estimated risk ratios are due entirely to random variation (Table 2.8). The model structure dictates this property since within all weight categories (strata) the influence of behavior type is the same (b = constant). For example, for individuals who weight more than 180 pounds ($j = 4$) and who exhibit type A behavior, the logarithm of the model probability of CHD is

$$\log (P_4) = a + b + c_4$$

and for type B individuals in the same weight category

$$\log (p_4) = a + c_4.$$

Then

$$\log (P_4) - \log (p_4) = b \quad \text{or} \quad \frac{P_4}{p_4} = e^b = rr$$

and the model-generated measure of association (b or rr) is identical for the other four weight categories.

Second, each count of individuals (cell frequency) must be an observation sampled from a Poisson distribution or at least an approximate Poisson distribution. Based on these two assumptions and the WCGS data (Table 2.7), model coefficients and their standard errors are estimated and given in Table 2.10.

Estimated probabilities of CHD follow directly from the Poisson model.

Table 2.10. Coefficients Estimated from the Additive Poisson Model Using Western Collaborative Group Study Data

	Coefficient	Estimate	Std. Error
intercept	a	−3.349	—
behavior type	b	0.774	0.135
150–160 lb	c_1	0.056	0.252
160–170 lb	c_2	0.329	0.226
170–180 lb	c_3	0.723	0.216
>180 lb	c_4	0.515	0.210

residual deviance = 3.601 with degrees of freedom = 4

For example, the log-probability reflecting the risk of CHD associated with type A individuals whose body weights are greater than 180 pounds is

$$\log(\tilde{P}_4) = -3.349 + 0.774 + 0.515 = -2.060$$

and for the corresponding type B individuals it is

$$\log(\tilde{p}_4) = -3.349 + 0 + 0.515 = -2.834$$

yielding model-estimated probabilities $\tilde{P}_4 = e^{-2.060} = 0.127$ (type A) and $\tilde{p}_4 = e^{-2.834} = 0.059$ (type B).

The model-based summary log-relative risk estimate is $\hat{b} = \log(\tilde{rr}) = 0.774$. The model-estimated common relative risk then becomes $\tilde{rr} = e^{\hat{b}} = e^{0.774} = 2.168$ and is necessarily identical for all five body weight categories. For example, $\tilde{rr} = \tilde{P}_4/\tilde{p}_4 = 0.127/0.059 = 2.168$ for individuals who weigh more than 180 lb. The nonmodel relative risk estimate ($\hat{rr} = 2.145$) and its standard error ($S_{\hat{rr}} = 0.131$) are essentially the same. Graphically, the plots of $\log(\tilde{P}_i)$ and $\log(\tilde{p}_i)$ form exactly parallel lines separated by a distance $|\hat{b}| = 0.774$ (Figure 2.4—solid lines) since the estimated values conform perfectly to the model (i.e., $\hat{b}$ and $\tilde{rr}_i$ are constant).

The estimated probabilities allow estimates of the cell frequencies based strictly on the Poisson model (Figure 2.5—solid lines = estimated probabilities and dotted lines = observed probabilities). For example, the expected number of CHD events among type A individuals who weigh more than 180 pounds is 0.127(437) = 55.670, and the estimated number of CHD events among type B individuals who weight more than 180 pounds is 0.059(380) = 22.330. The corresponding observed values are 59 and 19 CHD events, respectively. All 20 model-generated expected and observed values are given in Table 2.11.

Goodness-of-fit is again evaluated directly by comparing the observed and expected values (Table 2.11). A basic "fit" issue is the homogeneity of the

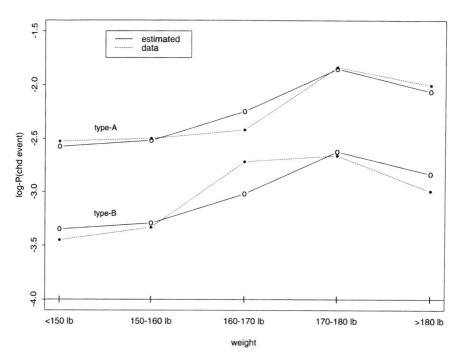

Figure 2.4. Log-probabilities (observed and Poisson model estimated) associated with a coronary event.

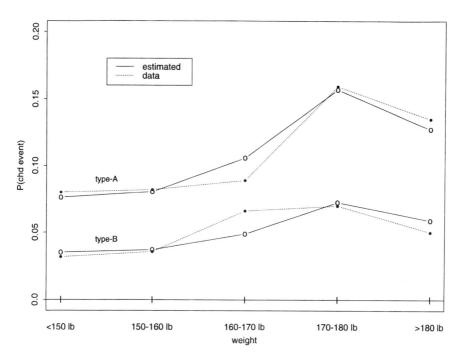

Figure 2.5. Probabilities (observed and Poisson model estimated) associated with a coronary event.

Table 2.11. The Observed ($\hat{p}_j$, $\hat{P}_j$ and o_j) and Expected ($\tilde{p}_j$, $\tilde{P}_j$ and e_j) Values from the Western Collaborative Group Study Coronary Heart Disease Data

Weight (lb)	A/B	$\hat{P}_j$	$\tilde{P}_j^*$	o_j	e_j	$n_j - o_j$	$n_j - e_j$
<150	A	0.080	0.076	22	20.937	253	254.063
150–160	A	0.082	0.080	21	20.604	235	235.396
160–170	A	0.089	0.106	29	34.484	297	291.516
170–180	A	0.159	0.157	47	46.305	248	248.695
>180	A	0.135	0.127	59	55.670	378	381.330
Weight (lb)	A/B	$\hat{p}_j$	$\tilde{p}_j^*$	o_j	e_j	$n_j - o_j$	$n_j - e_j$
<150	B	0.032	0.035	10	11.063	305	303.937
150–160	B	0.036	0.037	10	10.396	270	269.604
160–170	B	0.066	0.049	21	15.516	297	302.484
170–180	B	0.070	0.072	19	19.695	253	252.305
>180	B	0.050	0.059	19	22.330	361	357.670

*Probabilities estimated from the Poisson model.

relative risk measures (i.e., $rr_1 = rr_2 = rr_3 = rr_4 = rr_5 = rr$?). The Pearson test statistic is $X^2 = \sum (o_j - e_j)^2/e_j = 3.995$ and is a value from an approximate chi-square distribution with four degrees of freedom when the model is "correct," that is, when the observed values differ from the expected values only by chance. The significance probability generated by comparing observed cell frequencies to the model estimates is the p-value = $P (X^2 \geq 3.995 \mid$ homogeneous) $= 0.41$, indicating that the additive (b = constant) Poisson model adequately describes the CHD risk. The value of the residual deviance is similar (Table 2.10—residual deviance = 3.601) and has the same role in evaluating the goodness-of-fit. The fit evaluated visually, displayed in Figure 2.5 (dotted line versus solid line), also shows no remarkable differences between the observed and model-estimated probabilities.

Three small points:

1. The patterns of assessing the odds ratio and relative risk measures of association differ, by and large, only in detail. The issues, the estimation techniques, the testing, and confidence interval construction are the same in principle.
2. The relative risk measure is always closer to 1.0 (no association) than the odds ratio calculated form the same data. This property means that the relative risk measure is conservative: if the relative risk measure is extreme or significant, then the odds ratio is more extreme or more significant.
3. If the frequency of disease is rare in both the exposed and unexposed groups, the odds ratio approximately equals the relative risk ratio. For example, ignoring the body weight categories, the relative risk is $\hat{rr} = 2.219$ and the odds ratio calculated from the same data is $\hat{or} = 2.373$. Specifically,

Behavior	CHD	No CHD	Total
type A	178	1411	1589
type B	79	1486	1565
total	257	2897	3154

giving $\hat{rr} = (178/1589)/(79/1565) = 2.219$ and $\hat{or} = (178/1411)/(79/1486) = 2.373$. The odds ratio is expectedly a bit larger but not very different since a CHD event is relatively rare among both type A and type B individuals.

CONCLUSIONS

Part I

Maternal cigarette smoking is strongly associated with the likelihood of a low birth weight newborn infant, and the risk is similar regardless of the mother's race/ethnicity (white, African-American, Hispanic, or Asian). A summary odds ratio of 2.441 (95% CI: 1.996, 2.986) indicates substantially increased risk. A parallel analysis using a logistic model repeats this result. The model-generated summary odds ratio estimate is essentially the same as the model-free estimate ($\hat{or} = 2.423$). The logistic model additionally provides evidence that the relationship between smoking and low birth weight is homogeneous among the four race/ethnicity groups (p-value = 0.42).

Part II

The analysis of the WCGS data contained in five 2 by 2 tables indicates a strong association between a person's behavior and the risk of a CHD event. The relative risk for a type A versus a type B individual, accounting for the confounding influence of body weight, is 2.145 (95% CI: 1.658, 2.775). A summary relative risk estimated from an additive Poisson model is similar (2.168) and also accounts for the influence of differing body weight distributions between type A and type B individuals. Like the logistic model (Part 1), the Poisson model reinforces the model-free approach showing a homogeneous relative risk (p-value = 0.41) among the five weight categories.

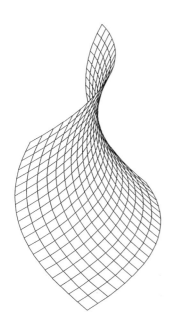

CHAPTER 3

Randomized Trial

OBJECTIVE

To evaluate the results of a randomized trial conducted to test the effectiveness of an experimental treatment in slowing the pathological changes in memory caused by Alzheimer's disease.

DATA

Individuals with Alzheimer's disease were randomly divided into two groups. One group received a placebo (26 patients), and the other received a treatment of lecithin (25 patients). However, three patients refused the treatment. It was hoped that the treated group would show a slower rate of cognitive loss. Each subject participated in the trial for six months. A memory recall test was administered to all 48 participants at the beginning of the trial period and at the end of the period, producing two scores for each participant.

METHODS

A series of control/treatment group comparisons are made using two-sample *t*-tests and Wilcoxon tests. Parallel computer intensive methods (bootstrap and randomization methods) are also used to make the same comparisons.

Data type: randomized trial
Reference: *Multivariate Analysis of Variance and Repeated Measures*, D. J.
        Hand and C. C. Taylor, Chapman and Hill (1961)

The variables are:

1. Treatment indicator: coded 1 for the treatment group and 0 for the placebo
   group
2. Score 1: test score at baseline (before treatment)
3. Score 2: test score after six months

Part of the data file of 48 Alzheimer's disease patients is:

```
file name = alzheimer.3.data
```

group	score1	score2
0	15	14
0	11	6
0	2	7
0	5	1
0	6	3
0	5	8
0	3	5
0	22	18
0	13	10
0	3	6
0	8	7
0	4	4
0	10	0
0	14	13
0	11	6
—	—	—
—	—	—
—	—	—

DISCUSSION

The early statistician R. A. Fisher and his contemporaries first recognized the importance of randomization, revolutionizing the design of experiments and analysis of data. A randomized trial, such as the trial of lecithin, starts with selecting individuals who are as similar as possible and dividing them randomly into two groups. The key word is *randomly*. When nothing but chance determines membership in one group or the other, any differences observed between the two groups must be due only to variation among the participants. Then the members of one group are assigned to a specific treatment, and the members of the other make up the control or placebo "treatment" group. If the treatment has an effect, a systematic difference should emerge between the two groups. If the treatment has no effect, then the two groups will continue to differ randomly only because of the original variation among the individuals participating in the trial.

In evaluating the lecithin treatment, all participants were given a memory test at the beginning of the trial (first score denoted x_i) and at the end of six months (second score denoted y_i). Randomization guarantees that differences between the placebo and lecithin groups at the baseline are strictly due to chance variation. However, three individuals dropped out of the lecithin group, possibly causing an important systematic difference between the two groups. To explore this potential selection bias, the mean scores at baseline between the placebo and lecithin groups are compared. The mean score for the control group $\bar{x}_c$ is 8.385 based on $n_c = 26$ patients (standard error = 1.086), and the mean score for the treatment group $\bar{x}_t$ is 7.591 based on $n_t = 22$ patients (standard error = 1.127), producing a mean difference of $\bar{x}_c - \bar{x}_t$ is 0.794 (standard error = 1.571). A 95% confidence interval, based on the observed difference in baseline test scores, of $(-2.369, 3.952)$ indicates that zero is a plausible underlying mean value, implying that the observed difference likely results from random variation. Alternatively, a t-statistic to evaluate the observed difference yields

$$T = \frac{(\bar{x}_t - \bar{x}_c) - 0}{S_{\bar{x}_t - \bar{x}_c}} = \frac{8.385 - 7.591}{1.571} = 0.505.$$

The test statistic T has a t-distribution with $n_c + n_t - 2 = 46$ degrees of freedom when the two mean values differ only by chance (i.e., the three individuals who left the study were no different from those who remained). The associated p-value $P(|T| \geq 0.505 \mid \text{no difference at baseline}) = 0.62$ also shows no evidence of a systematic difference between the control and treatment groups at baseline.

The two-sample t-test designed to compare two mean values requires the observations to be sampled from two normal distributions with the same variance. However, for sample sizes in the neighborhood of 20 or 30 observations, mean values and differences between mean values typically have at least approximate normal distributions unless the distributions sampled are extremely asymmetric. Furthermore, the requirement that the two variances be equal is not very important when the number of individuals in the compared groups is approximately the same. The mathematics of the t-distribution demonstrates that rather unequal variances have little effect on the accuracy of the test as long as the numbers in each group are about equal (i.e., $n_c \approx n_t$).[6]

Nevertheless, a nonparametric Wilcoxon rank test provides a distribution-free assessment of the observed difference. That is, the accuracy of the p-value does not depend on whether or not the observations are sampled from normal distributions. The Wilcoxon rank procedure yields a test statistic $z = 0.353$, which has an approximate standard normal distribution when only random differences exist between the control and treatment groups. The p-value for the lecithin trial data using this nonparametric approach is $P(|Z| \geq 0.353 \,|\, \text{no difference at baseline}) = 0.72$. Neither parametric nor nonparametric analysis provides convincing evidence that the baseline test scores are systematically influenced by the three individuals who declined to participate.

Figures 3.1 and 3.2 display a histogram of the test scores and a quantile plot for the placebo and lecithin groups. A histogram based on so few observations is not a very useful description of the distribution of the collected data, except to identify extreme and perhaps outlier observations. A quantile plot produces a straight line when the sampled data are normally distributed. For the lecithin trial data, the control group line is remarkably straight and that of the treatment group is reasonably straight.

A natural approach to assessing the impact of the lecithin treatment is to compare the mean scores observed after six months for the placebo and treatment groups. The mean test scores are $\bar{y}_c = 5.962$ (standard error = 0.874) and $\bar{y}_t = 7.091$ (standard error = 0.967) for the control and treatment groups, respectively. The mean difference $\bar{y}_c - \bar{y}_t = -1.129$ shows that the control patients did somewhat poorer on the memory test than the lecithin-treated

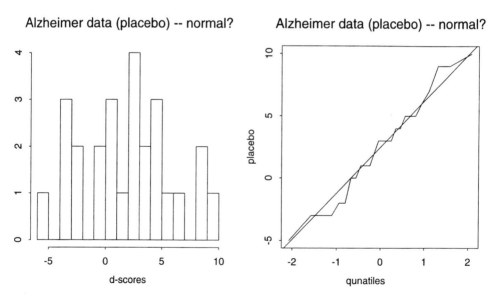

Figure 3.1. Histogram and quantile plots describing the scores for the placebo group from the lecithin trial data.

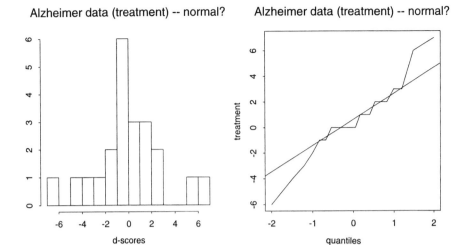

Figure 3.2. Histogram and quantile plots describing the scores for the treatment group from the lecithin trial data.

patients (scores are based on the number of correct answers). A two-sample t-test yields a test statistic of $T = 0.868$ (degrees of freedom $= 46$) with an associated p-value of 0.39.

A statistically more efficient approach capitalizes on the differences between each patient's six month test scores, sometimes called a *before/after* comparison (Figure 3.3). That is, the six month score y_i is subtracted from the baseline score x_i for each individual; in symbols, $d_i = x_i - y_i$. Positive values indicate the amount of each person's deterioration over the six month period. Therefore, the difference between the mean values for the placebo group $(\bar{d}_c)$ and the treatment group $(\bar{d}_t)$ measures the influence of the lecithin treatment on the rate of deterioration. The d_i-values make each person his or her own "control" so that the baseline level of each individual, estimated by the initial score, is removed for consideration. The variation among individuals, then, is no longer a factor in evaluating the treatment impact. As a result, the within-person differences in scores give a mean control/treatment difference $\bar{d}_c - \bar{d}_t$ with appreciably lower variance when compared to the variance of the mean difference between six month scores $\bar{y}_c - \bar{y}_t$ (variances: 1.065 versus 1.694, respectively—a 37% decrease). Reducing the variance of a comparison (the denominator of the t-statistic) increases the probability of detecting a treatment influence (increased statistical power).

The measured deterioration in the control group (mean score $\bar{d}_c = 2.423$ with standard error $= 0.789$) is greater than the deterioration observed in the treatment group (mean score $\bar{d}_t = 0.500$ with standard error $= 0.623$). The smaller amount of deterioration indicates a tendency for the treated individ-

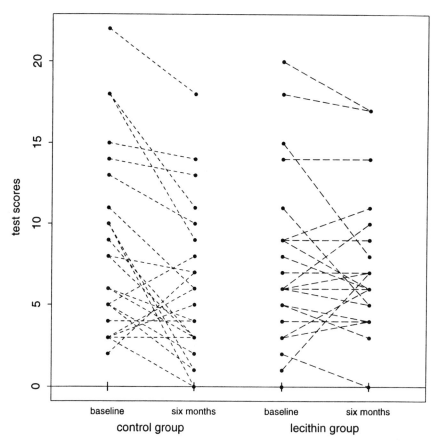

Figure 3.3. Graphic description of the lecithin trial data contrasting the change in scores for control and lecithin-treated individuals.

uals to remember more than the controls after a six month period. The mean difference between the placebo and lecithin groups is $\bar{d}_c - \bar{d}_t = 1.923$, yielding a 95% confidence interval of $(-0.154, 4.001)$. The t-test to evaluate formally the observed difference in treatment results is

$$T = \frac{(\bar{d}_c - \bar{d}_t) - 0}{S_{\bar{d}_c - \bar{d}_t}} = \frac{(2.423 - 0.500) - 0}{1.032} = 1.863.$$

The test statistic T has a t-distribution (degrees of freedom = 46) when only random differences exist between the control and treatment groups. The associated one-sided p-value is $P(T \geq 1.863 \mid \text{no treatment effect}) = 0.03$.

The parallel Wilcoxon test applied to observed differences (control versus treatment) is distribution-free (i.e., the sampled distribution of test score differences is not relevant to the calculation of the *p*-value) but slightly less efficient than the *t*-test. Nevertheless, this nonparametric approach gives almost identical results where the approximate, normally distributed test statistic based on ranks is $z = 1.830$, producing a *p*-value of $P\ (Z \geq 1.830\ |$ no treatment effect$) = 0.034$. The confidence interval, the *t*-test, and the Wilcoxon rank procedure all indicate some evidence of a benefit from the lecithin treatment, but the evidence is not overwhelming.

Computer-Intensive Approaches

The expression *computer-intensive* applies to statistical methods that require little or no statistical theory but instead rely on a repeated sampling strategy, implemented with a computer, to assess various issues arising from the observed data. Two such computer-intensive methods relevant to the lecithin trial involve a bootstrap estimated distribution[7] and a randomization test.[8]

A *bootstrap analysis* of the lecithin data begins by repeatedly sampling the collected data to estimate the distribution from which the observed mean difference, $\bar{d}_c - \bar{d}_t = 1.923$, was sampled. A sample of 26 observations is randomly selected from the control group. The observations are sampled with replacement so that some individuals are included in the bootstrap sample more than once and other individuals are not included at all. The only source of differences among a series of such bootstrap samples is the variation among the individuals within the control group. Thus, a series of estimated mean scores (denoted $\bar{D}_c$—capital letters denote results from the resampling process) each calculated from a bootstrap sample differ only because of the variation among the 24 sampled individuals. That is, each sample contains a different set of individuals producing differences among the $\bar{D}$-values, which then reflect the degree of sampling variation. A sample of 22 observations is similarly selected from the lecithin group and the mean score is calculated (denoted $\bar{D}_t$). These two samples are used to estimate the mean difference between the control and treatment test scores (denoted $\bar{D}_c - \bar{D}_t$). The bootstrap sampling is repeated a large number of times, producing a large number of estimated differences in mean scores. The variation among these bootstrap-replicated mean score differences estimates the variation associated with the observed mean difference, $\bar{d}_c - \bar{d}_t$. In fact, the distribution of these bootstrap mean differences estimates the distribution that produced the original observed mean difference (1.923). Figure 3.4 (left side) shows the estimated distribution of $\bar{d}_c - \bar{d}_t$ based on 6000 bootstrap samples $\bar{D}_c - \bar{D}_t$ from the lecithin trial data (mean = 1.921). The important point is that this estimated distribution provides an opportunity to assess the impact of random variation on the observed value $\bar{d}_c - \bar{d}_t = 1.923$. Furthermore, this assessment is free of assumptions or requirements.

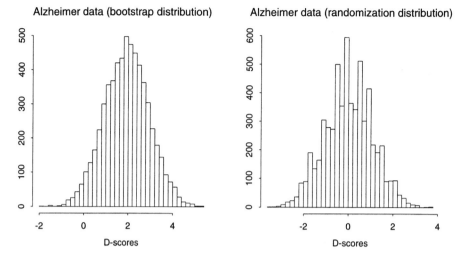

Figure 3.4. Bootstrap and randomization estimated distributions of the difference in mean scores (D-scores).

The mean of the bootstrap-estimated distribution is 1.921 with a variance of 0.965 and, as expected, resembles a normal distribution. A central issue concerns the value zero. If the lecithin treatment has no effect, then about half of the mean differences should be below zero and about half above zero. That is, in light of the variation associated with the observed difference in test scores, an important question becomes: *is an observed mean difference less than zero likely or not?* The bootstrap-estimated distribution directly addresses this question. The number of computer-generated differences $\overline{D}_c - \overline{D}_t$ less than zero is 144 out of the 6000 sampled, indicating that rarely would mean differences be less than zero. That is, rarely would the mean value for the control group be smaller than the value from the treated group. Quantitatively, a bootstrap-generated p-value is $P(\overline{D}_c - \overline{D}_t \leq 0 \mid \text{mean} = 1.921) = 144/6000 = 0.024$. The small p-value indicates that a negative difference between mean scores is not likely by chance alone, implying that it is probable that a nonrandom and positive difference exists between the placebo and lecithin groups measured by the mean test scores. The estimated bootstrap distribution is sufficiently shifted to the right (observed positive difference in mean values of 1.921) suggesting less deterioration in memory is associated with the lecithin treatment group.

A second computer-intensive approach to assessing the observed difference $\overline{d}_c - \overline{d}_t$ is called a *randomization test*. Unlike the bootstrap estimate, the distinction between control and treatment group status is temporarily ignored and the data are combined. A sample of 26 random observations is selected without replacement from the combined 48 observations. A random sample of 22 observations then remains unsampled. The comparison of the mean value of the sample observations to the mean value of the unsampled observations produces a randomized mean difference in test scores (denoted $\overline{D}_c' - \overline{D}_t'$). The expected difference between $\overline{D}_c'$ and $\overline{D}_t'$ is zero regardless of any treatment effect since control and treated individuals, in the long run, balance between the two compared groups. To the extent that a mean difference differs from zero, it measures the random variation associated with the collected data. In other words, the participants in the trial are randomly sampled disregarding their placebo/lecithin status, and differences between randomized mean values are, therefore, due strictly to the variation among participants. No other reason but chance exists to cause the observed differences. As always, the randomization process produces only random differences between the two randomized groups.

As with the bootstrap procedure, a large number of these randomized mean differences $\overline{D}_c' - \overline{D}_t'$ are computer-generated. The results of 6000 randomized samples are displayed in Figure 3.4 (right side). The mean value is -0.008 with variance 1.092. Again, the distribution of sampled values $\overline{D}_c' - \overline{D}_t'$ resembles at least an approximate normal distribution, with close to half of the observations below zero and half above. This distribution is an estimate of the distribution of $\overline{d}_c - \overline{d}_t$ as if the difference between control and treatment individuals arose only because of *background* variation (no treatment effect). Since only random variation influences the computer-generated distribution, it is called the *null distribution*. Questions about the observed mean difference $\overline{d}_c - \overline{d}_t$ are again directly addressed from this estimated distribution, but this time under the null hypothesis of "no treatment effect." The central question relevant to the specific mean difference observed in the lecithin trial is: *what is the likelihood that a mean difference of 1.923 or greater occurs by chance alone when the treatment has no influence?* More specifically, *what is the probability of observing a mean difference of 1.923 or greater sampled from the null distribution?* This probability is directly estimated by counting the computer-generated differences of $\overline{D}_c' - \overline{D}_t'$ that exceed 1.923. A total of 192 values from the null distribution of the 6000 randomized values are greater than 1.923. A randomization test *p*-value is then $P(\overline{D}_c' - \overline{D}_t' \geq 1.923 \mid \text{no difference}) = 192/6000 = 0.032$.

Each analytic approach provides an estimate of the variance associated with the test statistic $\overline{d}_c - \overline{d}_t$, which is the key element in detecting a treatment effect. These estimated variances estimate the same quantity and, thus, are expected to be similar (*t*-test: 1.065, bootstrap: 0.965, and randomization: 1.092). An estimated variance, as usual, allows the construction of statistical tests and confidence intervals.

The bootstrap and randomization approaches are related. Although the *p*-values differ (0.024 versus 0.032), this difference is due to the variation inherent in using computer-intensive methods based on 48 observations. Both approaches estimate the same significance probability (*p*-value). Since the bootstrap and randomization estimated distributions differ very little from a normal distribution (mean values based on moderately large samples have approximate normal distributions—central limit theorem), the two p-values are, theoretically,

$$p\text{-value (bootstrap)} = P\,(\overline{D}_c - \overline{D}_t \leq 0 \mid E\,(\overline{D}_c - \overline{D}_t) = \mu)$$

$$= P\!\left(Z \leq \frac{0 - \mu}{\sigma}\right)$$

and

$$p\text{-value (randomization)} = P\,(\overline{D}_c' - \overline{D}_t' \geq \mu \mid E\,(\overline{D}_c' - \overline{D}_t') = 0)$$

$$= P\!\left(Z \geq \frac{\mu - 0}{\sigma}\right) = P\!\left(Z \leq \frac{0 - \mu}{\sigma}\right)$$

$$= p\text{-value (bootstrap)}$$

where μ represents the mean difference between the control and treatment groups with associated variance σ^2 and Z represents a variable with a stan-

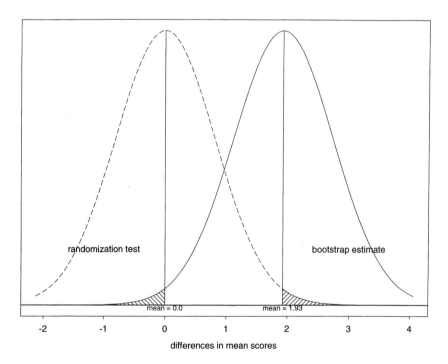

Figure 3.5. Comparison of idealized bootstrap and randomization distributions of the difference in mean scores (D-scores).

dard normal distribution. These two theoretical probabilities are equal when the differences in mean values have normal distributions with the same variances. Figure 3.5 shows idealized normal distributions of the bootstrap $(\overline{D}_c - \overline{D}_t)$-values and randomization $(\overline{D}_c' - \overline{D}_t')$-values for the lecithin trial data. The shaded areas are the two equal p-values.

CONCLUSIONS

Comparing "before" and "after" measures of memory among Alzheimer's disease patients indicates an important difference between the patients who received lecithin and the patients who received a placebo. Four statistical approaches (t-test, Wilcoxon, bootstrap, and randomization procedures) yield the same inference: the lecithin patients appear to have significantly less deterioration (smaller average differences between the "before" and "after" test scores). One-tailed statistical tests using the four approaches produce similar p-values, in the neighborhood of 0.03.

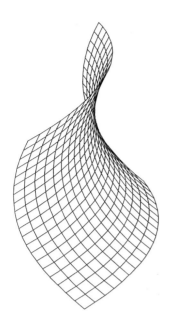

CHAPTER 4

Bias

PART I: REGRESSION TO THE MEAN

OBJECTIVE

To describe the regression to the mean incurred in measuring and remeasuring systolic blood pressure on the same individual.

DATA

The data analyzed are from the Buffalo Blood Pressure Study, designed to investigate the misclassification of blood pressure measurements, which are notoriously difficult to read accurately. The study consisted of a random sample of 1082 households made up of 2279 individuals who were interviewed and measured for blood pressure levels. A random subsample of 50 individuals was revisited and a second blood pressure measurement obtained approximately eight months later. The 50 measurement/remeasurement pairs provided a set of observations made on the same individual recorded at two different times, frequently referred to as *repeated measurement data*.

METHODS

The phenomenon called *regression to the mean* is described using simple linear regression techniques and evaluated primarily with mean values, *t*-tests, and correlation coefficients.

Data type: nested random sample (repeated measures)
Reference: *American Journal of Epidemiology*, 1966, 84(3): 510–23

The variables are:

1. First systolic blood pressure: recorded as measured in millimeters of mercury (mm Hg)
2. Second systolic blood pressure: recorded as measured in millimeters of mercury (mm Hg)

Part of the data file of the 50 study participants is:

```
file name = blood.4.data

     first      second
        98         104
       100         112
       102         108
       104         126
       106          94
       106         132
       108         138
       108         108
       108          98
       108         122
       108         126
       110         118
       110         108
       112         118
       114         104
         —           —
         —           —
         —           —
```

DISCUSSION

It is called the *sophomore jinx* in baseball. More formally, the phenomenon is called *regression to the mean*. It arises when repeated measurements are made on the same individual or related individuals and these measurements are subject to random variation. This phenomenon was first noticed in the early days of statistics when Francis Galton (b. 1822) described the heights of fathers and sons.[9] He observed that tall fathers tended to have sons shorter than themselves, on average, and short fathers tended to have sons taller than themselves, again on average. Galton called this property *regression to mediocrity*.

Karl Pearson (b. 1857) invented several analytic methods to study this regression phenomenon (regression in the sense of returning to the original level). These methods were subsequently applied to a much wider class of problems that had nothing to do with regression to the mean, but nevertheless, they retained the name regression analysis. Therefore, today the term *regression* in a statistical context identifies specific analytic techniques, but with a few exceptions it refers only to its historical origins and not to any particular statistical property.

The Buffalo blood pressure study contains 50 systolic blood pressure values recorded on two occasions on the same individual. The mean value of the first measurements is 133.240 (standard error = 3.992), and the mean value of the second measurements is 134.240 (standard error = 3.752). The mean difference of 1.0 is small and inconsequential (T-statistic = 0.426, yielding a p-value = 0.67).

More interestingly, for those individuals with first blood pressure levels above or equal to the median value (median = 130 based on all 50 participants), the second measurement is an average of 3.231 below the first measurement (standard error = 3.700). Also, for those individuals with first blood pressure levels below the median, the second measurement is on average 5.583 above the first measurement (standard error = 2.571). That is, for the 26 individuals with blood pressures greater than or equal to 130 on the first measurement ($\bar{y}_1 = 152.769$), the mean of their second measurement is lower ($\bar{y}_2 = 149.539$), producing a paired t-statistic of 0.873 (p-value = 0.39). For the 24 individuals with blood pressures less than 130 on the first measurement ($\bar{y}_1 = 112.083$), the mean of their second measurement is higher ($\bar{y}_2 = 117.667$), producing a paired t-statistic of -2.172 (p-value = 0.04). As with Galton's father/son pairs, the second blood pressure measurements tend to regress toward the overall mean ($\bar{y} = 133.740$). The pairs of observations (first versus second measurements) are plotted in Figure 4.1.

If the first and second blood pressure measurements made on each individual did not vary (variance (within pair difference) = 0), then the second measurement would be identical to the first. Geometrically, points representing the first and second blood pressure readings would fall on a straight line with a slope equal to 1.0 (dotted line in Figure 4.1). Within-pair variation is distinct from the variation among individuals, and whether the variation among individuals is large or small, the slope remains 1.0 when no within-individual variation exists.

The least squares estimated line summarizing the average relationship between the first and second observed blood pressure measurements has an

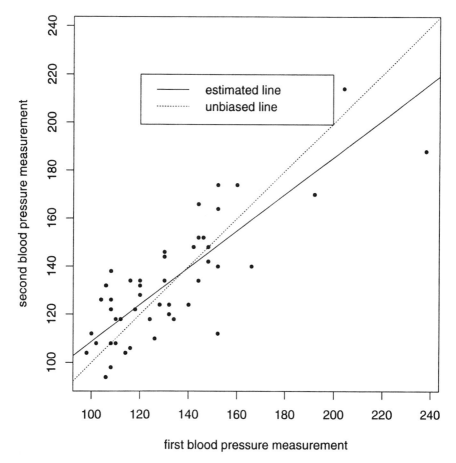

Figure 4.1. Repeated blood pressure levels from the Buffalo Blood Pressure study, first measurement versus second measurement—version 1.

estimated slope of $\hat{b} = 0.769$ (solid line in Figure 4.1). As forecast by the comparison of mean values of individuals above and below the median, the slope of the line determined by the 50 repeated blood pressure pairs is less than 1.0 ($\hat{b} = 0.769 < 1.0$). The reduction in the slope indicates the degree to which large first blood pressure measurements are followed by smaller second measurements and small first blood pressure measurements are followed by larger second measurements.

Formally comparing the estimated slope ($\hat{b}$) to the value expected in the absence of regression to the mean ($b = 1.0$) follows the usual pattern. The ordinary least squares estimated slope is $\hat{b} = 0.769$ (to repeat), and an estimate of the variance associated with this estimate, calculated as part of the estimation procedure, is $S_{\hat{b}}^2 = 0.00609$. To assess the conjecture that $b = 1$ (no within-individual variation), a t-statistic is

$$T = \frac{\hat{b} - 1.0}{S_{\hat{b}}} = \frac{0.769 - 1.0}{0.078} = -2.965.$$

The p-value = $P(T \le -2.965 \mid b = 1.0) = 0.002$ (degrees of freedom = 48) leaves little doubt that the underlying slope estimated by $\hat{b} = 0.769$ is less than 1.0. Thus, regression to the mean is a substantial issue when determining the true systolic blood pressure of an individual based on two measurements.

Figure 4.2 displays another view of the regression to the mean. The vertical lines represent the differences between the first and second blood pres-

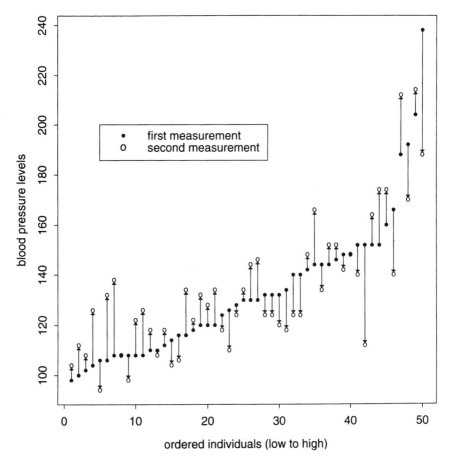

Figure 4.2. Repeated blood pressure levels from the Buffalo Blood Pressure Study, first measurement versus second measurement—version 2.

sure measurements for each individual (ordered from low to high by first values). These lines are generally down after a large first measurement and up after a small first measurement.

A large first measurement is probably followed by a smaller second measurement because random variation dictates that an extreme measurement is not likely to be repeated. It is more likely that a following measurement will be smaller, better reflecting an individual expected level (true mean). Similarly, a small first measurement is likely to be followed by a measurement closer to its expectation, yielding a larger second measurement. More extreme random second measurements are rare simply because extreme measurements in general are not as likely as moderate measurements. For this reason, regression to the mean always exists to some extent as long as repeated measurements are subject to random variation within pairs.

For a baseball player, a high batting average in the first half of the season is likely to be followed by a decreased average in the second half of the season because he is not likely to get all the "good breaks" again and have an equally good or better second half of the season. Nevertheless, the sports press inevitably projects at the all-star break (half of the season) that a player who hit 30 home runs is "on a pace" to hit 60 for the entire season (no regression to the mean). Similarly, but usually less noticed, players who do poorly during the first half of the season likely improve during the second half (i.e., there is nowhere to go but up).

Algebraically comparing the estimated regression line (regression to the mean) to a line with a slope equal to 1.0 (no regression to the mean) gives an expression to correct the second observation. Specifically,

$$\text{estimated correction} = (1 - \hat{b})(y_{1i} - \bar{y}_1)$$

where y_{1i} represents the first measurement on the ith individual. Then a corrected second measurement for the ith individual is estimated by $\hat{Y}_{2i} = y_{2i} +$ correction. If the first blood pressure measurement y_{1i} is greater than the mean $\bar{y}_1$, then the observed second value y_{2i} is likely too small because it is, on average, reduced by regression to the mean (*correction* > 0). Analogously, if the first blood pressure measurement y_{1i} is less than the mean $\bar{y}_1$, then the second measurement y_{2i} is likely too large because it is on average increased by regression to the mean (*correction* < 0). The corrected value $\hat{Y}_2$ is free of the bias caused by regression to the mean. In more statistical terms, the slope of the line describing y_1 and y_2 is less than the slope of the line based on y_1 and $\hat{Y}_2$, which is 1.0. A direct result of the relationship between slopes $\hat{b}$ and 1.0 is that, typically, the correlation between y_1 and y_2 is less than the correlation between y_1 and $\hat{Y}_2$. That is, regression to the mean reduces the within-pair correlation between the first and second measurements. Specifically, for the blood pressure data, the correlations are $r_{y_1 y_2} = 0.818$ (uncorrected) and $r_{y_1 \hat{Y}_2} = 0.880$ (corrected).

It is tempting to correct the observed second measurement, that is, to use $\hat{Y}_2$ in place of y_2. The gain is that the value $\hat{Y}_2$ is unbiased. The loss is that the corrected value has increased variability. The net result may be a loss in usefulness due to instability of the corrected but unbiased estimate. Therefore, correction of the second observation is not a straightforward matter of adding or subtracting the estimated bias. If individual observations are corrected for bias, the correction needs to be done cautiously, paying careful attention to the potential of substantially increased variation in the unbiased values.

Intraclass Correlation Coefficient

The total variation among the Buffalo Blood Pressure Study 100 blood pressure measurements is attributable to two sources. First, the 50 sampled individuals have different levels of blood pressure. This between-person variability in blood pressure levels is summarized by estimating the variance among their mean blood pressure values ($v_{between} = 612.431$). The second source of variation arises from differences between measurements within sampled individuals. Clearly, the two blood pressure measurements made on each person are not identical, and the degree to which these measurements differ reflects the within-person variation. For the blood pressure data, the within-person variability among the 50 differences $y_{1i} - y_{2i}$ is also statistically described by an estimated variance ($v_{within} = 137.898$). Figure 4.3 graphically characterizes these two sources of variation.

More technically, the between-person variance is estimated by

$$\text{between variance} = v_{between} = \text{variance} (\bar{y}_i) - \tfrac{1}{2} v_{within} = 612.431$$

where the within-person variance is estimated by

$$\text{within variance} = v_{within} = \frac{\text{variance} (y_1 - y_2)}{2} = 137.898.$$

The intraclass correlation coefficient (denoted c) is defined as the proportion of between-person variance relative to the total variance from these two sources, simply combining these two measures of variability into a single value between 0 and 1. Specifically, the intraclass correlation coefficient c is estimated by

$$\hat{c} = \frac{v_{between}}{v_{between} + v_{within}} = \frac{612.431}{612.431 + 137.898} = 0.816$$

from the blood pressure data.

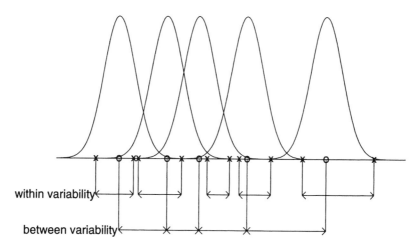

Figure 4.3. A schematic description of within-group and between-group variability for five hypothetical blood pressure distributions.

If the within-individual measurements are identical, then $c = 1.0$ ($v_{within} = 0$). If the sampled individuals all have the same mean level of the measured variable ($v_{between} = 0$), then $c = 0$. Values between 0 and 1 reflect a partitioning of the total variability into two meaningful pieces directly related to the amount of regression to the mean. For example, no regression to the mean occurs when the within-person variation is zero ($c = 1$ and $b = 1$).

In fact, the intraclass correlation coefficient is an alternative estimate of the slope relating the first blood pressure measurement to the second (i.e., $\hat{b} \approx \hat{c}$). The previously estimated slope $\hat{b} = 0.769$ and the intraclass correlation coefficient $\hat{c} = 0.816$ differ because of the random variation associated with these estimated quantities. Such differences diminish as the sample size increases. Demonstration of the equality of the slope of the regression line (b) and the intraclass correlation coefficient (c) rests on the requirements that each observed blood pressure is an estimate of the mean level of that person's distribution of blood pressures and is additionally subject to an independent and consistent within person variation (for example, measurement error). Viewed either as a slope of a regression line or as an intraclass correlation coefficient, the degree of the regression to the mean in a series of repeated measurements is a function of the relative variability between and within persons.

Additional Illustration

Another example of regression to the mean occurs when the scores on a midterm exam and the scores on a final exam are considered. The repeated measures are again two observations made on the same individual. Data from a beginning statistics class (196 students) provide a specific illustration. The students whose midterm scores were below the 30th percentile (score = 84) improved on the final exam by an average of 2.590 points (75.445 to 78.035). Those with scores above the 70th percentile (score = 93) on the midterm exam had scores that decreased on the final exam by an average of 8.074 points (96.333 to 88.259). These exam scores are displayed in Figure 4.4. The dotted line again has a slope of 1.0 representing the scores that would have occurred if the results on the midterm and final exams were identical (no within-individual variation). The solid line is the least squares estimated

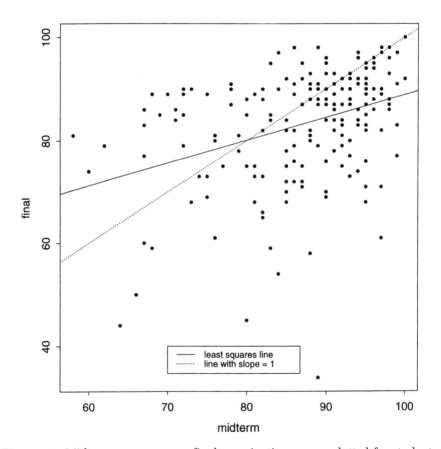

Figure 4.4. Midterm scores versus final examination scores plotted for students in an elementary statistics course.

line with estimated slope $\hat{b} = 0.442$ ($S_{\hat{b}} = 0.079$), which is considerably less than 1.0.

Based on the estimated line, students who scored 10 points above the mean on the midterm had their scores drop, on average, to about 4.4 points above the mean on the final. Conversely, students who scored 10 points below the mean on the midterm improved, on average, to about 4.4 points below the mean on the final exam. In symbols,

$$y_{2i} - \bar{y} \approx 0.442(y_{1i} - \bar{y}).$$

The source of this regression to the mean is likely not entirely statistical. Students who did poorly on the midterm may have increased their efforts for the final exam, and those who did well on the midterm may have become complacent. Such behavior also explains at least part of the observed regression to the mean (Figure 4.4).

The inability to distinguish regression to the mean from other influences that tend to curtail the extremes of the variable under study is a general problem. This issue becomes critically important, for example, when a clinical investigation is conducted to lower the level of a specific substance among individuals with particularly high levels. A trial might be conducted to lower the blood pressure of patients with systolic blood pressure levels over 180 mm Hg. These individuals are measured at baseline, then treated and measured again at a later time. This kind of trial suffers from the difficulty of distinguishing the reduction in blood pressure due to regression to the mean from reduction due to the influence of the treatment or intervention. The analysis of such trials typically depends on sophisticated statistical models to separate these two confounded affects.

In a less serious vein, a national television commercial states that eating a specific breakfast cereal (Quaker Oats) each morning for a week reduces cholesterol levels. To emphasize the claim, several people are presented whose high cholesterol levels notably decreased while eating Quaker Oats. These people are undoubtedly selected to illustrate the reduction; additionally, regression to the mean is part of, if not the whole, explanation of the decrease.

PART II: MISCLASSIFICATION

OBJECTIVE

To evaluate an experimental diet thought to decrease the severity of benign breast disease when the results are biased by misclassification of individuals assigned to treatment and control groups.

DATA

In 1979, it was reported (*Vogue* magazine) that a diet eliminating methylxanthines (primarily coffee, tea, cola, and chocolate) substantially reduced the severity of benign breast disease. To investigate this casually observed association, a randomized trial was conducted on women from the Breast Screening Clinic at the University of California, San Francisco. A total of 154 eligible women were randomly assigned to one of two groups: the members of one group (82 women) were encouraged to remove methylxanthines from their diets, and the members of the other group (82 women) received no dietary recommendations. At baseline each woman was examined by an experienced nurse, and the severity of her disease was scored on a scale from 0 to 4 for each quadrant of the breast, where 1 = slightly nodular, 2 = moderately nodular, 3 = firm dysplasia, and 4 = hard dysplasia. At the end of four months, this examination was repeated and these patients were classified as improved or not improved based on their severity scores. Additionally, the caffeine levels of most participants (132 women) were determined using radioimmunoassay techniques yielding a measure of the diet compliance for the treatment and control individuals. A determination of the participants' compliance status made it possible to estimate the number of women assigned to the diet group who did not maintain the diet and the number of women assigned to the control group who independently adopted a methylxanthine-free diet (i.e., the degree of misclassification). Ten women in the diet group and eight women in the control group were lost to follow-up. The analysis focuses on 124 women with moderate to severe disease (mean severity score ≥ 2).

METHODS

The association between treatment/control status and disease improvement is measured by an estimated odds ratio. A second odds ratio corrected to compensate for misclassification of control/case individuals is estimated to reflect more accurately the effectiveness of the diet. Computer simulation methods are used to conduct statistical tests and construct confidence intervals.

Data type: randomized trial
Reference: *Surgery*, 1982, 91(3): 263–7

The variables are:

1. Diet status: coded 1 if assigned to the treatment group and 0 if assigned to the control group
2. Outcome status: coded 1 for improved and 0 for failed to improve

The tabulated data for 124 trial participants are:

```
file name = breast.4.data

      x1       x2       count
      1        1         15
      1        0         48
      0        1         11
      0        0         50

x1 = diet(1) and no diet (0)
x2 = improved(1) and no improvement(0)

      y1       y2       count
      1        1         58
      1        0         15
      0        1         11
      0        0         48

y1 = diet(1) and no diet(0)
y2 = conformed(1) and failed to conform to the diet(0)
```

DISCUSSION

Even in a simple 2 by 2 table where misclassification takes the form of placing observations in the wrong cell, there are a variety of ways misclassification occurs. For the breast disease data, a special case is relevant. Improvement in the signs of benign breast disease can be determined with essentially no misclassification error. However, considerable misclassification occurs in the treatment (diet recommended) and control (no diet recommended) groups. A number of patients in the treatment group failed to stay on the diet, and a number of patients in the control group took up the diet without recommendation. Measures of the association between diet status and outcome are affected (biased) by this misclassification. A statistically corrected measure of association therefore reflects more accurately the efficacy of the diet in reducing benign breast disease severity.

Part of the data collected to study the value of a methylxanthine-free diet is given in Table 4.1 for the 124 women with the more severe signs of benign breast disease. Taken at face value, these data yield an estimated odds ratio of $\hat{or} = (15)(50)/[(11)(48)] = 1.420$. This approach to assessing the impact of the diet is sometimes referred to as an *intend-to-treat* analysis. The data are analyzed ignoring the misclassification bias in order to maintain the original randomization. The original 63 patients assigned to the diet are compared to the original 61 patients given no dietary recommendations. The intend-to-treat strategy produces an analysis subject to misclassification bias but free of the potentially more damaging selection bias caused by comparing non-randomized groups, that is, those who maintained the diet compared to those who did not.

If the probabilities of misclassification are the same for patients who improved and patients who failed to improve, the misclassification is said to be *nondifferential* with respect to the outcome. Additionally, when nondif-ferential misclassification is present, the odds ratio is biased toward 1.0 if the misclassification is not extreme. That is, the observed odds ratio is closer to 1.0 than the odds ratio that would have been observed in the absence of misclassification. Specifically, from the diet data, the estimated odds ratio (1.420) is likely too small, assuming that the probability a person assign to the diet maintains the diet is the same regardless of the outcome and assuming that the probability a control patient does not take up the diet is the same regardless of the outcome. These two nonmisclassification rates are measured by probabilities called *sensitivity* (denoted p_1) and *specificity* (denoted p_2), respectively. Nondifferential misclassification requires that p_1 and p_2 be the same for both outcomes. When the values $p_1 = 1$ (sensitivity) and $p_2 = 1$ (specificity), no misclassification of either kind occurs. This is not the case for the present data. Using evidence from the caffeine assay, the data in Table 4.2 indicate the degree of misclassification associated with assigned treatment/control status.

Therefore, from Table 4.2, the estimated sensitivity is $\hat{p}_1 = 58/69 = 0.841$ and the estimated specificity is $\hat{p}_2 = 48/63 = 0.762$. Both probabilities are important elements in evaluating the trial data (Table 4.1). The fact that the treatment group contains nondieters and the control group contains dieters

Table 4.1. Distribution of the 124 Severely Affected Women by Diet (Treatment/Control) and Outcome Status

	Diet	No Diet	Total
improved	15	11	26
failed to improve	48	50	98
total	63	61	124

Table 4.2. Distribution of 132 Women Tested for Conformity
(Caffeine Present/Absent) to their Original Treatment
and Control Assignments

	Diet	No Diet	Total
conformed	58	11	69
failed to conform	15	48	63
total	73	59	132

makes these two groups similar regardless of the influence of the diet, bias-
ing any association measured by the odds ratio toward 1.0. The odds ratio
that would have occurred if no misclassification was present can be estimated
based on estimates of sensitivity and specificity associated with classifying
the trial participants.

To describe such an estimate, the benign breast disease trial data are
denoted as follows:

	Diet	No Diet	Total
improved	a	b	$a + b$
failed to improve	c	d	$c + d$
total	$a + c$	$b + d$	n

Using this notation and a bit of algebra produces expressions for the four corrected cell frequencies (Table 4.3) when the misclassification is nondifferential. "Corrected" means that the four cell counts estimate those frequencies
that would have been observed if no misclassification had occurred.

The misclassified observations (Table 4.1) yield a table of data corrected
for treatment/control misclassification (Table 4.4) using the estimated probabilities for sensitivity and specificity (Table 4.2). These "data" then allow an
estimate of a corrected odds ratio that compensates for the misclassification,
where $\hat{or}_{corrected} = (14.622)(57.058)/[(11.378)(40.942)] = 1.791$. The assumption of nondifferential misclassification is important but not unequivocal. It
simply provides a starting point to explore the impact of misclassification bias
incurred in estimating the intend-to-treat odds ratio (1.420 versus 1.791).

Table 4.3. Cell Frequencies Taking Nondifferential Misclassification into
Account (p_1 = Sensitivity and p_2 = Specificity)

	Diet	No Diet	Total
improved	$[b - p_2(a + b)]/(1 - p_1 - p_2)$	$[a - p_1(a + b)]/(1 - p_1 - p_2)$	$a + b$
failed to improve	$[d - p_2(c + d)]/(1 - p_1 - p_2)$	$[c - p_1(c + d)]/(1 - p_1 - p_2)$	$c + d$
total	$[b + d - np_2]/(1 - p_1 - p_2)$	$[a + c - np_1]/(1 - p_1 - p_2)$	n

Note: if $p_1 = p_2 = 1.0$, then the cell frequencies are unchanged.

Table 4.4. Distribution of 124 Women by Diet and Outcome Status Taking Misclassification into Account ($\hat{p}_1 = 0.841$ and $\hat{p}_2 = 0.762$)

	Diet	No Diet	Total
improved	14.622	11.378	26
failed to improve	40.942	57.058	98
total	55.564	68.436	124

The corrected odds ratio is an estimate, and like all estimates it is subject to the impact of sampling variation. Assessing this impact is a necessary part of evaluating the results from a clinical trial. The statistical distribution of the corrected odds ratio can be estimated using a computer sampling strategy. To start, consider the values for sensitivity (p_1) and specificity (p_2) fixed (not subject to variation). To calculate a series of computer-generated corrected odds ratios, it is postulated that the members of the diet group have a binomial distribution (a.3) with parameters $N_1 = 63$ and probability of improvement equal to $P_1 = 15/63 = 0.238$, and the members of the control group also have a binomial distribution but with parameters $N_2 = 61$ and probability of improvement equal to $P_2 = 11/61 = 0.180$. Simulated data from each binomial distribution generate an observed number of "improved" and "failed to improve" individuals for the treatment and control groups, allowing the construction of a computer-generated 2 by 2 table. The variability among a series of replicate tables estimates the variability associated with the 2 by 2 table based on the observed 124 patients in the methylxanthine-free diet trial. Using these tables and sensitivity $= p_1 = 0.841$ and specificity $= p_2 = 0.762$ produces corrected cell frequencies. Computing the corrected odds ratios from 2000 computer-generated tables and taking the logarithms of these values creates an estimated distribution of the corrected log-odds ratio (Figure 4.5). The mean of this distribution is 0.570 yielding an estimated odds ratio of $\hat{or}_{\text{corrected}} = e^{0.570} = 1.768$. Using this estimated distribution, an estimated variance of the logarithm of the corrected odds ratio is also directly calculated ($S^2_{\log(\hat{or}_{\text{corrected}})} = 0.578$). Therefore, a test contrasting the observed $\log(\hat{or}_{\text{corrected}}) = 0.570$ (mean of the computer-generated distribution) with $\log(or_{\text{corrected}}) = \log(1) = 0$ (no impact of the diet) gives

$$z = \frac{\log(\hat{or}_{\text{corrected}}) - 0}{S_{\log(\hat{or}_{\text{corrected}})}} = \frac{0.570 - 0}{\sqrt{0.578}} = 0.750$$

yielding a p-value $= P(|Z| \geq 0.750 \mid or_{\text{corrected}} = 1) = 0.45$. Also, an approximate 95% confidence interval based on the estimated mean and variance from the computer-generated distribution is

$$\text{lower bound} = \log(\hat{or}_{\text{corrected}}) - 1.960 \, S_{\log(\hat{or}_{\text{corrected}})}$$
$$= 0.570 - 1.960\sqrt{0.578} = -0.919$$

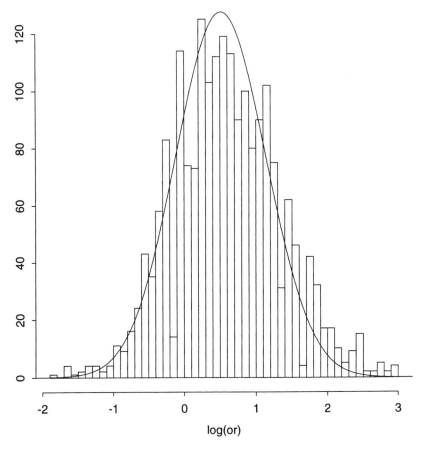

Figure 4.5. Computer-generated estimate of the distribution of the logarithm of the adjusted odds ratios from the methylxanthine-free diet data.

$$\text{upper bound} = \log\left(\hat{or}_{\text{corrected}}\right) + 1.960\ S_{\log\left(\hat{or}_{\text{corrected}}\right)}$$
$$= 0.570 + 1.960\sqrt{0.578} = 2.059$$

giving an approximate 95% confidence interval $(-0.919, 2.059)$ for the underlying corrected log-odds ratio. The approximate 95% confidence interval, based on the unbiased value estimated by $\hat{or}_{\text{corrected}} = e^{0.570} = 1.768$, is then

$$\left(e^{\text{lower}}, e^{\text{upper}}\right) = \left(e^{-0.919}, e^{2.059}\right) = (0.399, 7.836).$$

Again, using a computer simulation process, but incorporating the fact that the measures of sensitivity and specificity ($\hat{p}_1 = 0.840$ and $\hat{p}_2 = 0.762$) are themselves estimates and subject to sampling variation, gives similar results. The parallel test statistic $z = 0.731$ yields a p-value of 0.46, and the approximate 95% confidence interval (0.373, 8.709) is slightly larger. The reason for the similarity between the two computer simulation analyses is that the sensitivity and specificity probabilities p_1 and p_2 are estimated using sample sizes large enough (diet = 69 and controls = 63 observations) so that the additional sampling variation contributes only marginally to the assessment of the corrected odds ratio.

CONCLUSIONS

Part I

The analysis of the repeated blood pressure measurements shows substantial regression to the mean. Necessarily, an intraclass correlation coefficient indicates the same magnitude of regression to the mean. Specifically, the estimated slope is 0.769 from the regression analysis of the first and second blood pressure measurements, and the estimated intraclass correlation coefficient is 0.816. If no regression to the mean exists, both values would be close to 1.0.

Part II

The clinical trial to evaluate the influence of a methylxanthine-free diet on the signs of benign breast disease produces no strong evidence that the diet is effective. The analysis comparing the intend-to-treat individuals (maintaining the randomization) yields an odd ratio of 1.420. This odds ratio, however, is reduced by considerable misclassification bias. An adjustment based on the assumption that the misclassification is nondifferential allows an estimate free from this bias ($\hat{or}_{corrected}$ = 1.768). The impact of random variation on the adjusted odds ratio is described using a simulation strategy, but the analysis gives no indication of a systematic influence from the diet (p-value = 0.46 and 95% CI: 0.373, 8.709).

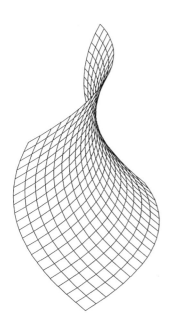

CHAPTER 5

Goodness-of-Fit

OBJECTIVE

To review Gregor Mendel's observations made on ornamental garden peas (*Pisum sativum*), particularly the correspondence to two specific ratios (3:1 and 2:1). In addition, to explore the question: *do Mendel's data correspond to these ratios too closely, indicating a bias in recording his experimental results?*

DATA

In 1866, Mendel reported on 14 now famous experiments.[10] Using ornamental plants, he observed characteristics of the seeds and plants in the offspring from specific parental generations. Two properties of the seeds were observed (shape and color), and observations on five properties of the plants were also made (plant color, pod shape, pod color, flower position, and stem length). These experiments were conducted under two conditions yielding two sets of seven experiments, and each experiment produced two outcomes.

THE GENETICS

Using modern genetic knowledge, Mendel's experiments can be described in terms of a simple model. The first seven experiments consist of crossing two heterozygotic plants (parental generation). In symbols, a heterozygotic cross is represented as $Aa \times Aa$ (A denotes one gene and a denotes a second gene). This mating produces three possible offspring, namely, AA, Aa, and aa. Today it is known that the probability of an AA plant is 1/4, that of an Aa plant is 1/2, and that of an aa plant is 1/4. However, Mendel could not distinguish directly between AA and Aa offspring and simply counted two kinds of plants, now called *dominant* (AA or Aa plants) and *recessive* (aa plants) *phenotypes*. The expected ratio of dominant to recessive phenotypes is then 3:1.

To further understand the properties of these offspring, Mendel crossed dominant offspring with themselves, yielding a second set of seven experiments. Two kinds of matings between identical-appearing dominant phenotypes occurred, which in modern genetic notation are represented as $Aa \times Aa$ and $AA \times AA$. The first kind of mating produces a mixture of dominant and recessive offspring (both dominant AA/Aa and recessive aa phenotypes), and the second kind of mating produces only one type of offspring (dominant—AA only). The probability of the first kind of mating is 2/3 and the probability of the second kind of mating is 1/3 among the dominant offspring. Mendel's second experiments demonstrated that among the identical-appearing dominant offspring of the first generation there were two kinds of plants, those that did not breed true and those that did. The expected ratio of these two kinds of plants is 2:1. Combining the results of these two experiments, Mendel deduced that three different offspring result from a heterozygotic mating in a ratio of 1:2:1 ($AA:Aa:aa$). These 14 experiments are fundamentally important because they were the first indication that genes are discrete units passed from one generation to the next, expressing their effects through different combinations.

METHODS

A variety of Pearson's chi-square goodness-of-fit tests are used to evaluate the correspondence between observed and expected frequencies for each seed/plant characteristic and combined sets of seed/plant characteristics. Simulation techniques are also used to describe the correspondence between the first set of experiments and a 3:1 ratio and the correspondence between the second set of experiments and a 2:1 ratio without approximations or a parametric-based analysis.

Data type: experimental
Reference: *The Origin of Genetics*, C Stern and E. R. Sherwood, W. H. Freeman and Co. (1966)

The variables are:

1. Total number of seeds/plants
2. Number of seeds/plants expressing a specific trait
3. Number of seeds/plants expressing an alternative specific trait

The tabulated data file from Mendel's 14 experiments is:

```
                  file name = mendel.5.data
```

seed:	shape	7324	5474	1850
seed:	color	8023	6022	2001
plant:	color	929	705	224
plant:	pod shape	1181	882	299
plant:	pod color	580	428	152
plant:	position	858	651	207
plant:	stem length	1064	787	277
seed:	shape	565	372	193
seed:	color	519	353	166
plant:	color	100	64	36
plant:	pod shape	100	71	29
plant:	pod color	100	60	40
plant:	position	100	67	33
plant:	stem length	100	72	28

DISCUSSION

It might be argued that the theory of genetics began when Gregor Mendel presented the results of his plant breeding experiments in 1866.[10] In 1936, statistician/geneticist R. A. Fisher[11] concluded that Mendel or his co-workers had intentionally or unintentionally manipulated these experiments to favor the expected outcomes. Fisher's conclusion was based on a series of chi-square analyses indicating that the Mendel's plant data lacked the expected variability, causing the observed values to be too close to their theoretical values.[12,13]

A natural way to start to explore Mendel's experimental data and R. A. Fisher's suggestion that the data were too-good-to-be-true is to compute the expected counts for all 14 experiments (28 values) and compare them to the observed counts (also 28 values). For example, the first experiment produced 7324 seeds, 5474 of which were round or roundish and 1850 were angular. The corresponding expected numbers based on a 3:1 ratio are $(3/4)7324 = 5493$ round seeds and $(1/4)7324 = 1831$ angular seeds. Similarly, for all 14 of Mendel's experiments, the observed counts (o_i) and the calculated expected counts (e_i) are given in Table 5.1. The classic Pearson chi-square statistic pro-

Table 5.1. Mendel's Data (o_i), Expected Values (e_i) and Contributions to the Chi-Square Statistic (residual$_i$)

Experiment	Type	Ratio	o_i	e_i	$o_i - e_i$	residual$_i$
1	seed	3:1	5474	5493.000	−19.000	−0.256
	seed	3:1	1850	1831.000	19.000	0.444
2	seed	3:1	6022	6017.250	4.750	0.061
	seed	3:1	2001	2005.750	−4.750	−0.106
3	plant	3:1	705	696.750	8.250	0.313
	plant	3:1	224	232.250	−8.250	−0.541
4	plant	3:1	882	885.750	−3.750	−0.126
	plant	3:1	299	295.250	3.750	0.218
5	plant	3:1	428	435.000	−7.000	−0.336
	plant	3:1	152	145.000	7.000	0.581
6	plant	3:1	651	643.500	7.500	0.296
	plant	3:1	207	214.500	−7.500	−0.512
7	plant	3:1	787	798.000	−11.000	−0.389
	plant	3:1	277	266.000	11.000	0.674
8	seed	2:1	372	376.667	−4.667	−0.240
	seed	2:1	193	188.333	4.667	0.340
9	seed	2:1	353	346.000	7.000	0.376
	seed	2:1	166	173.000	−7.000	−0.532
10	plant	2:1	64	66.667	−2.667	−0.327
	plant	2:1	36	33.333	2.667	0.462
11	plant	2:1	71	66.667	4.333	0.531
	plant	2:1	29	33.333	−4.333	−0.751
12	plant	2:1	60	66.667	−6.667	−0.816
	plant	2:1	40	33.333	6.667	1.155
13	plant	2:1	67	66.667	0.333	0.041
	plant	2:1	33	33.333	−0.333	−0.058
14	plant	2:1	72	66.667	5.333	0.653
	plant	2:1	28	33.333	−5.333	−0.924

vides an overall summary of the goodness-of-fit (a.5). In addition, the individual contributions to the chi-square statistic provide information on the closeness of the fit for each experiment (also Table 5.1—labeled "residual$_i$"). Algebraically, these residual values measure the relative correspondence between each observed and expected count as

$$\text{residual}_i = \frac{o_i - e_i}{\sqrt{e_i}}.$$

The test statistic X^2 has an approximate chi-square distribution with 14 degrees of freedom if the theory generating the expected values is correct. Additionally, when the observed values differ from the expected values only because of random variation, the observed chi-square statistic X^2 is expected to be about equal to its degrees of freedom. For the 28 comparisons, this property translates into a rule of thumb that each residual value should be roughly

$\sqrt{14/28} = \pm 0.7$. Therefore, as a guide, residual values greater than 1.4 or less than -1.4 indicate experiments with exceptional lack of fit. Based in this ad hoc guideline, Mendel's data certainly show no evidence of a lack of fit to either the 3:1 or 2:1 ratio. The largest residual is 1.155.

Using Mendel's plant data, Fisher focused on the left tail of the chi-square distribution. Hypotheses that direct attention to small values of a chi-square statistic are extremely unusual but address the conjecture that the observed data fit the expected values too well. That is, a chi-square value of $X^2 = 0$ means that the observed values correspond exactly to the expected values and the data show no (random) variation. Furthermore, unlikely values of X^2 in the neighborhood of zero imply an unlikely lack of random variability. The question then becomes; *is the chi-square test statistic too small (improbably little?), implying that the observed results lack sufficient random variation?*

The chi-square test statistic summarizing the fit of all 28 experimental results (Table 5.1) is $X^2 = 7.187$ (degrees of freedom $= 14$) and the association left-tail significance probability is p-value $= P(X^2 \leq 7.187 \mid$ random variation only$) = 0.07$. This moderately small probability hints at a lack of random variation when the 14 experiments are combined into one analysis, but it is certainly not exceptionally strong evidence of a too-good fit. This inference is supported by the observation that among the 28 residual values a few (5) values exceed the expected range of ± 0.7 but, on the other hand, a few (3) are remarkably small (less than 0.1). Incidentally, the usual p-value calculated to assess lack of fit (right-tail significance probability) is the complementary probability or 0.93, clearly indicating that no evidence exists of important deviations from the 3:1 and 2:1 ratios, which is the primary genetic issue.

Alternatively, and perhaps more naturally, an observed proportion summarizes each of Mendel's 14 experiments. For example, the seed data from the first experiment produce a proportion of round seeds of $5474/7324 = 0.747$ ($\hat{p}_1 = 0.747$), and the expected proportion is 0.750 ($p_0 = 0.750$). The 14 observed and expected proportions are recorded in Table 5.2.

To identify closeness, the probability that by chance alone a value would occur as close as or closer to the expected value as the value observed is one effective description. For example, the number of round seeds observed for the first experiment is 5474 and the expected value is 5493. The probability is 0.401 that a random value would be as close as or closer to the expectation, that is, between 5474 and 5512 or would deviate from 5493 by 19 or fewer round seeds. If Mendel's data fit too well, these closeness probabilities should be small (unusually close). Alternatively, if the data have the expected amount of variation (a binomial distribution), these probabilities would reflect only random differences within the 14 experiments.

Table 5.2. Mendel's 14 Experimental Results Expressed in Terms of Proportions

Experiment	$\hat{p}_i$	p_0	Exact	Approx.	z_i	p-Value
1	0.747	0.750	0.401	0.401	0.526	0.599
2	0.751	0.750	0.109	0.108	0.135	0.892
3	0.759	0.750	0.496	0.493	0.663	0.507
4	0.747	0.750	0.225	0.225	0.286	0.775
5	0.738	0.750	0.528	0.528	0.719	0.472
6	0.759	0.750	0.472	0.472	0.631	0.528
7	0.740	0.750	0.584	0.584	0.814	0.416
8	0.658	0.667	0.355	0.355	0.461	0.645
9	0.680	0.667	0.515	0.515	0.698	0.485
10	0.640	0.667	0.497	0.498	0.672	0.502
11	0.710	0.667	0.694	0.695	1.025	0.305
12	0.600	0.667	0.871	0.872	1.510	0.128
13	0.670	0.667	0.140	0.140	0.177	0.860
14	0.720	0.667	0.783	0.784	1.237	0.216

The binomial probability of observing by chance a random value as close as or closer to the expectation than the one observed among n_i observations is

$$P(\text{close}) = \sum_{k=x_0}^{x_1} \binom{n_i}{k} p_0^k (1 - p_0)^{n_i - k}$$

where $x_0 = n_i p_0 - x$, $x_1 = n_i p_0 + x$ and x is the distance between the observed and expected counts (absolute value of the difference—column 6, Table 5.1). For the first experiment, for example,

$$P(\text{close}) = \sum_{k=5474}^{5512} \binom{7324}{k} 0.75^k (1 - 0.75)^{7324 - k} = 0.401.$$

These probabilities are given in Table 5.2 (column labeled "Exact").

Using a standard normal distribution as an approximation of the exact binomial distribution, the same closeness probability is approximately

$$P(\text{close}) = P\left[Z \le \frac{|\hat{p}_i - p_0| + 0.5/n_i}{\sqrt{\text{variance }(\hat{p}_i)}}\right] - P\left[Z \le -\frac{|\hat{p}_i - p_0| + 0.5/n_i}{\sqrt{\text{variance }(\hat{p}_i)}}\right]$$

where the variance of the observed proportion $\hat{p}_i$ is variance $(\hat{p}_i) = p_0(1 - p_0)/n_i$. The term $0.5/n_i$ is a continuity correction factor that increases the accuracy of the approximation. These probabilities are also given in Table 5.2 (column labeled "Approx."). No exceptionally close observations occur among the 14 probabilities (minimum = 0.109).

An alternative assessment of the difference between $\hat{p}_i$ and p_0 is achieved with another normal approximation where

$$p\text{-value} = 2 \times P\left[Z \geq \frac{|\hat{p}_i - p_0| + 0.5/n_i}{\sqrt{\text{variance} (\hat{p}_i)}}\right].$$

The value Z again has an approximate standard normal distribution when the underlying probability estimated by $\hat{p}_i$ is p_0. Large probabilities again indicate unlikely small deviations from the expected values. For the first experiment, $\hat{p}_1 = 0.747$ and $p_0 = 0.750$, yielding $z_1 = 0.526$ (Table 5.2). Then, from a standard normal distribution, the p-value is $2P(Z \geq 0.526 \mid$ random difference$) = 0.60$. Therefore, the probability of a more extreme value than the one observed is 0.60 when only random variation influences the difference between observed and expected proportions (i.e., $\hat{p}_i$ has expected value p_0). These 14 approximate p-values are listed in Table 5.2 (column labeled "p-Value") and are directly related to the closeness probabilities also listed in Table 5.2. They sum to 1.0.

Either comparison (Table 5.2) provides 14 separate perspectives, one for each experiment, on the likelihood that $\hat{p}_i$ differs from p_0 by chance. Evaluated one experiment at a time, Mendel's data show no clear pattern of closeness.

A chi-square statistic summarizing all 14 experiments (Table 5.2) is $\sum z_i^2 = 7.256$, which is not appreciably different from the previous Pearson chi-square value, $X^2 = 7.187$. The two chi-square statistics differ only because of the correction factor $0.5/n_i$ used in the normal approximation; without the correction factor the two summaries are identical (a.5).

Mendel's data can be analyzed where similar experiments are considered together rather than as 14 separate sets of observations. Six possibilities based on natural combinations of the z_i-values follow from Table 5.2 and are summarized with a chi-square statistic:

1. Seed properties and a 3:1 ratio, where
   $X_1^2 = z_1^2 + z_2^2 = 0.295$ (degrees of freedom = 2), giving a p-value = 0.14.
2. Plant properties and a 3:1 ratio, where
   $X_2^2 = z_3^2 + \cdots + z_7^2 = 2.099$ (degrees of freedom = 5), giving a p-value = 0.17.
3. Seed properties and a 2:1 ratio, where
   $X_3^2 = z_8^2 + z_9^2 = 0.700$ (degrees of freedom = 2), giving a p-value = 0.30.
4. Plant properties and a 2:1 ratio, where
   $X_4^2 = z_{10}^2 + \cdots + z_{14}^2 = 5.376$ (degrees of freedom = 5), giving a p-value = 0.63.
5. Summary for a 3:1 ratio, where
   $X_5^2 = z_1^2 + \cdots + z_7^2 = 2.394$ (degrees of freedom = 7), giving a p-value = 0.06.
6. Summary for a 2:1 ratio, where
   $X_6^2 = z_8^2 + \cdots + z_{14}^2 = 6.077$ (degrees of freedom = 7), giving a p-value = 0.47.

These specific chi-square statistics and p-values (left-tail probabilities) show a mixture of results with regard to the fit of the data. It could be argued that the seven experiments with expected 3:1 ratios indicate some lack of the expected random variation (p-value $= 0.06$). The results from the summary analyses of the 2:1 ratio data show rather usual correspondence between observed and expected values (p-value $= 0.47$). However, the combined results are rather unlikely. The likelihood associated with both the 3:1 and 2:1 experiments is $0.06(0.47) = 0.028$.

Simulation Approach

Using computer simulation techniques, Mendel's data from the 14 plant breeding experiments can be re-created. A sample of n_i values is randomly selected (with replacement) from a population consisting of $n_i p_0$ values of 1 and $n_i (1 - p_0)$ values of 0. The observed number of ones (denoted X) simulates Mendel's experimental results except that the computer-generated data conform perfectly to the theoretical binomial distribution with parameters n_i and p_0. The computer sample produces a simulated proportion (denoted $\hat{P}_i = X/n_i$) and then a test statistic z_i where

$$ z_i = \frac{\hat{P}_i - p_0}{\sqrt{\text{variance}\,(\hat{P}_i)}}. $$

The z_i-values for each experiment conform perfectly to the underlying hypothetical situation, namely, a sample size n_i with probability 0.75 (3:1) or 0.667 (2:1) with exactly the expected random variation.

To explore the issues surrounding Mendel's data, simulated z_i-values are generated for seven 3:1 computer experiments based on the seven sample sizes from his original data and $p_0 = 0.75$. The seven z_i-values combined into a single chi-square-like test statistic give

$$ Y_3^2 = z_1^2 + z_2^2 + \cdots + z_7^2. $$

The subscript 3 indicates a 3:1 ratio or $p_0 = 3/4$. The process is repeated a large number of times to estimate the distribution of Y_3 without theory or assumptions. Such a distribution is shown in Figure 5.1 based on 2000 simulated values of Y_3^2.

The mean of this simulated chi-square-like distribution is 7.220, with a variance of 14.561. Incidentally, the corresponding theoretical chi-square distribution has a mean of 7 and a variance of 14 (solid line in Figure 5.1). The left-tail empiric p-value associated with this simulated distribution is the

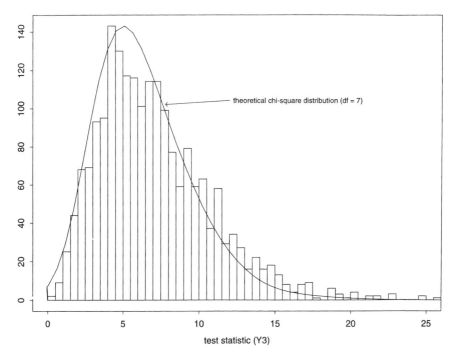

Figure 5.1. The simulated distribution of the chi-square statistic summarizing Mendel's 3:1 experiments (line = theoretical chi-square distribution).

number of Y_3^2-values smaller than 2.394 (the corresponding summary value observed from Mendel's first set of seven experiments). Among the 2000 experiments 104 values are less than 2.394, yielding an empiric left-tail p-value of $P(Y_3^2 \le 2.394 \mid p_0 = 3/4) = 104/2000 = 0.052$.

The same process repeated for the seven experiments with an expected 2:1 ratio produces an analogous empiric p-value. That is, the simulation process creates 2000 values of Y_2^2 based on a 2:1 ratio ($p_0 = 2/3$) and the binomial distribution where

$$Y_2^2 = z_1^2 + z_2^2 + \cdots + z_7^2.$$

The estimated distribution of Y_2^2 is displayed in Figure 5.2. The observed mean of these simulated Y_2^2-values is 7.036, with a variance of 12.966 (as before, the corresponding chi-square distribution has a mean of 7 and a variance of 14). The empiric p-value is again the count of the simulated test statistics smaller than the observed value of 6.077 (the corresponding value from

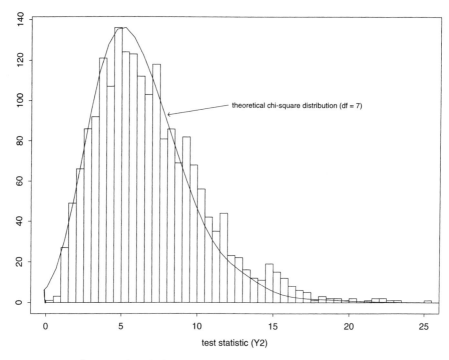

theoretical chi-square distribution (df = 7)

test statistic (Y2)

Figure 5.2. The simulated distribution of the chi-square statistic summarizing Mendel's 2:1 experiments (line = theoretical chi-square distribution).

Mendel's second set of seven experiments). The observed count of 652 yields an empiric p-value of $P(Y_2^2 \leq 6.077 \mid p_0 = 2/3) = 652/2000 = 0.326$. Both simulation experiments accurately reproduce the analysis based on the theoretical chi-square distribution. Although the similarity is not surprising, it is reassuring that the approximate and parametric chi-square results hardly differ from the nonparametric simulation results.

The simulated Y^2-distributions provide an answer to another question. The combined results estimate the overall likelihood associated with both the 3:1 and 2:1 experiments. That is, the joint probability associated with the combined 3:1 and 2:1 data sets is

$$\text{joint } p\text{-value} = P(Y_3^2 \leq 2.394 \text{ and } Y_2^2 \leq 6.077).$$

Again, it is simply a matter of counting the pairs of simulated Y^2-values that are simultaneously less than the observed values 2.394 and 6.077, respectively. Figure 5.3 shows all 2000 (Y_3^2, Y_2^2) pairs, and 44 pairs occur where both simulated Y^2-values are simultaneously less than the observed values, making the empiric joint p-value = 44/2000 = 0.022.

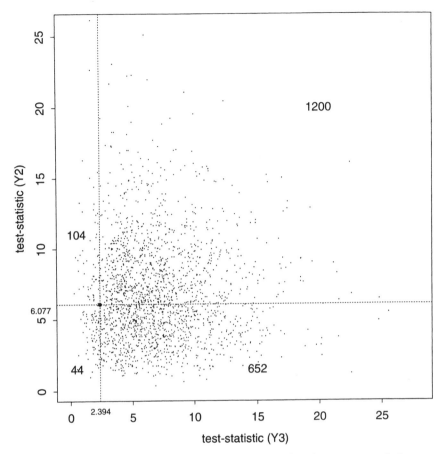

Figure 5.3. The simulated bivariate distribution of the chi-square statistics summarizing Mendel's 3:1 and 2:1 experiments.

Two last points:

The second set of experiments designed to identify the two kinds of dominant characteristics (AA from Aa) has the potential to be slightly biased. The heterozygotic matings ($Aa \times Aa$) among the dominant offspring do not necessarily produce an aa-type offspring, distinguishing the AA-type from the Aa-type plants. The probability of a series of matings between two Aa plants not producing an aa offspring is $(3/4)^n$, where n represents the number of matings. For example, if $n = 10$, then $(3/4)^{10} = 0.06$ is the probability that an Aa plant (heterozygotic) will not be recognized. To the extent that Mendel's experiments failed to identify the Aa-type plants, the 2:1 ratio is understated. Inspection of Mendel's data, however, shows no evidence of this subtle bias.

Another potential bias arises from the fact that a chi-square analysis requires the observations to be sampled independently. It is likely that many of Mendel's plants were grown from seeds of a single pair of parents ("sibs"). Again, the bias from this lack of independence is not likely a substantial influence on the observed experimental results.

CONCLUSIONS

The analysis of Mendel's data illustrates a concern in most analyses of categorical data. The results are influenced, sometimes substantially, by how the categories are defined and tables constructed. R. A. Fisher chose to classify the observations into tables that tend to indicate a lack of random variation in the collected data.[11] Other geneticists, based on different tabulations, found less good fits and concluded that no strong evidence exists that the data were collected in a biased manner.[12,13] The important principle illustrated by the "too-good-to-be-true" controversy is that results based on categorical data frequently depend on sometimes subjective and sometimes arbitrary choices made to classify the observations. This problem is frequently an issue in dealing with tabular data in general and is not easily solved. The variety of results that emerge from the present analyses of Mendel's garden pea data as well as other published analyses[11–13] clearly illustrate this concern.

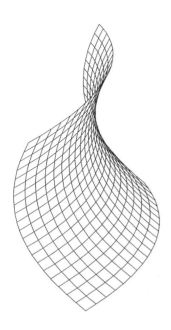

CHAPTER **6**

Analysis of a
Two-Way Table

OBJECTIVE

To describe the relationship between marital status and the incidence of cancer of the rectum among white and African-American males.

DATA

Incident cases of rectal cancer were abstracted from the Third National Cancer Survey data and classified by gender, age, and marital status for whites and African-Americans for ages ranging from 35 to 64 years. The Third National Cancer Survey consists of data collected from nine selected areas (21 million population) over a three year period (1969–71). Cancer incidence rates were calculated using population counts derived from 1970 U.S. Census Bureau enumerations. A total of 2,905,825 white and 294,940 black males yielded 569 and 60 cancer cases, respectively. The data were classified into three 10-year age groups (35–44, 45–54, and 55–64 years). Grouping disease or mortality data generally reduces the heterogeneity of risk of disease and is particularly important for cancer incidence data, where considerable heterogeneity is typically found associated with age. Furthermore, rectal cancer in individuals under the age of 35 is extremely rare. Five marital status groups were used: single, married, separated, divorced, and widowed. Marital status was unreported in only a small proportion of cases, about 1% among white males and about 1.2% among black males.

METHODS

Incidence rates are tabulated forming a two-way table (a 6 by 5 table—six age/race categories by five marital status categories). The table is analyzed by a distribution-free technique (median polish) to describe differences in risk of rectal cancer with respect to marital status among white and black race/ethnicity groups. A parallel analysis is conducted based on a linear model where the number of cases within each cell of the table is assumed to have a Poisson distribution (Poisson regression analysis).

Data type: survey/incidence (surveillance records)
Reference: *Journal of the National Cancer Institute*, 1979, 63(3): 567–85

The variables are:

1. White population: white population person-years at risk
2. Black population: black population person-years at risk
3. White cases: counts of white incidence cases
4. Black cases: counts of black incidence cases

The tabulated data file of 629 rectal cancer cases is:

file name = rectal.6.data

white	black	wcases	bcases
74457	12374	3	1
923669	79874	33	5
12317	9788	1	1
42984	8407	2	1
4787	1959	1	1
61665	7569	17	1
929227	75641	146	14
12276	8967	2	1
45574	8643	11	1
13662	4666	3	1
46009	4492	29	5
670266	54154	287	21
8465	5534	2	2
32917	5768	17	2
27550	7104	15	3

row order:
ages 35–44; single, married, separated, divorced, widowed
ages 45–54; single, married, separated, divorced, widowed
ages 55–64; single, married, separated, divorced, widowed

DISCUSSION

Tables are fundamental to understanding collected data. They come in a variety of shapes and kinds. An important distinction is based on their contents. The cells of a table can contain a count or a continuous measure such as a mean or a rate. The kind of data dictates the statistical approach. The investigation of the relationship between marital status and the risk of rectal cancer focuses on an r by c table containing rates. The symbol r stands for the number of rows and c stands for the number of columns. The rectal cancer data form an $r = 6$ by $c = 5$ table of 30 cancer incidence rates. The age/race-specific incidence rates of rectal cancer per 100,000 persons-years at risk are given in Table 6.1 and displayed in Figure 6.1 (left side) for each marital status category. Age and race are combined into a single six-level variable to produce a parsimonious two-way table. Incidentally, almost no difference exists in the overall race-specific incidence rates. These incidence rates (*crude rates*—ignoring age and marital status) are 19.6 cases/100,000 among whites and 20.3 cases/100,000 among blacks.

When the levels of a categorical variable have multiplicative influences on the risk of disease or death, an additive model based on the logarithm of the rates is frequently an appropriate statistical structure (a.13). Even if an additive model is not appropriate, it remains a good place to start the analysis of an r by c table. An additive model describing log-rates classified into a two-way table is

$$\log (R_{ij}) = a + r_i + c_j.$$

The logarithm of the expected cancer incidence rate (denoted R_{ij}) in the (ith, jth) cell is represented as a function of a background level (denoted a) plus an influence from the row variable (denoted r_i) plus an influence from the column variable (denoted c_j). An additive model describes the row and column variables as independent in the sense that row influences are unaffected by the level of the column variable and, conversely, the column influences

Table 6.1. Incidence Rates of Rectal Cancer (Cases per 100,000 Person-Years) by Age/Race and Marital Status

Age	Race	Single	Married	Separated	Divorced	Widowed
35–44	white	4.0	3.6	8.1	4.7	20.9
45–54	white	27.6	15.7	16.3	24.1	22.0
55–64	white	63.0	42.8	23.6	51.6	54.4
35–44	black	8.1	6.3	10.2	11.9	51.0
45–54	black	13.2	18.5	11.2	11.6	21.4
55–64	black	111.3	38.8	36.1	34.7	42.2

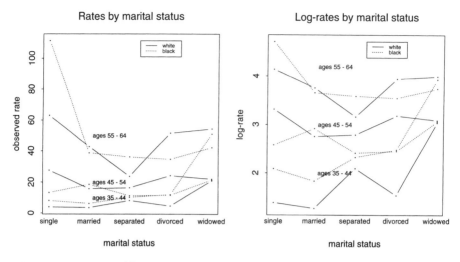

Figure 6.1. Rates and log-rates of the incidence of rectal cancer among white and black males by marital status for three age groups.

are unaffected by the level of the row variable. In terms of the model parameters, comparing additive log-rates between two age/race groups (the ith and kth rows) gives

$$\log (R_{ij}) - \log (R_{kj}) = (a + r_i + c_j) - (a + r_k + c_j) = r_i - r_k.$$

The column variable does not affect the comparison of log-rates between rows. The same property applies to comparing columns. The validity (goodness-of-fit) of the additive model then becomes an essential issue in the analysis because row and column influences are not necessarily independent. The log-rates from the rectal cancer incidence data contained in the 6 by 5 table are also displayed in Figure 6.1 (right side).

Conjecturing that the row and column categorical variables have additive influences on the log-rates is the same as postulating that the categorical variables have independent multiplicative influences on the incidence rates themselves. In symbols, the two equivalent model are

$$\log (R_{ij}) = a + r_i + c_j \quad \text{and} \quad R_{ij} = e^{a+r_i+c_j} = AR_iC_j$$

making the expected rate R_{ij} a multiplicative function of a background level (denoted A), a row variable influence (denoted R_i), and a column variable influence (denoted C_j).

Like most statistical analyses, the analysis of an r by c table can be descriptive (distribution-free), analytic, or both. A descriptive approach, called the

median polish,[14] allows estimates of the additive and nonadditive components of the model based on the observed log-rates and is distribution-free
in the sense that no statistical distribution is postulated as underlying the
sampled data.

For the rectal cancer incidence data, each log-rate is partitioned into two
pieces where

$$\log (\text{rate}) = \text{additive component} + \text{residual component}.$$

The additive component, as might be suspected, conforms perfectly to the
additive model structure. In other words, a residual value of zero indicates
that the row and column influences are exactly additive and, therefore, completely unrelated. The extent to which the residual values are not zero measures either random variation or both random variation and the degree of
association between the influences of the row and columns variables (also
called an *interaction* or *nonadditivity*).

A description of the mechanics of applying the median polish smoothing
process to a two-way table follows:[15]

A median polish provides estimates of the residual values by an iterative
process. First the row influences are estimated by the median value of each
row. Each row median is then subtracted from each cell value in the corresponding row of the table, producing a revised value for each cell. The
additive row effect is thus "removed." Then, column medians are found for
each column of the revised table. The estimated column influences are subtracted from each cell value in the corresponding column. This process is
repeated a number of times (usually about five or so) until the residual values no longer appreciably change (i.e., until all row and column medians
are zero or approximately zero). When the cell residual values become stable, they reflect the non-additivity among components of the table. The differences between these residual values and the original data yield "data"
that perfectly conform to the additive model. The process partitions the
original cell values into an additive piece and a residual piece (*data = additive "data" + residual*). Cells with large residual values show the areas of
lack of fit to the additive structure and are potentially important in understanding of the joint effects of the row and column categorical variables.
The median polish process can also begin by estimating the column influences (column medians) and iterating to a set of stable residual values. The
results will slightly differ from those where the row median is used to begin
the median polish but generally it makes little difference whether the process begins with the rows or the columns.

The residual values generated from the median polish applied to the marital status log-rates are given in Table 6.2.

The smallest residual value is −0.631 and the largest is 1.177. The two
largest residual values are associated with the rectal cancer rates for the

Table 6.2. Residual Values Based on the Marital Status Data (Log-Rates)
Estimated from a Median Polish

Age	Race	Single	Married	Separated	Divorced	Widowed
35–44	white	−0.253	−0.077	0.708	0.000	1.177
45–54	white	0.266	0.000	0.000	0.242	−0.177
55–64	white	0.091	0.000	−0.631	0.000	−0.272
35–44	black	−0.494	−0.454	0.000	0.001	1.133
45–54	black	−0.091	0.543	0.000	−0.115	0.177
55–64	black	0.865	0.107	0.000	−0.193	−0.320

young, widowed whites (1.177) and blacks (1.133). These residual values and the other 28 residual values are small relative to the original rates, and many values are zero or nearly zero. A more statistically rigorous assessment of the residual values is possible but requires a parametric model (to follow). That is, the lack of fit can be assessed formally when it is postulated that the data are sampled from a specific underlying statistical distribution.

As mentioned, residual values are frequently indicators of important systematic influences. The 30 marital status residual values summarized by a "+", "−", or zero (Table 6.3) is one way to recognize possible patterns. The table of pluses and minuses shows no remarkable pattern. The lack of large residual values and the absence of any pattern are necessary to use an additive relationship meaningfully to summarize the influence of age/race and marital status on the incidence of rectal cancer.

The estimated rates based on the assumption of additivity are given in Table 6.4, where estimated log-rate = observed log-rate − residual and the estimated *additive rate* is then rate = $e^{\text{estimated log-rate}}$. For example, for single white males aged 35–44, the residual value is −0.253 (Table 6.2) and the estimated additive log-rate follows as $\log(3/74{,}457 \times 100{,}000) - (-0.253) = \log(4.029) - (-0.253) = 1.394 + 0.253 = 1.647$. The estimated additive rate is then rate = $e^{1.647} = 5.189$ cases/100,000 (Table 6.4). The observed rate is 4.0 cases per 100,000 person-years. The median polish estimated rates in Table 6.4 are perfectly multiplicative, and all residual values are exactly zero.

Table 6.3. Rectal Cancer Residual Values where "+" Indicates a Positive Value, "−" Indicates a Negative Value, and "0" Indicates a Zero or Near-Zero Value

Age	Race	Single	Married	Separated	Divorced	Widowed
35–44	white	−	−	+	0	+
45–54	white	+	0	0	+	−
55–64	white	+	0	−	0	−
35–44	black	−	−	0	+	+
45–54	black	−	+	0	−	+
55–64	black	+	+	0	−	−

Table 6.4. Estimated Rates of Rectal Cancer Incidence Cases per 100,000
from the Median Polish—Perfect Additivity

Age	Race	Single	Married	Separated	Divorced	Widowed
35–44	white	5.2	3.9	4.0	4.7	6.4
45–54	white	21.1	15.7	16.3	18.9	26.2
55–64	white	57.6	42.8	44.3	51.3	71.3
35–44	black	13.3	9.9	10.2	11.9	16.4
45–54	black	14.5	10.8	11.2	12.9	17.9
55–64	black	47.0	34.9	36.1	42.0	58.2

As noted, additivity of the log-rates requires that the estimated column "rates" be constant multiple for any two rows. For example, the ratio of single to married "rates" is 1.345 for all six age/race groups (all rows). The row rates have the same property. For example, the ratio of the estimated rate of older (55–64) white males to younger (35–44) white males is 11.027 for all five marital status groups (all columns). As a consequence, the impact of one variable can be described without considering the influence of the other. Specifically, the influence of marital status can be described without regard to age/race status.

The perfectly additive estimated log-rates are displayed in Figure 6.2 by age/race and marital status. Additivity between age/race and marital status variables translates geometrically into parallel lines representing the log-rates (Figure 6.2—left side). The distances between log-rates among the five marital status categories (columns) are, therefore, equal for any two age/race groups (rows). In other words, the same U-shaped curve describes the rectal

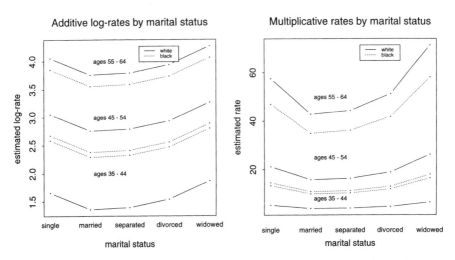

Figure 6.2. Median polish rates and log-rates of the incidence of rectal cancer among white and black males by marital status for three age groups.

cancer incidence pattern by marital status for any or all of the six age/race groups, differing only by risk level associated with age/race category. From a geometric perspective, the residual values measure the deviation from the parallel. The estimated and exactly multiplicative rates are also displayed (Figure 6.2—right side).

Parametric Model Approach

Adding theoretical structure to an analysis has both advantages and disadvantages. The advantages include estimation and assessment of the model components relevant to the understanding of the data, construction of rigorous statistical tests and confidence intervals, formal statistical analysis of the residual values (goodness-of-fit), and the ability to evaluate analytically many of the underlying assumptions. A major disadvantage is that the additional assumptions are frequently not verifiable, adding uncertainty to subsequent inferences. For the marital status data, the assumption is made that rectal cancer incidence is a multiplicative function of age, race, and marital status. Furthermore, the number of rectal cancer cases in each category (each cell of a table) is postulated to have at least an approximate Poisson distribution. That is, a Poisson distribution is assumed to describe accurately the random variation associated with the counts of rectal cancer cases among individuals with the same age, race, and marital status (30 categories). These two assumptions then allow a model-based analysis of rectal cancer risk.

A model postulating that age, race, and marital status have multiplicative influences on rectal cancer risk is

$$\text{rate} = B_0 \times B_1^{\text{age}_i} \times B_2^{\text{race}_j} \times B_3^{z_{1k}} \times B_4^{z_{2k}} \times B_5^{z_{3k}} \times B_6^{z_{4k}}$$

or

$$\log(\text{rate}) = b_0 + b_1 \text{age}_i + b_2 \text{race}_j + b_3 z_{1k} + b_4 z_{2k} + b_5 z_{3k} + b_6 z_{4k} \quad \text{note: } B_j = e^{b_j}$$

or

$$\log(\text{cases}) = b_0 + b_1 \text{age}_i + b_2 \text{race}_j + b_3 z_{1k} + b_4 z_{2k}$$
$$+ b_5 z_{3k} + b_6 z_{4k} + \log(\text{number of persons-years at risk}).$$

All three models are different algebraic versions of the same relationship. Again, the influences of age, race, and marital status on the log-rates are additive, making the influences on the rates multiplicative. The variable age (age_i; $i = 1, 2, 3$) is coded 1, 2, or 3. In fact, any equally spaced values could represent the ages 40, 50, and 60 without changing the properties of the model.

In general, the variable $(x - a)/b$ gives the same analytic results as the variable x in an additive model when a and b represent constants. Race is represented by a binary variable taking on the value $race_j = 0$ for whites and $race_j = 1$ for blacks. The five marital status categories are represented by a four-component design variable $(z_{1k}, z_{2k}, z_{3k}, z_{4k})$ consisting of zeros and ones. Specifically, the design variable that identifies the five marital status categories is

	z_{1k}	z_{2k}	z_{3k}	z_{4k}
single	0	0	0	0
married	1	0	0	0
separated	0	1	0	0
divorced	0	0	1	0
widowed	0	0	0	1

For example, the expected log-cases among middle-aged (45–54), white, married individuals is represented by

$$\log(\text{cases}) = b_0 + b_1(2) + b_2(0) + b_3 + \log(\text{number of persons-years at risk})$$

or, equivalently, the incidence rate is represented by

$$\text{rate} = B_0 \times B_1^2 \times B_3.$$

Probably the most influential and the least interesting component of the model is the person-years at risk. The number of cases of rectal cancer depends directly on the number of persons at risk. The more individuals at risk, the more cases, regardless of other factors. Therefore, the person-years at risk is included in the model directly (independent variable) or indirectly (denominator of the rates). The estimated coefficients based on a multiplicative/additive Poisson model and the 30 observed rates (Table 6.1) of rectal cancer incidence are given in Table 6.5.

Table 6.5. Estimated Coefficients from the Multiplicative/Additive
Poisson Model and their Standard Errors

	Coefficient	Estimates	Std. Error
intercept	b_0	-10.602	—
age	b_1	1.098	0.060
race	b_2	0.042	0.138
married	b_3	-0.442	0.141
separated	b_4	-0.578	0.361
divorced	b_5	-0.214	0.217
widowed	b_6	-0.156	0.245

Residual deviance = 16.752 with 23 degrees of freedom.

Comparing the model-generated cases of rectal cancer to the number of observed cases provides a clear view of the adequacy of the estimated model to represent the relationships under investigation. The estimated coefficients lead to an estimated number of cases, which, in turn, leads to an estimated rate. For example, for white individuals aged 45 to 54 who are married, the estimated logarithm of the number of cases and the estimated cancer incidence rate follow from the model since

$$\log(\text{cases}) = \hat{b}_0 + \hat{b}_1(2) + \hat{b}_2(0) + \hat{b}_3 + \log(\text{number of person-years at risk})$$

and, specifically,

$$\log(\text{cases}) = -10.602 + 1.098(2) + 0.042(0) - 0.442 + \log(929{,}227) = 4.894.$$

Then the estimated number of cases is $e^{4.894} = 133.487$ and the estimated rate is $(133.487/929{,}227) \times 100{,}000 = 14.365$ cases per 100,000. The corresponding observed number of cases is 146, with an observed rate of 15.712 cases per 100,000. The model-estimated and observed number of incidence cases are given in Table 6.6 for the 30 cells in the original rectal cancer two-way table.

The 30 observed cases compared to the 30 estimated cases calculated from the model directly indicate the goodness-of-fit of the additive/multiplicative model. The summary Pearson chi-square test statistic is $X^2 = \sum(o_i - e_i)^2/e_i = 20.803$, which is an observation from a chi-square distribution when the model is correct. As before, "correct" means that all observed values differ from the expected values by chance alone. The degrees of freedom are the number of cells in the table minus the number of parameters used to define the model (i.e., degrees of freedom $= 30 - 7 = 23$).* The p-value is $P(X^2 \geq 20.803 \mid \text{model is correct}) = 0.59$. The chi-square analysis indicates that no convincing evidence exists to suspect that the influences of age, race, and marital status do not have multiplicative (additive) influences on the rate (log-rate) of rectal cancer. Therefore, an additive/multiplicative model that dictates independent influences from the three risk factors likely provides a simple and useful description of the relationships of age, race, and marital status to rectal cancer risk. The chi-square statistic (20.803) is not very different from the residual deviance value (16.752), which is typical. The residual deviance also measures the goodness-of-fit of the estimated model, and these two quantities become increasingly similar as the sample size increases.

---

*The degrees of freedom are in general a difficult concept, best explained in terms of n-dimensional geometry. However, for most analyses, calculation of the degrees of freedom reduces to applying a simple rule. For models used to analyze tabular data, the degrees of freedom are typically the number of cells in the table minus the number of independent parameters necessary to define the model.

Table 6.6. Observed Number and Estimated Number of Incidence Cases
of Rectal Cancer by Age, Race, and Marital Status

Age	Race		Single	Married	Separated	Divorced	Widowed
35–44	white	observed	3	33	1	2	1
		expected	5.55	44.27	0.51	2.59	0.31
45–54	white	observed	17	146	2	11	3
		expected	13.78	133.49	1.54	8.22	2.61
55–64	white	observed	29	287	2	17	15
		expected	30.81	288.58	3.18	17.79	15.78
35–44	black	observed	1	5	1	1	1
		expected	0.96	3.99	0.43	0.53	0.13
45–54	black	observed	1	14	1	1	1
		expected	1.76	11.34	1.17	1.63	0.93
55–64	black	observed	5	21	2	2	3
		expected	3.14	24.33	2.17	3.25	4.24

Figure 6.3 displays a plot of the model-estimated log-rates by age and race for the five marital status categories. The estimated log-rates necessarily exhibit perfect additivity (no interaction) and necessarily form parallel lines. As before, estimated additive log-rates make the row rate ratios the same for all columns and the column rate ratios the same for all rows (Table 6.7) when the log-rates form parallel lines.

The degree of influence of marital status on the risk of rectal cancer is assessed directly by comparing two models. The first model contains the four-level design variable (z-values) accounting for marital status (an unordered categorical variable), and the second model does not. That is, the model

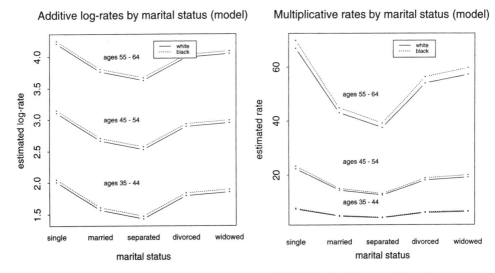

Figure 6.3. Rates and log-rates (Poisson model) of the incidence of rectal cancer among white and black males by marital status for three age groups.

Table 6.7. Estimated Rates of Rectal Cancer per 100,000 by Age, Race, and Marital Status from the Poisson Model—Perfect Additivity of Log-Rates

Age	Race	Single	Married	Separated	Divorced	Widowed
35–44	white	7.5	4.8	4.2	6.0	6.4
45–54	white	22.3	14.4	12.5	18.0	19.1
55–64	white	67.0	43.1	37.6	54.0	57.3
35–44	black	7.8	5.0	4.4	6.3	6.7
45–54	black	23.3	15.0	13.1	18.8	19.9
55–64	black	69.9	44.9	39.2	56.4	59.8

including the influence of marital status (Table 6.5) is compared to the model with the influence of marital status removed ($b_3 = b_4 = b_5 = b_6 = 0$) or, in symbols, the additive model becomes

$$\log(\text{rate}) = b_0 + b_1 \text{age}_i + b_2 \text{race}_j.$$

The role of marital status is reflected by the change in goodness-of-fit, as measured by the difference in the residual deviances. For the model including marital status, the residual deviance is 16.752 with 23 degrees of freedom. The model with marital status excluded produces a residual deviance of 28.158 with 27 degrees of freedom. If marital status has no systematic influence on the incidence of rectal cancer, then the difference between these two measures of fit results from only random variation and has a chi-square distribution with degrees of freedom equal to the difference in the degrees of freedom associated with each model. Equivalently, the degrees of freedom are equal to the number of terms removed (coefficients set to zero) from the more extensive model. Specifically, the chi-square test statistic $X^2 = 28.158 - 16.752 = 11.406$ comes from a chi-square distribution with four degrees of freedom when marital status is unrelated to the risk of rectal cancer. The p-value $P(X^2 \leq 11.406 \mid b_3 = b_4 = b_5 = b_6 = 0) = 0.022$ implies that the difference in goodness-of-fit between these two additive Poisson models is not likely due to chance and, therefore, marital status likely has an important impact on the risk of rectal cancer. Geometrically, the curves are U-shaped and not horizontal (Figure 6.3).

Frequently, the individual influence of a variable in a linear model is evaluated statistically by dividing the corresponding regression coefficient by its standard error (i.e., t-statistic $= \hat{b}_i/S_{\hat{b}_i}$), producing an assessment of its impact on the outcome variable. For the components of a design variable, the values of the coefficients and the resulting t-statistics depend on how the design variable is constructed. There are a number of equally valid ways to describe an unordered categorical variable such as marital status with a design variable. The choice does not influence the overall assessment but does affect the relative magnitudes of the individual *t*-statistics associated with each component of the design variable. That is, different choices give different *t*-statistics. The design variable made up of zeros and ones used for the rectal cancer data, however, is interpreted directly, and the *t*-statistics are useful assessments of the impact of each level of the categorical variable. Other kinds of design variables (for example, orthogonal polynomial and Helmert parameterizations) do not have the same straightforward interpretations. The total influence of a categorical variable, as noted, is evaluated by comparing the change in goodness-of-fit induced by deleting the design variable (all components) from the model and gives identical results, regardless of the kind of design variable used.

CONCLUSIONS

The results from the median polish approach show that widowed men have the highest estimated rate of rectal cancer, followed by single men. The lowest estimated rates are observed in married men. Blacks have lower estimated rates than whites in the age categories 45–54 and 55–64. The parametric model gives somewhat different results. The highest estimated cancer rates are found among single men, followed by widowed men. The lowest estimated rates are found in men from separated couples. Whites and blacks have almost identical estimated rectal cancer incidence rates within each of the three age categories.

The question immediately arises: *which analysis is correct?* This question is not easily answered. The two approaches (median polish versus Poisson model) are fundamentally different. The median polish analysis, for example, treats all rates equally, regardless of the number of observations. That is, black rates based on sparse data are treated identically to white rates based on substantially more data. The fact that the median polish method does not account for the precision of the observed rates is one possible source of the observed differences between these two approaches. Additionally, race and age are combined in the distribution-free approach, forming a simple two-way table. On the other hand, if assumptions of a model-based approach are not fulfilled, the analysis produces biased and potentially misleading results (*wrong model bias*). For the marital status model, if the number of cases in each category is not described accurately by a Poisson distribution or if the influences from age, race, or marital status do not act in a multiplicative fashion, then the inferences made from the model become suspect. However, if the assumptions are fulfilled, a parametric analysis is typically more precise, parsimonious, and often leads to a deeper understanding of the relationships within the data than does a descriptive approach. Since the results from the two analyses of rectal cancer data appear to differ, it is certain that the choice of approach is a sensitive issue. Not surprisingly, statistical analysis does not answer every question, and frequently, whether to use or not use a model-based approach is one of these questions. What is clear is that the approach chosen can substantially affect the analytic results, so the choice requires considerable care and effort.

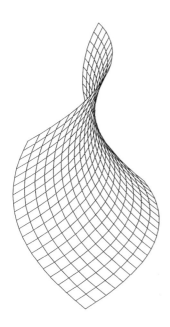

CHAPTER 7

Cluster Analysis

OBJECTIVE

To identify the similarities and differences among a series of human populations based on variations in genetic frequencies.

DATA

The frequencies of genetic variants within three major red blood cell systems (ABO-system, Rh-system, and MN-system) for 26 race/ethnicity groups were collected from a variety of sources. The presence of genetic variation in human blood was first established by Lansteiner in 1901 with the identification of different blood group types, now called the ABO-system. The Rh- and MN-systems also contain well-known and reliably identified genetic variants. Using these three red blood cell systems (a total of 13 variants), the *genetic distances* between the members of the 26 populations can be estimated (325 distances). Data consisting of summary values (such as genetic frequencies) rather than individual measurements are commonly referred to as *aggregate* or *ecologic data*.

METHODS

Graphic displays called *dendrograms* based on Euclidean distance and a nearest-neighbor criterion describe a hierarchical classification process and pinpoint clustering based on genetic distance. Principal component summaries provide a bivariate measure of genetic variation, allowing a two-dimensional graphic display of clustering. Identification of these clusters is further enhanced by a spatial contour plot.

Data type: aggregate or ecologic
Reference: *Systematic Zoology*, 21(2): 174–86 and *Handbook for Forensic Individualization of Human Blood and Blood Stains*, B. W. Grunbaum (ed.) (1972).

The variables are:

1. Race/ethnicity group: 26 groups,
2. ABO frequencies: observed phenotypic frequencies of four red blood cell types (labeled A, B, AB, and O)
   Rh frequencies: observed gene frequencies of seven red blood cell types (labeled CDE, CDe, Cde, cDE, cdE, cDe, and cde)
   MN frequencies: observed gene frequencies of two red blood cell types (labeled M and N)

Part of the file of 26 race/ethnicity group names is:

file name = gnames.7.data

french czech german basque chinese ainu aborigine - - -

Part of the data file of 13 genetic frequencies from 26 race/ethnicity groups is:

file name = gene.7.data

A	B	AB	O	CDE	CDe	Cde	–	–
0.21	0.06	0.06	0.67	0.00	0.43	0.01	–	–
0.25	0.04	0.14	0.57	0.01	0.42	0.01	–	–
0.22	0.06	0.08	0.64	0.02	0.38	0.03	–	–
0.19	0.04	0.02	0.75	0.00	0.38	0.01	–	–
0.18	0.00	0.15	0.67	0.00	0.74	0.00	–	–
0.23	0.00	0.28	0.49	0.00	0.56	0.00	–	–
0.22	0.00	0.00	0.78	0.03	0.63	0.04	–	–
0.22	0.00	0.14	0.64	0.00	0.95	0.00	–	–
0.34	0.00	0.00	0.66	0.00	0.48	0.01	–	–
0.13	0.06	0.06	0.75	0.00	0.43	0.00	–	–
0.30	0.00	0.06	0.64	0.03	0.59	0.00	–	–
0.00	0.00	0.00	1.00	0.03	0.55	0.00	–	–
0.10	0.08	0.11	0.71	0.00	0.08	0.05	–	–
0.17	0.06	0.15	0.62	0.00	0.43	0.00	–	–
0.16	0.03	0.22	0.59	0.01	0.57	0.00	–	–
–	–	–	–	–	–	–	–	–
–	–	–	–	–	–	–	–	–
–	–	–	–	–	–	–	–	–

13 columns: {A, B, AB and O},
{CDE, CDe, Cde, cDE, cdE, cDe and cde}, {M and N}

26 rows: race/ethnicity groups

DISCUSSION

The complete genetic frequency* data set is displayed in Table 7.1—a 26 by 13 array where the rows are 26 race/ethnicity groups and the columns are 13 frequencies of genetic variants from the three red cell blood systems (ABO, Rh, and MN). The 13 observed frequencies allow each of the 26 race/ethnicity groups to be characterized by their genetic similarities/differences, which become the basis for classifying race/ethnicity groups in terms of genetic distance. Two fundamental components of the classification process are a definition of distance and, once distance is defined, a method to group successively similar distances into fewer and fewer subdivisions (a hierarchical classification scheme).

The distance between two points (x_1, y_1) and (x_2, y_2) is given by

$$d_{12} = \sqrt{(x_1 - x_2)^2 + (y_1 + y_2)^2} \quad \text{(Pythagorean theorem)}.$$

This classic geometric definition of distance is directly extended to multidimensional points. The distance between one p-dimensional point represented as $\{x_{i1}, x_{i2}, x_{i3}, \ldots, x_{ip}\}$ and another represented as $\{x_{j1}, x_{j2}, x_{j3}, \ldots, x_{jp}\}$ is

$$d_{ij} = \sqrt{\sum (x_{ik} - x_{jk})^2} \quad k = 1, 2, 3, \ldots, p.$$

This distance between the ith and jth points is usually referred to as *Euclidean distance*. For example, if *point i* is $\{x_{i1}, x_{i2}, x_{i3}, x_{i4}\} = \{1,2,3,4\}$ and if *point j* is $\{x_{j1}, x_{j2}, x_{j3}, x_{j4}\} = \{4,3,2,1\}$, then the Euclidean distance between these two four-dimensional points becomes

$$d_{ij} = \sqrt{(1 - 4)^2 + (2 - 3)^2 + (3 - 2)^2 + (4 - 1)^2} = \sqrt{20} = 4.472.$$

Euclidean distance reflects, somewhat arbitrarily but effectively, the differences between race/ethnicity groups. Summarizing genetic differences in terms of Euclidean distance yields a useful numeric comparison among the compared groups but is only one of a number of choices for measuring genetic distance.[16] However, it is perhaps the simplest.

To illustrate, the 13 genetic frequencies in Chinese born in the United States (Table 7.1—row 20) are

$$\{0.21, 0.0, 0.18, 0.61, \ldots, 0.42\}$$

---

*Note: the gene frequency data are technically a combination of phenotypic (ABO) and gene frequencies (Rh and MN).

Table 7.1. Gene Frequencies for 26 Race/Ethnicity Groups

Group	ABO-system				Rh-system							MN-system	
	A	B	AB	O	CDE	CDe	Cde	cDE	cdE	cDe	cde	M	N
French	0.21	0.06	0.06	0.67	0.00	0.43	0.01	0.14	0.01	0.02	0.39	0.55	0.45
Czech	0.25	0.04	0.14	0.57	0.01	0.42	0.01	0.15	0.00	0.01	0.40	0.53	0.47
German	0.22	0.06	0.08	0.64	0.02	0.38	0.03	0.12	0.01	0.03	0.41	0.55	0.45
Basque	0.19	0.04	0.02	0.75	0.00	0.38	0.01	0.07	0.00	0.01	0.53	0.54	0.46
Chinese	0.18	0.00	0.15	0.67	0.00	0.74	0.00	0.19	0.00	0.03	0.04	0.62	0.38
Ainu	0.23	0.00	0.28	0.49	0.00	0.56	0.00	0.21	0.19	0.00	0.04	0.40	0.60
Aborigine	0.22	0.00	0.00	0.78	0.03	0.63	0.04	0.14	0.00	0.16	0.00	0.22	0.78
Guinea	0.22	0.00	0.14	0.64	0.00	0.95	0.00	0.04	0.00	0.01	0.00	0.21	0.79
Maori	0.34	0.00	0.00	0.66	0.00	0.48	0.01	0.48	0.00	0.03	0.00	0.51	0.49
Icelander	0.13	0.06	0.06	0.75	0.00	0.43	0.00	0.16	0.02	0.02	0.37	0.57	0.43
Eskimo	0.30	0.00	0.06	0.64	0.03	0.59	0.00	0.33	0.00	0.05	0.00	0.83	0.17
Indian (Brazil)	0.00	0.00	0.00	1.00	0.03	0.55	0.00	0.40	0.00	0.02	0.00	0.74	0.26
Bantu	0.10	0.08	0.11	0.71	0.00	0.08	0.05	0.06	0.00	0.61	0.20	0.56	0.44
North African	0.17	0.06	0.15	0.62	0.00	0.43	0.00	0.14	0.00	0.09	0.34	0.54	0.46
India	0.16	0.03	0.22	0.59	0.01	0.57	0.00	0.14	0.00	0.04	0.24	0.69	0.31
Spanish	0.27	0.04	0.06	0.63	0.02	0.44	0.01	0.11	0.00	0.04	0.38	0.53	0.47
Norwegian	0.26	0.06	0.06	0.62	0.00	0.43	0.01	0.13	0.01	0.02	0.40	0.55	0.45
Indian (Mex.)	0.02	0.00	0.01	0.97	0.00	0.68	0.00	0.30	0.00	0.02	0.00	0.79	0.21
Egyptian	0.21	0.05	0.20	0.54	0.00	0.46	0.01	0.14	0.00	0.24	0.15	0.52	0.48
Chinese (U.S.)	0.21	0.00	0.18	0.61	0.00	0.71	0.00	0.20	0.00	0.02	0.07	0.58	0.42
Japanese (U.S.)	0.28	0.00	0.18	0.54	0.00	0.63	0.00	0.32	0.00	0.00	0.05	0.56	0.44
Navaho	0.03	0.00	0.00	0.97	0.04	0.38	0.09	0.31	0.01	0.17	0.00	0.91	0.09
white (U.S.)	0.20	0.07	0.07	0.66	0.01	0.38	0.01	0.14	0.01	0.04	0.41	0.56	0.44
black (Calif.)	0.13	0.04	0.13	0.71	0.01	0.16	0.03	0.11	0.00	0.40	0.30	0.41	0.59
Mexican (U.S.)	0.11	0.02	0.06	0.81	0.06	0.50	0.01	0.24	0.02	0.04	0.14	0.70	0.30
Asian (U.S.)	0.24	0.01	0.17	0.58	0.00	0.63	0.01	0.26	0.00	0.02	0.06	0.56	0.44

and the frequencies of the same 13 genetic variants in Chinese born in China (Table 7.1—row 5) are

$$\{0.18, 0.0, 0.15, 0.67, \ldots, 0.38\}$$

making the genetic distance between these two groups

distance (Chinese [U.S.], Chinese [China])
$$= \sqrt{(0.21 - 0.18)^2 + \cdots + (0.42 - 0.38)^2} = 0.103.$$

For contrast, the 13 frequencies of the same genetic variants in white Americans (Table 7.1—row 23) are

$$\{0.20, 0.07, 0.07, 0.66, \ldots, 0.44\}$$

and the genetic distance between white Americans and Chinese born in the United States is

distance (white [U.S.], China [US])
$$= \sqrt{(0.21 - 0.20)^2 + \cdots + (0.42 - 0.44)^2} = 0.499.$$

The obvious point is that, in terms of genetic distance, the U.S.-born Chinese are closer to the Chinese born in China than to U.S.-born white Americans.

For the genetic frequency data set, there are $\binom{26}{2} = 325$ possible distances between the race/ethnicity groups. The distribution of all 325 Euclidean distances is displayed in Figure 7.1. The smallest genetic distance is 0.047, between U.S. whites and Germans. The largest genetic distance is 1.256, between the populations of Guinea and India. The median distance is 0.546.

To classify multivariate observations, it is necessary to define similarity. A natural definition of similarity is closeness, as measured by Euclidean distance. More formally, the 325 distances are reduced to 26 nearest-neighbor genetic distances to characterize proximity between race/ethnicity groups. The nearest-neighbor measure is no more than the name suggests. One of the 26 race/ethnicity groups is chosen, and the Euclidean distances to the other 25 race/ethnicity groups are calculated. Then the smallest distance (nearest) is the nearest-neighbor distance. For example, if the Spanish race/ethnicity group is selected, then among the genetic distances to the 25 other race/ethnicity groups, the smallest distance is to the Norwegians (nearest-neighbor distance = 0.057). Table 7.2 lists the ordered 26 nearest-neighbor genetic distances.

White and German genetic frequencies, as before, produce the smallest nearest-neighbor distance (0.047—rank 1). The largest nearest-neighbor dis-

Distribution of gene distances (Euclidean)

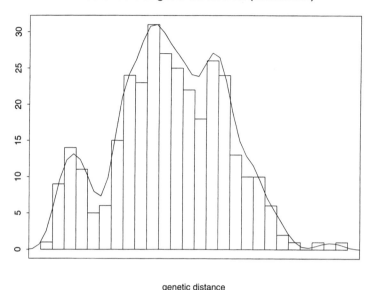

genetic distance

Figure 7.1. Distribution of all possible genetic distances used to classify the 26 race/ethnicity groups based on Euclidean distance.

tance is from Guinean to Aborigine genetic frequencies (0.420—rank 26), and both groups are a large distance from the Europeans. The nearest-neighbor distance from group A to group B is not necessarily the nearest-neighbor distance from group B to group A. The nearest-neighbor distance from the Czechs to the Norwegians is 0.105, but the nearest-neighbor distance associated with the Norwegians is 0.057, which is the genetic distance to the Spanish population.

Calculating the nearest neighbor distances is the first step in sorting out the similarities and differences among the 26 race/ethnicity groups. The next step is to construct a specialized plot displaying the classification process. Plots of hierarchical classification strategies are called *dendrograms* (*dendro*- from the Greek meaning "tree"). Dendrograms describing the hierarchical classification of the 26 nearest-neighbor genetic distances are displayed in Figures 7.2 (each blood group system separately) and 7.3 (all these blood group systems combined).

An illustration of the mechanics used to construct a dendrogram follows:

The dendrogram plot using all three genetic variants (Figure 7.3) is constructed by first identifying the closest pair of race/ethnicity groups (German-U.S. whites). This pair forms the first cluster. The next race/

Table 7.2. Nearest Neighbor Distances for the 26 Race/Ethnicity
Groups Ordered from Smallest to Largest

From	To	Distance
German	white (U.S.)	0.047
white (U.S.)	German	0.047
Spanish	Norwegian	0.057
Norwegian	Spanish	0.057
French	white (U.S.)	0.063
Japanese (U.S.)	Asians (U.S.)	0.087
Asians (U.S.)	Japanese (U.S.)	0.087
Chinese	Chinese (U.S.)	0.103
Chinese (U.S.)	Chinese	0.103
Czech	Norwegian	0.105
Icelander	French	0.121
North Africa	French	0.141
Basque	white (U.S.)	0.181
Indian (Brazil)	Indian (Mex.)	0.185
Indian (Mex.)	Indian (Brazil)	0.185
Egyptian	North Africa	0.266
India	Chinese (U.S.)	0.287
Mexican (U.S.)	India	0.324
Maori	Japanese (U.S.)	0.327
Bantu	Black (Calif.)	0.334
black (Calif.)	Bantu	0.334
Ainu	Asians (U.S.)	0.341
Navaho	India (Brazil)	0.357
Eskimo	Mexican (U.S.)	0.369
Aborigine	Guinean	0.420
Guinean	Aborigine	0.420

ethnicity group to be classified is either nearest to the first cluster or nearest to another race/ethnicity group. The latter is the case, creating a second cluster (Spanish-Norwegian). This same comparison is repeated. The French genetic frequencies are closer to the first cluster than any other pair of race/ethnicity groups are to each other, forming two classification clusters (German–U.S. white–French and Spanish-Norwegian). On the fourth step, these two clusters are closer to each other than any other two race/ethnicity groups and therefore, become a single cluster. The fifth step produces a new cluster between the Japanese and Asians born in the United States. The sixth step produces an additional member of the first cluster, the Czech population. The process continues until the least similar race/ethnicity group or groups are added (Aboriginal-Guinean). The classification process begins with 26 groups and ends with one. The dendrogram is a graphic record. It shows which race/ethnicity groups are close and which are not. Euclidean nearest-neighbor distance is recorded on the vertical axis.

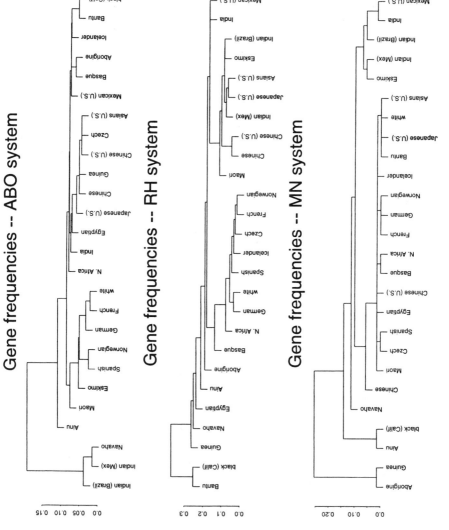

Figure 7.2. Dendrogram of genetic distances (Euclidean distances) classifying the 26 race/ethnicity groups—separate blood group systems.

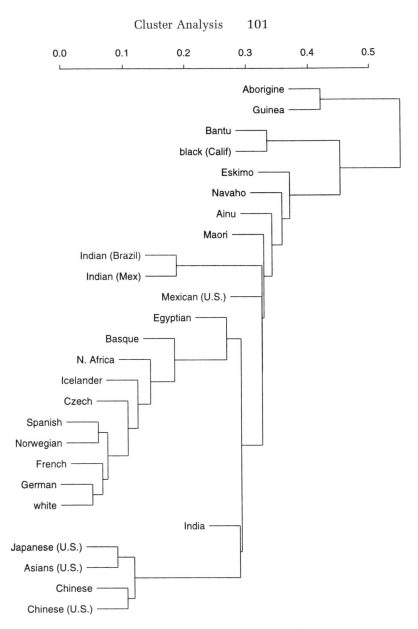

Figure 7.3. Dendrogram of genetic distances (Euclidean distances) classifying the 26 race/ethnicity groups—combined blood group systems.

Several properties of the multivariate genetic data are directly identified from the dendrogram in Figure 7.3:

1. The closest race/ethnicity groups are the Germans and U.S. whites (smallest nearest-neighbor distance).

2. Europeans are members of a tight cluster (Germans-French-Norwegian-Spanish-Czech).
3. Asian also form a rather tight cluster [Japanese (U.S.)-Asian (U.S.)-Chinese (U.S.)-Chinese (China)].
4. One focus of clustering is centered in Europe, starting with France and Germany, and the genetic distance smoothly increases as geographic distance from Central Europe increases (Germany < France < Spain-Norway < Czechoslovakia < Iceland < North Africa).
5. The most distance race/ethnicity groups are the European and the Aboriginal-Guinean groupings.

The end product of the grouping process is not only a frequently instructive classification of multivariate data but also the identification of very similar, similar, different, and very different observations within a multivariate data set. Choices other than Euclidean distance are available for describing distance. Furthermore, a variety of definitions of closeness other than nearest-neighbor distance exist. Therefore, a number of possibilities are available for classifying multivariate data and constructing the dendrogram plots that describe the classification process.[17] It is not guaranteed, however, that these alternative approaches will give the same or even similar results.

Principal Component Summaries

A dendrogram operates on a measure of similarity. Another approach to classifying multivariate data uses canonical variables and, in the case of comparing race/ethnicity groups based on genetic frequencies, yields similar results. A canonical variable summarizes a multivariate observation by combining the components that make up the observation creating a simpler summary variable. Mathematically, it is said that the dimensionality of the multivariate observation is reduced. For the genetic data, a multivariate observation with 13 components is reduced to a summary made up of two components (a 13-dimensional multivariate observation is reduced to a 2-dimensional bivariate observation).

One choice of a canonical variable (denoted P_i) is a linear combination of the genetic components given by

$$P_i = a_1 A_i + a_2 B_i + a_3 AB_i + \cdots + a_{12} N_i + a_{13} M_i$$

where A_i, B_i, AB_i, . . . , N_i and M_i represent the 13 genetic frequencies (rows of Table 7.1) for the ith race/ethnicity group. The 13 coefficients a_j are determined, so the canonical variate has the maximum variability among all possible linear combinations of the 13 genetic frequencies. This particular canonical variable is called the *first principal component*.[18] Variability is a desirable feature of a summary statistic. Clearly, a summary measure with little or no variability is not much use. If a summary takes on essentially the same value under all circumstances, it is a poor indicator of a multivariate observation. If the Dow-Jones index (summary), for example, barely changed when the component stocks themselves changed, it would not usefully reflect stock market prices. A highly variable summary potentially captures, with a single number, much of the information contained in a multivariate observation, particularly when the components within the observation are highly correlated.

A second principal component is analogously created. Again, a linear combination of the multivariate components yields another canonical summary, denoted

$$Q_i = b_1A_i + b_2B_i + b_3AB_i + \cdots + b_{12}N_i + b_{13}M_i.$$

The second principal component is again a linear combination of the genetic frequencies, but the 13 coefficients b_j are chosen so that the second principal component has two properties. First, the second principal component Q is the second most variable of all possible linear combinations (variance $(P) >$ variance $(Q) >$ variance (R), where R is any other linear combination of the multivariate components). Additionally, the correlation between the 26 values of P_i and Q_i is exactly zero (correlation $(P, Q) = 0$). The second principal component is not only an additional summary of the genetic frequencies but also potentially summarizes characteristics of the multivariate observation not summarized by the first principal component. These two uncorrelated linear combinations are designed to reflect different aspects of a multivariate observation. Table 7.3 contains the coefficients for the first two principal components calculated from the gene frequency data.

Table 7.3. The Coefficients for the Two Principal Components
P and Q Summarizing the 26 Gene Frequencies

j	Gene	a_j	b_j
1	A	−0.16	0.14
2	B	−0.06	−0.08
3	AB	−0.11	0.10
4	O	0.33	−0.15
5	CDE	0.03	−0.01
6	CDe	0.17	0.69
7	Cde	0.01	−0.04
8	cDE	0.32	0.10
9	cdE	−0.02	0.03
10	cDe	−0.12	−0.30
11	cde	−0.39	−0.47
12	M	0.53	−0.27
13	N	−0.53	0.27

For example, the 13 French genetic frequencies (row 1 in Table 7.1) reduce to the two summary values given by

$$P_1 = -0.16(0.21) - 0.06(0.06) - 0.11(0.06) + \cdots + 0.53(0.55)$$
$$- 0.53(0.45) = 0.191$$

and

$$Q_1 = 0.14(0.21) - 0.08(0.06) + 0.10(0.06) + \cdots - 0.27(0.55)$$
$$+ 0.27(0.45) = 0.021.$$

The point $(P_1, Q_1) = (0.191, 0.021)$ succinctly summarizes the information contained in the 13 French genetic frequencies as a bivariate measurement. The other 25 bivariate measurements are similarly calculated $(P_i, Q_i$—Table 7.4) and are plotted in Figure 7.4. The correlation between these 26 pairs of principal component values is exactly zero. The resulting principal component summaries provide a simple characterization of much of the information contained in the 26 genetic frequencies using only two values.

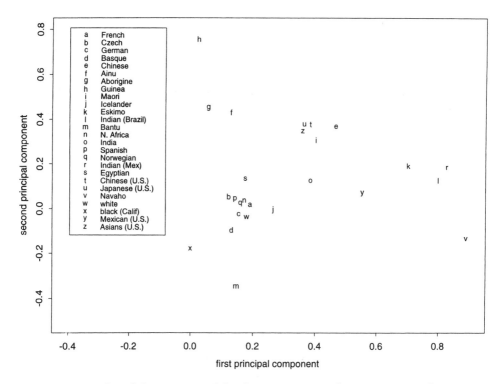

Figure 7.4. Plot of the 26 pairs of the first two principal components indicating the clustering among the race/ethnicity groups.

Table 7.4. The 26 Values of the First Two Principal
Components, P and Q

i	Group	P_i	Q_i
1	French	0.191	0.021
2	Czech	0.123	0.054
3	German	0.154	-0.021
4	Basque	0.131	-0.095
5	Chinese	0.467	0.371
6	Ainu	0.130	0.430
7	Aborigine	0.058	0.458
8	Guinean	0.025	0.756
9	Maori	0.402	0.307
10	Icelander	0.265	-0.001
11	Eskimo	0.702	0.192
12	Indian (Brazil)	0.799	0.127
13	Bantu	0.146	-0.344
14	North African	0.172	0.039
15	India	0.385	0.129
16	Spanish	0.143	0.050
17	Norwegian	0.159	0.030
18	Indian (Mex.)	0.827	0.188
19	Egyptian	0.175	0.137
20	Chinese (U.S.)	0.385	0.378
21	Japanese (U.S.)	0.365	0.381
22	Navaho	0.889	-0.131
23	white	0.180	-0.034
24	black (Calif)	-0.001	-0.175
25	Mexican (U.S.)	0.553	0.076
26	Asian (U.S.)	0.359	0.351

The magnitude of the principal component coefficients (Table 7.3) indicates which gene frequencies are important and which are not in producing
the summary values P_i and Q_i. The first principal component is dominated
by the MN-system ($a_{12} = a_{13} = \pm 0.53$). The largest coefficients in the second
principal component are associated with the Rh-system (CDe-gene: $b_6 = 0.69$
and the cde-gene: $b_{11} = -0.47$). These gene variants are, therefore, the most
influential elements of the multivariate measurement in a classification process based on the (P_i, Q_i) pairs.

Many of the same properties of the blood group data seen in the dendrograms are also apparent from the principal components plot (Figure 7.4). The
cluster containing the Europeans and the U.S. whites once again is a dominant feature ({c, w, q, a, b, p, and n} = {Germany, United States (white), Nor-
way, France, Czechoslovakia, Spain, and North Africa}). The Asian cluster is
similarly observed ({u, t, z, e, and i} = {Japanese (U.S.), Chinese (U.S.), Asians
(U.S.), Chinese (China), and Maori}). However, a cluster not obvious from the
dendrogram plot (Figure 7.3) is more apparent with the principal components
approach. Three North American Indian groups ({k, l, and r} = {Eskimo,

Indian (Brazil), and Indian (Mexico)}) form not an extremely tight cluster but, nevertheless, a notable cluster that has some historical basis. The genetically most different race/ethnicity groups lie on the perimeter of the plot ({m, v, and h} = {Bantu, Navaho, and Guinean}).

The principal components plot is further enhanced by using a smoothing algorithm producing a three-dimensional representation of the principal component summaries P and Q (Figure 7.5). The "floor" of the three-dimensional smoothed histogram represents race/ethnicity groups located by values of the two principal component summaries. The "hills" indicate areas of high concentration of the race/ethnicity groups, and the "valleys" indicate areas of low or no concentration. As in a two-dimensional histogram, the degree of clustering is proportional to the heights of the hills. The two tallest hills reflect the dominant European and Asian clusters, which contain a large number of genetically similar race/ethnicity groups.

To further describe the membership of the race/ethnicity clusters, a contour map of the three-dimensional representation is constructed (Figure 7.6). A contour plot contains no new information but is an alternative and visually simple representation of a three-dimensional display. The contour plot of the genetic distances combines the three-dimensional plot (Figure 7.5) and the principal components plot (Figure 7.4). Contours readily identify the groups that make up specific clusters (the hills) but are only one of a number of ways to display a three-dimensional relationship.

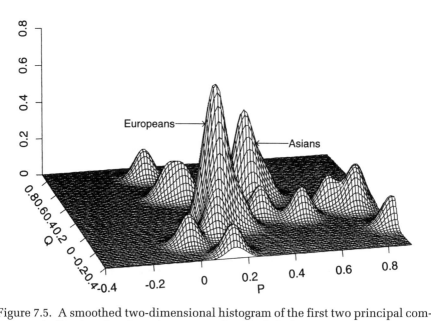

Figure 7.5. A smoothed two-dimensional histogram of the first two principal components indicating the clustering among the race/ethnicity groups.

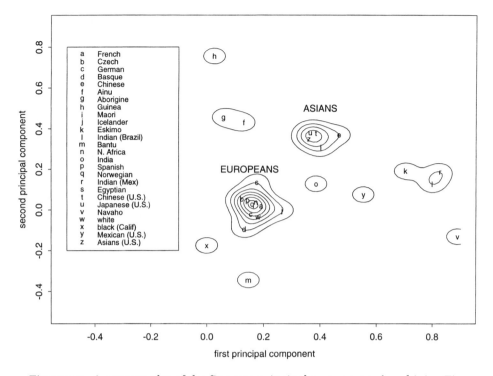

Figure 7.6. A contour plot of the first two principal components (combining Figures 7.4 and 7.5) to better identify the clustering in the genetic data.

CONCLUSIONS

Using gene frequency data from 26 race/ethnicity groups provide a basis for classifying these groups into a series of categories indicating genetic similarity/dissimilarity. Similarity defined by a nearest-neighbor criterion based on Euclidean distance allows two approaches to classification, one based on a dendrogram and the other on the first two principal components. Both approaches produce rather similar results when applied to the genetic variant data made up of 13 genetic frequencies. This similarity will not always occur, and the two descriptive approaches can differ substantially.

Starting from the closest groups (U.S. whites and Germans), the description of closeness continues until the most dissimilar groups are identified (Bantu, Navaho, and Guinean). The two descriptive approaches clearly identify two and, perhaps, three definite clusters based on gene frequencies. The results are more qualitative (graphic) than quantitative, which is typical of many cluster analysis techniques.

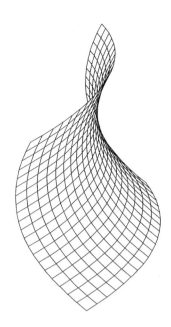

CHAPTER 8

Matched Analysis (One Case and Two Controls)

OBJECTIVE

To determine if exposure to electromagnetic radiation is associated with the risk of a birth defect. More specifically, *does a newborn infant whose mother lives near high-voltage power lines have an increased risk of a congenital anomaly?*

DATA

Of the infants born in the east-central region of France (1988–1991) and observed during the first year of life, 118 had major congenital anomalies. Each of these 118 infants were matched to two randomly selected controls who were of the same gender and born approximately on the same date in the same municipality. For all 354 study subjects, the distance from their mother's residence (home/apartment during pregnancy) was measured to the nearest 225 or 400 kilovolt high-voltage power line. These data were derived entirely from birth records and detailed maps. To reflect risk, two measures of maternal/infant exposure to electromagnetic field (emf) radiation were used—the distance as measured directly in meters and the distance dichotomized into less than or equal to 100 meters and more than 100 meters. The motivation for the matched design was to equalize, at least partially, comparisons between the case and the two controls for any interfering influences of general socioeconomic and demographic differences that could not be measured without personal interviews.

METHODS

Paired *t*-tests, bootstrap sampling, and analysis of variance are used to explore the association between distance to high-voltage lines and risk of a birth defect. Defining *exposed* as a pregnant woman living within 100 meters or less of a high-voltage power line and *unexposed* as residing more than 100 meters away provides a binary measure of exposure. Both model-free and conditional logistic model approaches are used to estimate and assess risk, as measured by this binary exposure variable.

Data type: Matched sets (sampled population-based vital records)
Reference: *Paediatric and Perinatal Epidemiology*, 1996, 10: 32–8

The variables are:

1. Distance: as recorded in meters
2. Case/control status: coded 0 for case, 1 for first control, and 2 for second control

Part of the data file of 354 infants (118 matched sets) is:

file name = defects.8.data

distance	case/control
750	0
300	1
1150	2
650	0
100	1
100	2
50	0
2150	1
2000	2
450	0
1350	1
350	2
700	0
800	1
400	2
–	–
–	–
–	–

DISCUSSION

The defining characteristic of matched data is that each matched set is a stratum of observations—a stratum with a small number of observations but, nevertheless, a stratum. The observations within each matched set are purposely made as similar as possible, except that one member is a case and the other members are controls. All of the 118 sets of one malformed infant and two control infants born in east-central France were made as similar as possible with regard to gender, date of birth, and residential location. The distance to the nearest electrical power lines is used to reflect exposure for each member of the matched set. The analysis focuses on identifying case/control differences in exposure.

Although the language of matched data analysis tends to be specialized and the statistical expressions often appear unfamiliar, the basic strategy in the analysis of matched data, like that of stratified case/control studies in general, is to measure the within-set (stratum) differences in exposure between cases and controls. Then, combining these measurements over all sets (strata) produces a single summary value reflecting risk. The summary measure is only minimally affected by the matching variables since the levels of these variables are the same or nearly the same within each set (for example, gender, date of birth, and location). A matched strategy is effective for continuous measurements as well as counts of binary events. For the emf radiation data, whether the within-set differences are measured as distance in meters (a continuous measure—comparisons of mean distances) or as a binary risk variable (exposed or not exposed—comparison of 2 by 2 tables), the approach is the same in principle. Statistical measures are constructed to assess differences between cases and the two controls in distance (mean values) or risk of exposure (odds ratios) within each matched set. These stratum-specific measures are then combined into a single summary measure describing the association between exposure and case/control status. The overall measure of association then reflects the risk of a congenital anomaly while eliminating to a large extent the confounding influences from the variables used to construct the matched sets.[19,20]

A First Approach: Recorded Distance (*t*-Test)

The average distances from each study subject's residence to the nearest high-voltage line are given in Table 8.1 for the cases and controls. The distributions of these distances are displayed in Figure 8.1. The three histograms show similar asymmetric (right-skewed—means > medians) distributions containing several extreme distances. Ten distances exceed 2500 meters. Figure 8.2 shows

Table 8.1. Description of Distances (meters) to High-Power Electric Lines
for Case and Control Infants

	n	Mean	Median	Std. Dev.	Minimum	Maximum
cases	118	745.2	600.0	591.9	50	3550
controls$_1$	118	825.0	650.0	682.8	50	3250
controls$_2$	118	819.5	625.0	653.7	50	3250

the same data in another form. Frequency polygons are plotted on the same scale for comparison (left side). These distributions are once again displayed (right side) but smoothed to estimate more realistically the continuous underlying nature of distance to the nearest high-power line.

A natural within-set measure of exposure is the difference between the distance to the nearest high-power line for the case and the mean distance observed for the two controls. That is, within each matched set, the difference (denoted d_i) is

$$d_i = d_{0i} - \frac{1}{2}(d_{1i} + d_{2i})$$

where d_{0i} represents case (*case*) distance, d_{1i} represents the first control (*control$_1$*) distance, and d_{2i} represents the second control (*control$_2$*) distance within the ith matched set. Figure 8.3 displays the distribution of the 118 within-set measures of exposure (d_i-values).

A single summary of these 118 within-set differences (exposure measures) is a mean value or

$$\bar{d} = \frac{1}{n}\sum d_i = \bar{d}_0 - \frac{1}{2}(\bar{d}_1 + \bar{d}_2) \quad i = 1, 2, 3, \ldots, n = 118.$$

Large negative values of $\bar{d}$ reflect shorter distances to the nearest power lines (higher exposures) among the cases. The observed mean difference $\bar{d}$ is -77.034. The 118 cases are on average 77.034 meters closer to high-power lines (emf radiation) than the 236 controls. This difference could have arisen strictly because of random variation or it could represent a systematic influence, leading to the suspicion that emf radiation is associated with the risk of a birth defect. A t-test is designed to help choose between these two alternatives (random versus systematic influences).

To calculate a t-statistic to assess the observed mean difference $\bar{d}$, it is necessary to estimate the variance of this summary contrast between cases and controls. The variance of $\bar{d}$ is clearly related to the variances and covariances

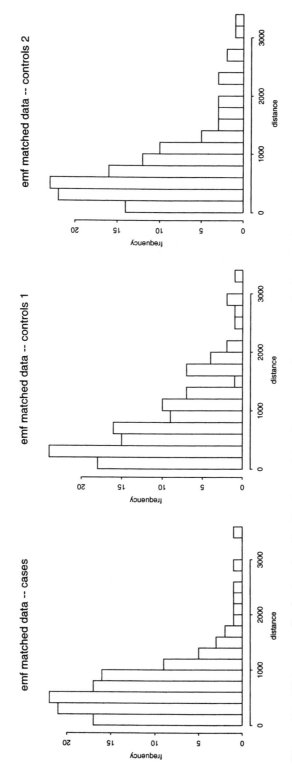

Figure 8.1. Histograms displaying the distributions of the distances to the nearest high-power line (emf exposure) for case and control groups.

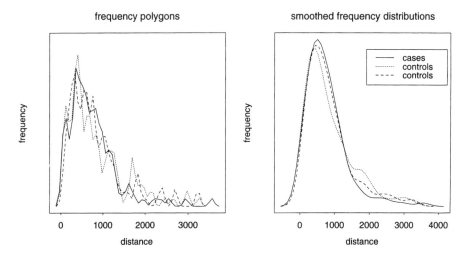

Figure 8.2. Frequency polygons and smoothed frequency distributions of the distance to the nearest high-power line for case and control groups.

of its components, $\overline{d}_0$, $\overline{d}_1$, and $\overline{d}_2$ (a.2). A straightforward estimate of the variance of $\overline{d}$ based on the observed d_i-differences is

$$\text{variance}(d) = S_d^2 = \frac{1}{n-1}\sum(d_i - \overline{d})^2 \quad\text{and}\quad S_{\overline{d}}^2 = \frac{1}{n}S_d^2.$$

Therefore, for the emf data, the estimated variance of the mean $\overline{d}$ is $S_{\overline{d}}^2 = 3431.342$.

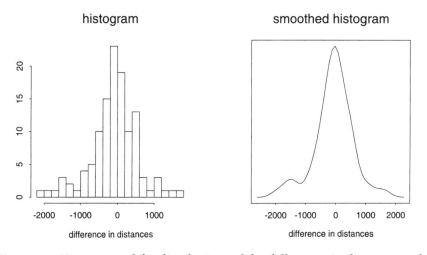

Figure 8.3. Histograms of the distributions of the differences in distances to the nearest high-power lines within matched sets.

The variance of the estimated mean difference $\bar{d}$ depends on the degree of correlation among the three within-set measured distances (a.2). The larger the correlations, the smaller the variance. Reducing the variance yields a greater likelihood that an observed difference (for example, -77.034) between cases and controls provides evidence of an underlying systematic influence. In general, the greater the correlations among the observations within a matched set, the more powerful the analysis (a fundamental feature of a matched design).

Although the sampled distance distributions (Figures 8.1 and 8.2) are not symmetric (not approximately normal), the distribution of the d_i-values is approximately symmetric (Figure 8.3), ensuring that the estimate $\bar{d}$ has an approximately normal distribution. Mean values have approximately normal distributions when the sample size is large, regardless of the distribution sampled (central limit theorem). This approximation is extremely accurate when the sampled distribution is symmetric, such as the distribution of the d_i-values. A sample of 118 is more than large enough to guarantee that the distribution of the mean value $\bar{d}$ is sufficiently close to a normal distribution to use a t-test accurately. The test statistic is

$$T = \frac{\bar{d} - 0}{S_{\bar{d}}} = \frac{-77.034 - 0}{58.578} = -1.315.$$

The test statistic T has a t-distribution with degrees of freedom equal to $n - 1 = 118 - 1 = 117$ when the sample mean $\bar{d}$ randomly differs from zero. The associated one-tail p-value is $P(T \leq -1.315 \mid$ no difference in distances$) = 0.09$.

A parallel assessment of the impact of random variation on the summary contrast $\bar{d}$ comes from a confidence interval. An approximate 95% confidence interval is

$$\bar{d} \pm 1.960 S_{\bar{d}} = -77.034 \pm 1.960(58.578)$$

yielding the interval $(-191.846, 37.778)$. The confidence interval indicates that a difference of zero (contained in the confidence interval) is not an unlikely candidate for the true underlying mean difference within the matched sets. Both statistical evaluations yield only a slight hint of an association between distance and the risk of a birth defect.

A Second Approach: Transformed Distance (Bootstrap Sampling)

A t-test requires the knowledge or assumption that the observations are normally distributed with equal variances within the two compared groups (cases versus combined controls). A more critical issue concerns the influence of the extreme distances observed among the 118 matched sets. A distance of more than 1000 or so meters provides no information on the risk from emf radiation (Figure 8.3). Such distances are so great that they have no credible impact on risk, but they substantially influence the comparison of mean values. One solution is to eliminate all but "credible" observations. The choice of a credible distance potentially flaws the analysis. The analytic results change, sometimes substantially, depending on which observations are eliminated and which are not.

An alternative to analyzing the measured distance directly is to use the reciprocal values of the distance to summarize exposure to emf radiation. This transformation emphasizes small distances (large values) and deemphasizes noninformative large differences (small values). The strategy avoids defining which distances are relevant and which distances are not relevant to the association between emf radiation exposure and case/control status. Therefore, instead of directly analyzing the within matched set case/control distance d_i, the reciprocal values $1/d_i$ are used. Following the same pattern as the t-test, a summary of the 118 within-set differences is

$$\bar{h} = \bar{h}_0 - \frac{1}{2}(\bar{h}_1 + \bar{h}_2)$$

where $\bar{h}_k$ is a harmonic mean given by

$$\bar{h}_k = \frac{n}{\Sigma(1/d_{ki})} \quad k = 0, 1, 2 \quad \text{and} \quad i = 1, 2, 3, \ldots, 118$$

and again d_{0i} represents the distance associated with the ith case, d_{1i} represents the distance associated with the ith first control, and d_{2i} represents the distance associated with the ith second control. The values of the three harmonic mean values for the emf data are listed in Table 8.2.

The observed mean difference between the case and control harmonic mean values is $\bar{h} = -47.795$ based on the 354 observed reciprocal distances. That is, the cases have a smaller harmonic mean than the average value of the two control groups.

Table 8.2. Harmonic Mean Values Summarizing the Distances to High-Power Electric Lines for Cases and Controls

	Symbol	n	Mean
cases	$\bar{h}_0$	118	320.400
controls$_1$	$\bar{h}_1$	118	330.857
controls$_2$	$\bar{h}_2$	118	405.531

At this point it might be assumed that the mean $\bar{h}$ has an approximate normal distribution, then estimate the variance of $\bar{h}$ and apply a t-test. This approach likely gives accurate and useful results. However, bootstrap replicate sampling estimates the distribution of $\bar{h}$ without assumptions or theory directly producing an estimated variance. Sampling the observed reciprocal distances with replacement from the 118 cases and each of the two sets of 118 controls produces three replicate harmonic mean values (denoted $\bar{H}_0$, $\bar{H}_1$, and $\bar{H}_2$), which are combined to give a bootstrap replicate contrast $\bar{H} = \bar{H}_0 - \frac{1}{2}(\bar{H}_1 + \bar{H}_2)$, where again

$$\bar{H}_k = \frac{n}{\sum(1/D_{ki})} \qquad k = 0,\ 1,\ 2 \quad \text{and} \quad i = 1,\ 2,\ 3,\ \ldots,\ n = 118.$$

Uppercase H and D denote "observations" resulting from the bootstrap replicate sampling. Repeating the bootstrap sampling of the 118 matched sets a large number of times yields an estimate of the distribution that produced the observed harmonic mean value $\bar{h} = -47.795$. Such an estimate is displayed in Figure 8.4 based on the 5000 replicate values of $\bar{H}$.

The mean of the estimated $\bar{H}$-distribution is -47.694 (median $= -48.791$), with a minimum value of -294.695 and a maximum value of 201.347. Estimating the variance associated with the contrast $\bar{h}$ directly from 5000 bootstrap-sampled mean values gives an estimated standard deviation of $S_{\bar{H}} = 52.493$. Additionally, the distribution appears close to symmetric.

The principal purpose for generating this bootstrap-estimated distribution is to describe the impact of random variation on the observed difference between harmonic mean values calculated from 118 matched sets. If only random variation causes within-set differences, then the expected value of $\bar{h}$ is zero. The number of replicated bootstrap mean values greater than zero (901 out of the 5000 simulated $\bar{H}$-values) indicates that it is rather usual for a value of $\bar{h}$ to exceed zero by chance alone (case risk greater than control). A one-sided "p-value" calculated from the estimated bootstrap distribution is then $P(\bar{H} \geq 0 \mid$ no case/control difference$) = 901/5000 = 0.18$. Additionally, assuming that the estimated distribution of $\bar{H}$-values is approximately normal (as indicated by the histogram—Figure 8.4), then

$$z = \frac{h_0 - (-47.694)}{S_{\bar{H}}} = \frac{0 - (-47.694)}{52.493} = 0.908$$

and $P(\bar{H} \geq 0 \mid$ no case/control difference$) = P(Z \geq 0.908) = 0.18$. Both results suggest that about 20% of sample harmonic mean distances associated with the cases would be greater than the harmonic mean values of the combined controls by chance alone (evidence against an association). That is, the

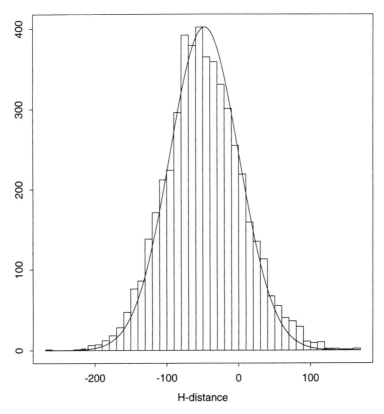

Figure 8.4. Bootstrap-estimated distribution of the differences in harmonic mean distances to the nearest high-power lines within matched sets.

bootstrap-estimated distribution is not sufficiently shifted toward the negative values of $\bar{h}$ to provide convincing evidence that the case distances are systematically smaller within the matched sets.

The bootstrap-estimated distribution of $\bar{h}$ also allows the construction of a confidence interval in the usual way. An approximate 95% confidence interval reflecting the impact of random variation on the estimate of $\bar{h} = -47.795$ is

$$\overline{H} \pm 1.960 S_{\overline{H}} = -47.694 \pm 1.960(52.493)$$

yielding the confidence interval $(-150.578, 55.190)$. The fact that zero is contained in the interval again shows that a harmonic mean of zero or greater is not an unlikely candidate for the underlying true difference between harmonic mean distances.

A Third Approach: Recorded Distance (Analysis of Variance)

Although no reason exists to suspect that the two controls differ in any systematic way, the emf radiation data can be analyzed without combining the control distances. To start, the data are classified into a two-way table. The cases and controls make up the columns, and the rows consist of the matched sets. For the emf radiation data, the table consists of three columns (case, $control_1$, and $control_2$) and 118 rows (matched sets). The cells of the 118 by 3 table contain the 354 measured distances. Matched data arranged in this form can be analyzed using analysis of variance techniques.

Differences among the rows result from differences among the matched sets and are typically not of much interest. For matched data, comparing the column mean values is important since these values summarize the 118 differences within rows and are, as before, summarized by $\bar{d}_0 = 745.2$, $\bar{d}_1 = 825.0$, and $\bar{d}_2 = 819.5$ (Table 8.1). Figure 8.5 displays the mean distance for the case and each control group (columns), as well as their associated 95% confidence intervals.

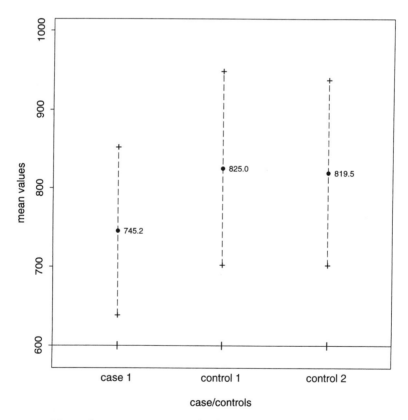

Figure 8.5. Mean distances to nearest high-power lines for the case group and both control groups with their associated 95% confidence intervals.

When the underlying population mean values (denoted μ_0, μ_1, and μ_2) do not differ among the cases and controls ($\mu_0 = \mu_1 = \mu_2 = \mu$), the differences among the observed mean values ($\bar{d}_0$, $\bar{d}_1$, and $\bar{d}_2$) result from random variation alone. To the extent that the variability among the observed column mean values increases, the hypothesis of equality among the population mean values becomes less plausible. A statistically convenient measure of the variation among the column mean values is $n\sum(\bar{d}_j - \bar{d})^2$, where $\bar{d}$ is the mean of all 358 distances, $\bar{d}_j$ is the mean of the jth column ($j = 0$, 1, and 2), and $n = 118$ is the number of rows (matched sets).

Analysis of variance techniques applied to a matched-set two-way table use an f-test to assess formally the "no-difference" hypothesis. For the matched emf radiation data, the primary issue is the variability among the distances within matched sets (Table 8.1) summarized by the differences among the column mean values. The statistics of an analysis of variance are given in Table 8.3.

The analysis of variance summary reflecting the differences among the column mean values (column sum of squares $= n\sum(\bar{d}_j - \bar{d})^2 = 0.469$) is small and entirely consistent with random variation. The p-value is $P\,(F \geq 0.717 \mid \mu_0 = \mu_1 = \mu_2 = \mu) = 0.49$. This result is no surprise in light of the overlapping confidence intervals (Figure 8.5), which also strongly indicate that no evidence of systematic differences exists among the three mean distances.

The assumptions underlying an analysis of variance of a two-way table are as follows:

1. The observed values have normal distributions.
2. The variances in each of the sampled populations are the same.
3. The matched sets are sampled independently.
4. The underlying relationship among the three column values is the same within all rows (no interaction).

The term *robust* in a statistical context means that the analysis continues to give accurate results even when the assumptions are not entirely fulfilled. The analysis of variance, applied to the emf radiation data is particularly robust with respect to the first two requirements (1 and 2) because the number of observations that make up the compared mean values is large and equal

Table 8.3. Analysis of Variance Table for the emf Radiation Data

	Sum of Squares*	Degrees of Freedom	Mean Square	F	p-Value
matched sets (rows)	69.077	117	0.590	1.806	<0.001
case/control (columns)	0.469	2	0.234	0.717	0.489
residual	76.459	234	0.327	—	—
total	146.005	353	—	—	—

*Distance is converted to kilometers to reduce the magnitude of the sums of squares.

($n = 116$). The large sample sizes essentially guarantee that the column mean values have approximately normal distributions (central limit theorem). When the compared mean values are based on the same sample size, the mathematics of the f-test is such that unequal variances have only a minimal impact on the analysis of a two-way table[6] unless the variability is extremely unequal.

The third and fourth requirements are much more critical for accurate inferences. *Independence* refers to the way the sample is collected and is usually under the control of the investigator. Without independent sampling of the matched sets, the accuracy of the f-test can be substantially biased.

The fourth requirement, that the relationship between case/control status and emf radiation exposure be the same within each matched set, is perhaps the most important. If the observed values (columns) within each matched set (rows) vary randomly from the same three mean values, μ_0, μ_1, and μ_2, respectively, then the overall mean values (column mean values) estimate the underlying mean values, namely, μ_0, μ_1, and μ_2 (no interaction). In other words, the underlying structure of the data contained in a two-way table of matched sets is required to be additive (a.13). For additive variables, the differences among the column values are the same, give or take random variation, within all rows. The comparison of column mean values, then, accurately summarizes these consistent differences. Otherwise, the column mean values do not reflect a single pattern within the rows, leading to a relatively meaningless summary estimate of the within-set case/control differences. This "no interaction" requirement becomes more explicit in the context of a statistical model (to be discussed).

A Fourth Approach: Dichotomized Exposure (Combining 2 by 2 Tables)

Another strategy that minimizes the impact of noninformative large distances involves defining a binary variable *exposed* and *unexposed* in terms of observed distance. A distance of 100 meters is chosen. *Exposed* is defined as a mother living within 100 meters or less of a high-power line (E), and *unexposed* is defined as a mother living more than 100 meters from the nearest high-power line ($\bar{E}$) during pregnancy. Distance is transformed into a binary measure of exposure. Thus, all values greater than 100 meters are treated the same way. A residence 150 meters from a high-voltage line is treated the same way as a residence 1500 meters away. Both observations are classified as unexposed, removing the impact of large, noninformative distances. The matched sets of French birth defects data, then, become a series of 2 by 2 tables, namely, 118 tables each made up of three individuals (one case and two controls). General notation for one of these 2 by 2 tables is

ith set	E	$\overline{E}$	Total
case	a_i	b_i	1
control	c_i	d_i	2
total	$a_i + c_i$	$b_i + d_i$	3

where a_i and b_i take on the values 0 or 1 and c_i and d_i take on the values 0, 1, or 2 in the ith table (stratum) for $i = 1, 2, 3, \ldots, 118$. The three infants, as before, are the same gender and were born on the same date in the same municipality, essentially eliminating any influences from these variables on the case/control differences observed within each matched set (a 2 by 2 table).

When two controls are collected for each case, six different matched sets (2 by 2 tables) are possible. The case can be exposed or not {1, 0}, and the two controls can both be exposed, or one control can be exposed, or neither control can be exposed {2, 1, or 0}. Since there are two possibilities for the cases and three possibilities for the controls, there are a total of six different kinds of 1:2 matched data sets or six kinds of 2 by 2 tables. These six 2 by 2 tables are displayed in Table 8.4. The observed counts of each kind of matched set (table) are represented by n_{ij}; specifically:

Table type 1 occurs n_{12}
Table type 2 occurs n_{11}
Table type 3 occurs n_{10}
Table type 4 occurs n_{02}
Table type 5 occurs n_{01}
Table type 6 occurs n_{00}

The first subscript indicates the number of exposed cases (residence ≤ 100 meters) in each matched set. The second subscript indicates the number of exposed controls (residence ≤ 100 meters). For example, there are n_{02} matched sets in which no cases are exposed and both controls are exposed. The data from the emf radiation study (one 2 by 2 table per matched set from 118 total strata) are summarized in Table 8.5. The sum of the six n_{ij}-values is the total number of matched sets ($n = n_{12} + n_{11} + n_{10} + n_{02} + n_{01} + n_{00} = 0 + 1 + 10 + 2 + 10 + 95 = 118$). To further describe the 118 matched sets:

Type	a_i	b_i	c_i	d_i	$a_i d_i/n_i$	$b_i c_i/n_i$	Number of Tables	Count
1	1	0	2	0	0	0	n_{12}	0
2	1	0	1	1	1/3	0	n_{11}	1
3	1	0	0	2	2/3	0	n_{10}	10
4	0	1	2	0	0	2/3	n_{02}	2
5	0	1	1	1	0	1/3	n_{01}	10
6	0	1	0	2	0	0	n_{00}	95

Table 8.4. The Six Possible 1:2 Matched Sets Tables (Strata)

TYPE 1	E	$\bar{E}$	Total
case	1	0	1
control	2	0	2
total	3	0	3
TYPE 2	E	$\bar{E}$	Total
case	1	0	1
control	1	1	2
total	2	1	3
TYPE 3	E	$\bar{E}$	Total
case	1	0	1
control	0	2	2
total	1	2	3
TYPE 4	E	$\bar{E}$	Total
case	0	1	1
control	2	0	2
total	2	1	3
TYPE 5	E	$\bar{E}$	Total
case	0	1	1
control	1	1	2
total	1	2	3
TYPE 6	E	$\bar{E}$	Total
case	0	1	1
control	0	2	2
total	0	3	3

A Mantel-Haenszel summary odds ratio is commonly used to combine the information from each matched set (stratum), producing a single measure of risk. The Mantel-Haenszel estimate of the summary odds ratio (a.6) is ($n_i = 3$ for all 118 matched sets)

$$\text{odds ratio} = \hat{or}_m = \frac{\sum(a_i d_i / n_i)}{\sum(b_i c_i / n_i)} = \frac{(1/3)n_{11} + (2/3)n_{10}}{(2/3)n_{02} + (1/3)n_{01}} = \frac{n_{11} + 2n_{10}}{2n_{02} + n_{01}}.$$

Table 8.5. The Frequency of the Six Kinds of 2 by 2 Tables for the 118 emf Radiation Matched Sets

	Control: E and E	Control: E or $\bar{E}$	Control: $\bar{E}$ and $\bar{E}$
case: E	$n_{12} = 0$	$n_{11} = 1$	$n_{10} = 10$
case: $\bar{E}$	$n_{02} = 2$	$n_{01} = 10$	$n_{00} = 95$

Treating the 1:2 matched sample of emf data as 118 observed 2 by 2 tables produces an estimated summary odds ratio of

$$\hat{or}_m = \frac{1 + 2(10)}{2(2) + 10} = \frac{21}{14} = 1.5 \quad (m \text{ for matched}).$$

A chi-square assessment of the association between exposure and case/control status employs the test statistic

$$X_m^2 = \frac{[(n_{11} + 2n_{10}) - (n_{01} + 2n_{02})]^2}{2(n_{11} + n_{10} + n_{02} + n_{01})}.$$

The test statistic X_m^2 has an approximate chi-square distribution with one degree of freedom when case/control status is unrelated to exposure (a.7). For the emf radiation data (Table 8.5), the chi-square statistic $X_m^2 = (21 - 14)^2/46 = 1.065$ yields the corresponding p-value of $P(X_m^2 \geq 1.065 \mid$ no association with exposure) = 0.30, indicating that emf exposure is not likely related to case/control status. The expression denoted by X_m^2 is a specific application of the Mantel-Haenszel-Cochran chi-square statistic[21] constructed to identify associations within a series of independent 2 by 2 tables (a.7). Two kinds of tables (types 1 and 6) consist of matched sets in which all members are exposed or all members are not exposed. The counts (n_{12} and n_{00}) of these concordant tables do not play a role in the estimation of the summary odds ratio or the test of association since no within-set case/control differences in exposure occurred.

An approximate 95% confidence interval is constructed from 1:2 matched data in the usual way, employing the estimated variance[21]

$$v = \text{variance (log } [\hat{or}_m]) = \left[2\hat{or}_m \left(\frac{n_{10} + n_{01}}{(2 + \hat{or}_m)^2} + \frac{n_{11} + n_{02}}{(1 + 2\hat{or}_m)^2} \right) \right]^{-1}.$$

An approximate 95% confidence interval for the underlying odds ratio is

$$or_{\text{lower}} = \hat{or}_m e^{-1.960\sqrt{v}} \quad \text{and} \quad or_{\text{upper}} = \hat{or}_m e^{1.960\sqrt{v}}.$$

From the emf radiation data, the estimated odds ratio $\hat{or}_m = 1.5$ and the estimated associated variance $v = 0.183$ become the basis of the approximate 95% confidence interval (0.648, 3.470), again giving no indication that distance (exposure) measured as a binary variable is related to the risk of a birth defect.

Statistical tests and confidence intervals exist for any number of controls per case. Even when the data consist of matched sets with different numbers of controls per case, estimates of the odds ratio are found with specialized expressions based on the Mantel-Haenszel summary odds ratio and tested to evaluate the influence of a risk factor (for example, emf exposure). An alternative approach uses regression techniques and a linear logistic model (next section).

A Fifth Approach: Dichotomized Exposure (Conditional Logistic Regression)

Since a matched design with a binary exposure classification is no more than a series of 2 by 2 tables, applying a logistic regression model also produces an estimated summary odds ratio. A logistic model representing 118 matched sets (2 by 2 tables) in terms of the log-odds is

$$\text{log-odds}_{ij} = a_i + bE_j \quad j = 0 \text{ or } 1 \quad \text{and} \quad i = 1, 2, 3, \ldots, 118.$$

The outcome variable is the log-odds associated with case/control status. The binary variable represented by E_j indicates exposed or unexposed ($E_j = 0 =$ unexposed and $E_j = 1 =$ exposed). The parameter a_i represents the baseline log-odds for the ith matched set or 2 by 2 table (stratum). Specifically, for the ith matched set

$$\text{log-odds}_{i0} = a_i \quad \text{(unexposed)} \quad \text{and} \quad \text{log-odds}_{i1} = a_i + b \quad \text{(exposed)}$$

where b represents the change in log-odds associated with exposure to emf radiation.

This logistic model explicitly requires that the impact of exposure on the outcome be the same within each matched set ($b = $ constant—no interaction). The analogous assumption of no interaction was required for the previous four approaches to analyzing the matched emf data but was less explicit. Frequently, a statistical model more dramatically defines the necessary underlying requirements of an analysis.

For matched data or any data classified into a large number of strata, estimates obtained from the application of standard logistic regression techniques are biased, sometimes seriously biased.[22] To analyze matched data accurately, an approach is needed that allows estimates of the important within-set relationships but avoids the bias associated with estimating the relationships among the large number of strata. Such a technique is called *conditional logistic regression analysis*.[22] Since 118 strata parameters (a_i-values) and one exposure parameter (b) are required to describe the emf data with a logistic model, conditional logistic regression techniques are necessary to provide an unbiased estimate of the within-set influence of emf exposure. A conditional logistic regression analysis yields an accurate estimate of the parameter for the postulated relationship between risk factor and case/control status, namely, the coefficient b, but does not supply estimates of the large number of parameters necessary to identify differences among strata, namely, the a_i-parameters. The differences among strata are rarely an important issue when the data are matched. Conceptually, the conditional logistic analysis of the emf data is based on 118 differences in log-odds values, eliminating the parameters a_i and combining the 118 differences to estimate the parameter b. Therefore, a conditional logistic analysis of the matched emf radiation data focuses on the single parameter b, and no estimates of the 118 model parameters a_i are possible. Then $\hat{or}_{model} = e^{\hat{b}}$ is the estimated summary odds ratio measuring the association between emf exposure and case/control status, since $\hat{b}$ represents the estimated difference in log-odds for all 118 matched sets.

Using the 118 cases and 236 controls, the estimate of the conditional logistic model parameter b is $\hat{b} = 0.438$, and its associated estimated standard error is $S_{\hat{b}} = 0.427$. The estimate of the summary odds ratio follows as $\hat{or}_{model} = e^{\hat{b}} = e^{0.438} = 1.549$.

To evaluate the estimated coefficient $\hat{b}$ against the conjecture of no association ($b = 0$), then, as usual,

$$z = \frac{\hat{b} - 0}{S_{\hat{b}}} = \frac{0.438 - 0}{0.427} = 1.025$$

and z has an approximate standard normal distribution when emf exposure is unrelated to the risk of a birth defect ($b = 0$). Since $z^2 = (1.025)^2 = 1.050$ has an approximate chi-square distribution with one degree of freedom when $b = 0$, the p-value is $P(Z^2 \geq 1.050 \mid b = 0) = 0.31$.

The construction of a 95% confidence interval also follows the usual pattern. An approximate 95% confidence interval based on the estimate $\hat{b}$ is $\hat{b} \pm 1.960\ S_{\hat{b}}$ or $(-0.400, 1.276)$. An approximate 95% confidence interval for the common odds ratio based on the estimate $\hat{or}_{model} = e^{\hat{b}} = 1.549$ is then (e^{lower}, e^{upper}) where $(e^{-0.400}, e^{1.276})$ yields the confidence interval $(0.671, 3.582)$.

The odds ratio estimated from the conditional logistic model, the test of the coefficient $\hat{b}$, and the 95% confidence interval are essentially the same as those estimated from the nonmodel approach. However, as always, a parametric model can be extended to address a variety of additional and sometimes complex issues. For example, the conditional logistic model can be extended to include variables with possibly confounding influences not accounted for by the matched design. Also, interactions between matching variables and other measured variables can be included in the model, yielding estimates and statistical tests.

CONCLUSIONS

Two definitions of exposure show no important association between the proximity to high-power lines (emf) and the risk of a birth defect among newborn infants. Matched analyses using the directly observed distance show a slight but not significantly smaller distance to power lines among the cases compared to controls. A t-test (p-value = 0.09), a bootstrap analysis (p-value = 0.18), and an analysis of variance (p-value = 0.49) provide little evidence that this association is not entirely due to random variation. Defining risk as a binary variable (distance $\leq$ 100 meters and distance $>$ 100 meters), matched analyses again provide little evidence of an association (model-free: p-value = 0.30; conditional logistic model: p-value = 0.31).

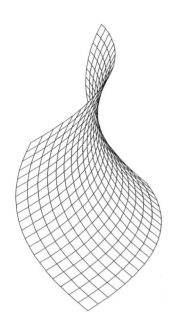

CHAPTER 9

Multivariable Linear Regression

OBJECTIVE

To examine the influence of maternal weight gained during pregnancy on the birth weight of a newborn infant while controlling for a variety of possibly important confounding factors.

DATA

The Department of Obstetrics, Gynecology, and Reproductive Science Perinatal Database maintained at the University of California, San Francisco (UCSF) contains data on a large number of characteristics of mothers and their newborn infants. Information on maternal age, smoking exposure, pre-pregnancy weight, parity, height, and rate of weight gained during pregnancy was abstracted, forming a cohort of 427 Hispanic mothers who gave birth during the eleven year period 1980 to 1990. In addition, length of gestation and birth weight were recorded for each mother's newborn infant. Birth weight was measured immediately at delivery. The length of the gestation period was determined by a rigorous process combining information from the last menstrual period and Dubowitz scores. Mothers were routinely weighed at every prenatal visit, allowing an estimate of the rate of weight gained during each trimester based on simple linear regression interpolation. Race, age, pre-pregnancy weight, and smoking history were self-reported values, reported by the mother at her first prenatal visit. When a mother appeared more than once in the sample, a random pregnancy was selected.

METHODS

Multivariable linear regression is used to assess the influence of maternal weight gain on the weight of a newborn infant. Since other variables influence the relationship between birth weight and a mother's weight gained during pregnancy, these variables are also included as part of a linear regression analysis. Standardized regression coefficients are used to rank the relative importance of each variable included in the analysis. Polynomial representations of the independent variables are additionally employed in regression models to describe more specifically the role of each independent variable, particularly maternal weight gain.

Data type: cross-sectional (hospital database)
Reference: *Obstetrics and Gynecology*, 1995, 86(2): 170–6

The variables are:

1. Maternal age: self-reported in years
2. Parity: count of previous live births
3. Gestation: reported days
4. Gender: male coded 1 and female coded 2
5. Birth weight: measured in grams
6. Smoking: self-reported number of cigarettes smoked per day
7. Maternal height: measured in centimeters
8. Maternal weight: self-reported prepregnancy weight in kilograms
9. Rate of weight gained during the first trimester: estimated kilograms per day
10. Rate of weight gained during the second trimester: estimated kilograms per day
11. Rate of weight gained during the third trimester: estimated kilograms per day

Part of the data file of 427 mother/infant measurements is:

```
file name = birthwt.9.data
```

age	parity	gest	sex	bwt	cigs	ht	wt	r1	r2	r3
29	0	294	2	3860	0	160.0	63.6	0.056	0.107	0.045
25	0	294	2	3870	0	170.2	65.2	−0.017	0.108	0.096
34	0	252	2	2440	0	175.3	58.6	0.007	0.057	0.053
29	2	280	1	3400	20	162.6	57.3	0.033	0.082	0.059
19	1	266	2	3480	0	162.6	69.1	−0.037	0.063	0.083
23	1	280	2	2820	1	157.5	65.9	−0.022	0.092	0.088
26	0	266	2	2940	3	162.6	59.1	0.063	0.159	0.032
30	4	245	1	2400	20	150.0	49.1	0.038	0.092	0.049
27	1	273	2	3080	0	175.0	69.5	0.000	0.101	0.075
26	1	273	2	3600	0	165.1	75.0	0.049	0.058	0.058

40	1	287	1	3600	0	170.2	82.0	−0.001	0.090	0.054
19	0	287	1	3930	0	157.0	58.3	0.043	0.095	0.091
20	0	294	2	3380	0	157.5	50.0	0.052	0.088	0.085
30	1	280	1	3440	0	152.4	65.5	0.051	0.056	0.081
41	0	287	1	3000	0	162.6	61.4	0.014	0.028	0.067
—	—	—	—	—	—	—	—	—	—	—
—	—	—	—	—	—	—	—	—	—	—
—	—	—	—	—	—	—	—	—	—	—

DISCUSSION

Perhaps the most important and one of the most popular statistical methods used to estimate and evaluate the influence of a series of variables on a single outcome is based on the multivariable linear regression model. Several books are devoted to this topic.[23,24] The reasons for this popularity include the following:

1. A linear model is mathematically simple.
2. Its properties are understood with a minimum of statistical theory.
3. The components of the model are easy to interpret.
4. A linear model appears to be appropriate for a large number of situations.
5. A linear model naturally serves as a point of departure for more sophisticated analyses.

For the UCSF birth weight data, eight variables are continuous (bwt, age, gest, ht, wt, wt1, wt2, and wt3), two are binary (sex and smk), and one is discrete (parity). Table 9.1 provides a brief description of these variables.

The comparison of the mean and median values gives some idea of the symmetry of the distribution of the independent variables. Standard deviation refers to the population from which the sample was selected and is sometimes confused with the standard error of the mean. The weight gained during each trimester is based on weights recorded at the mother's prenatal visits and calculated from the estimated rate of daily gain for each trimester (weight gained = 90 days × daily rate). The minimum and maximum values are a good check of the data, revealing outlier or errors (for example, a minimum value such as −999 is likely to be an unknown code and not a data value). These 10 variables can be used exactly as measured or transformed into more useful forms because the classic regression analysis allows the form of the explanatory variables to be completely unconstrained.

A multivariable linear regression model in a narrow mathematical sense is defined by the expression

$$y_i = b_0 + b_1 x_{i1} + b_2 x_{i2} + b_3 x_{i3} + \cdots + b_k x_{ik} + e_i$$

Table 9.1. Description of the Variables Recorded for 427 Hispanic Women and their Newborn Infants

Continuous Data

Variable	Symbol	Unit	Mean	Median	Std. dev.	Minimum	Maximum
birth weight	bwt	kilograms	3.5	3.5	0.5	1.6	5.7
age	age	years	27.8	27.0	5.5	15.0	42.0
gestation	gest	days	276.4	280.0	11.5	224.0	308.0
height	ht	centimeters	159.7	160.0	6.4	142.2	180.3
prepregnancy weight	wt	kilograms	58.4	56.8	10.2	40.9	123.6
weight gain/first*	wt1	kilograms	2.7	2.4	3.0	−4.0	11.4
weight gain/second*	wt2	kilograms	7.2	7.1	0.1	0.0	17.7
weight gain/third*	wt3	kilograms	6.7	6.7	0.1	−1.2	16.1

Discrete Data

parity (parity)	0	1	2	3	≥4	total	
frequency	185	143	66	24	9	427	

gender (sex)	male	female	total				
frequency	231	196	427				

smoking** (smk)	yes	no	total				
frequency	35	392	427				

*Rate of trimester maternal weight gain per day multiplied by 90 days.

**no = never smoked or past smoker; yes = one or more cigarettes/day.

where x_{ij} represents one of the k independent variables (ith observation of the jth independent variable). The variables omitted from the regression model are assumed to have nonsystematic (random) influences on the y-variable, represented by the error term e_i. The error term is the stochastic component of the linear model. These error terms are further required to be independent, to have a normal distributions with the same variance over the range of the dependent variables, and to be unrelated to the independent variables.

For the UCSF data, the birth weight of the ith infant is represented by such a linear model where

$$y_i = b_0 + b_1 age_i + b_2 parity_i + b_3 gest_i + b_4 sex_i + b_5 smk_i + b_6 ht_i$$
$$+ b_7 wt_i + b_8 wt1_i + b_9 wt2_i + b_{10} wt3_i + e_i \qquad i = 1, 2, 3, \ldots, n = 427.$$

The symbol y_i represents the dependent variable, which is a linear function of 10 ($k = 10$) measured quantities (also called *predictor* or *explanatory variables*). No restrictions are placed on these 10 variables, and they are analyzed exactly as reported. However, an important question is whether these variables have additive or multiplicative influences on infant birth weight. For the present analysis, a multiplicative model is chosen. That is, the logarithm of the birth weight is employed as the dependent variable, making the influences of the independent variables on birth weight multiplicative ($y_i = \log (bwt_i)$ instead of $y_i = bwt_i$). For example, if a mother gains one kilogram during the second trimester of pregnancy, the logarithm of the birth weight is increased by 0.007, which means that the birth weight itself is increased by a factor of $e^{0.007} = 1.007$. The distribution of the log-birth weights is displayed in Figure 9.1. This logarithmic transformation also serves to make the distribution of the error term (e_i) more symmetric (normal-like).

Employing the 427 mother/infant observations, the regression coefficients for the linear log-birth weight model are estimated (Table 9.2) to explore the relationships between the 10 independent variables and infant birth weight, with a primary focus on the influence of maternal weight gained during pregnancy. An estimated log-birth weight based on the regression model (denoted $\hat{y}_i$) is found using these coefficients (Table 9.2). Specifically, the estimated ith log-birth weight is

$$\hat{y}_i = -0.7842 + 0.0021 age_i + 0.0088 parity_i + \cdots + 0.0073 wt2_i - 0.0001 wt3_i.$$

These 427 estimated values are useful in a variety of ways. One important use is for the estimation of the error terms e_i by $\hat{e}_i = y_i - \hat{y}_i$, called a *residual value*.

Since a linear regression model in the broad sense requires the error term (e_i terms in the regression model) to have a normal distribution with the same

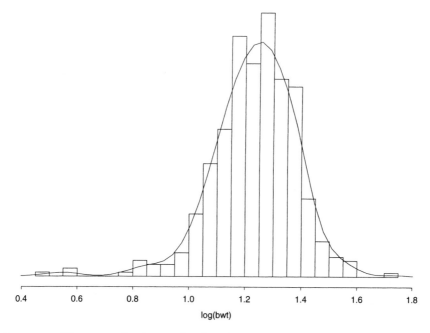

log(bwt)

Figure 9.1. Histogram displaying the distribution of the log-birth weights of newborn infants with Hispanic mothers.

variance for all values of the dependent variables, the estimated values $\hat{e}_i$ should reflect these two properties. Figure 9.2 is a quantile plot of the standardized estimated error terms $(\hat{e}_i/S_{\hat{e}_i})$. Normally distributed data displayed on such a plot deviate from a straight line only because of random variation. Inspection of Figure 9.2 gives no indication of nonnormality of the error terms

Table 9.2. Estimated Coefficients from the Multivariable Regression Model, where the Dependent Variable is the Logarithm of the Infant's Birth Weight

Variable	Coefficient	Estimate	Std. Error	t-Statistic	p-Value
intercept	b_0	−0.7842	—	—	—
age	b_1	0.0021	0.001	1.895	0.06
parity	b_2	0.0088	0.006	1.407	0.16
gestation	b_3	0.0067	0.001	13.220	<0.001
gender	b_4	−0.0342	0.012	−2.972	0.01
smoking	b_5	−0.0356	0.021	−1.704	0.09
height	b_6	−0.0004	0.001	−0.404	0.69
prepregnancy weight	b_7	0.0024	0.001	3.816	<0.001
weight gain/first	b_8	0.0040	0.002	2.055	0.04
weight gain/second	b_9	0.0073	0.002	3.208	<0.001
weight gain/third	b_{10}	−0.0001	0.002	−0.042	0.97

Residual deviance = 5.748 with degrees of freedom = 416.

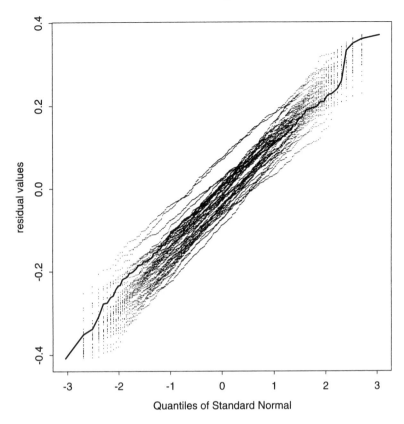

Figure 9.2. Residual values from the linear regression analysis of log-birth weights and simulated values reflecting random variation (dotted lines).

(solid line). The only remarkable deviation from a straight line occurs more than 2.5 standard deviations below the mean, an area where few observations occur and estimated residual values are subject to considerable sampling variation.

To explore further these residual values in light of the random variation, Figure 9.2 includes 40 sets of 427 points (small dots) randomly generated from a standard normal distribution. The simulated *standardized residual values* have mean = 0 and variance = 1, which are the same mean and variance associated with the standardized estimated $\hat{e}_i$-values. The spread of the computer-generated residual values gives a direct indication of the impact of sampling variation on the model-generated quantile plot (dots). The estimated residual values from the birth weight regression model are generally within the empiric limits defined by simulated normally distributed residual values, providing further evidence of the normality of the error terms.

Figure 9.3 displays the 427 pairs of points $(y_i, \hat{y}_i)$ = (observed values, estimated values). A plot of these points reflects the accuracy of the model in predicting the dependent variable, log-birth weight. If the model perfectly predicts the observed values, the plotted pairs of points would fall on a straight line with slope 1.0 ($y_i = \hat{y}_i$ when $\hat{e}_i = 0$ for all observed values). Therefore, the lack of fit of a linear model is a function of the degree to which the estimated values are not described by a straight line. A correlation coefficient provides a single summary of this lack of fit. In this context, the Pearson correlation applied to the n pairs of values y_i and $\hat{y}_i$ is called the *multiple correlation coefficient* (denoted R). For the birth weight data, the multiple correlation coefficient is R = correlation$(y_i, \hat{y}_i)$ = 0.610.

The multiple correlation coefficient relates to two other important sum-

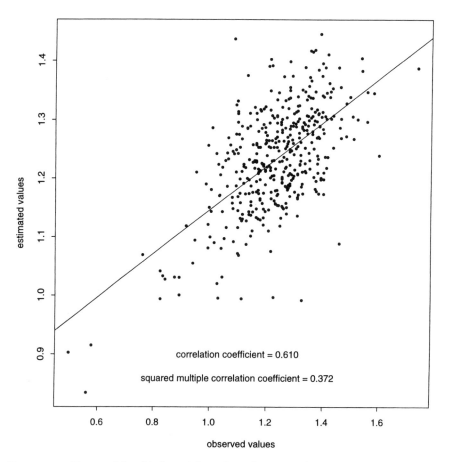

Figure 9.3. Observed log-birth weights plotted against the values estimated from the linear regression equation.

mary quantities—the residual deviance and the null deviance. The residual deviance is defined as

$$\text{residual deviance} = D_{\text{residual}} = \sum \hat{e}_i^2 = \sum (y_i - \hat{y}_i)^2$$

and the null deviance as

$$\text{null deviance} = D_{\text{null}} = \sum (y_i - \bar{y})^2.$$

The residual deviance reflects the differences between the observed values and the model-estimated values based on the independent variables. The null deviance reflects the difference between the observed values and the estimated values completely ignoring any influence of the independent variables. Thus, the difference between these two quantities measures the total impact of the independent variables. From the birth weight regression model, $D_{\text{residual}} = 5.748$ and $D_{\text{null}} = 9.156$. The reduction $D_{\text{null}} - D_{\text{residual}} = 3.408$ is achieved by using the information contained in the 10 independent variables to estimate infant log-birth weight. The ratio $D_{\text{residual}}/D_{\text{null}} = 5.748/9.156 = 0.628$ is directly related to the squared multiple correlation coefficient where

$$\text{square multiple correlation coefficient} = R^2 = 1 - \frac{D_{\text{residual}}}{D_{\text{null}}} = 1 - 0.628 = 0.372$$

and $R = \sqrt{0.372} = 0.610$, as before. Since $(1 - R^2)D_{\text{null}} = D_{\text{residual}}$, it is frequently said that R^2 indicates the proportion of variation explained by the linear model. Therefore, based on a linear model, the 10 maternal/infant independent variables explain 37.2% of the variation in the log-birth weight observations. The word *explain* is used in the rather narrow sense of a linear model referring primarily to goodness-of-fit and not in the usual sense of a given reason or cause.

The estimated model coefficients are the key elements of a regression analysis. The regression coefficient $\hat{b}_j$ estimates the change in the dependent variable y_i for a one unit increase in the jth independent variable accounting for the other $k - 1$ variables in the model. However, like all estimates, these estimated coefficients are subject to sampling variation. An estimated coefficient may reflect only random deviation from a value of zero or, on the other hand, it may indicate a significant contribution to the variability of the dependent variable. A fundamental question then becomes: *is the estimated regression coefficient relative to its standard error large enough to imply that a specific variable has a systematic influence on the outcome variable?*

The t-statistic constructed to evaluate the jth estimated regression coefficient $\hat{b}_j$ is

$$T_j = \frac{\hat{b}_j - 0}{S_{\hat{b}_j}}$$

and the test statistic T_j has a t-distribution with $n - (k + 1)$ degrees of freedom when the underlying regression coefficient equals zero ($b_j = 0$). That is, the likelihood associated with T_j is calculated (p-value) as if the jth independent variable has no impact on the dependent variable after accounting for the influences of the other $k - 1$ independent variables. A series of t-tests typically sorts out those independent variables that make small contributions (consistent with sampling variation) and those that make large contributions (over and above the influence of sampling variation) to the variability of the dependent variable. For example, the influence on log-birth weight associated with maternal age is reflected by the estimated regression coefficient $\hat{b}_1 = 0.0021$. Just because a coefficient is small does not mean that the associated independent variable is an insignificant contributor. The magnitude of a regression coefficient depends primarily on the units of measurement of the independent and dependent variables. A t-test to evaluate the role of maternal age in the estimated regression equation is

$$T_{age} = \frac{0.0021 - 0}{0.0011} = 1.895$$

and T_{age} has a t-distribution with $n - (k + 1) = 427 - (10 + 1) = 416$ degrees of freedom when the underlying coefficient is zero ($b_1 = 0$). The p-value is $P(|\ T_{age}\ | \geq 1.895\ |\ b_1 = 0) = 0.06$, indicating that maternal age likely influences (nonrandomly) the birth weight of an infant. Furthermore, the t-test procedure does not depend on the units of measurement.

The structure of the additive model requires each influence to be unaffected by the levels of the other nine independent variables. For example, the influence measured by b_1 is the same regardless of the mother's height or weight or the magnitude of any of the other variables, frequently called an *independent* effect. The independence of effects is a property of the model, not of the data. That is, independent variables are not necessarily *independent*.

The identical statistical test arises from comparing two models, one with all k independent variables included and another with a selected independent variable deleted. Each model has a residual deviance. The difference between the two residual deviances is caused only by the influence of the deleted variable. Specifically, the full model (all 10 variables) has the residual deviance of $D_{residual} = 5.748$. When the age variable is deleted, the nine-variable regression model has a residual deviance of $D'_{residual} = 5.797$. The difference $D'_{residual} - D_{residual} = 5.797 - 5.748 = 0.049$ directly measures only the influence of maternal age. An F-statistic provides a statistical evaluation of the difference. For the variable age, the difference in residual deviances is transformed to have an f-distribution where

$$F = \frac{D'_{residual} - D_{residual}}{D_{residual}/[n - (k + 1)]} = \frac{5.797 - 5.748}{0.014} = \frac{0.049}{0.014} = 3.592.$$

When $b_1 = 0$, the quantity F has an f-distribution with 1 and 416 degrees of freedom. The associated p-value is $P(D'_{residual} - D_{residual} \geq 0.049 \mid b_1 = 0) = P(F \geq 3.592 \mid b_1 = 0) = 0.06$. The two-tail t-test and the f-test are identical ($T^2 = F$ or $(1.895)^2 = 3.592$). The individual t-test of a single coefficient and the f-test contrasting two regression models that differ by a single variable are identical in general. Columns 5 and 6 in Table 9.2 give the t-statistics (square root of the F-statistics) and associated p-values assessing, one at a time, the independent influences on the log-birth weight from each of the 10 maternal/infant variables.

To assess statistically the simultaneous impact of more than one independent variable, the t-test no longer applies. The t-statistics associated with each of several variables may give a rough idea of the combined influences. However, this is only a rough indication since the interrelationships among the variables can cause deceptive impressions. It is entirely possible and not infrequent that the T_j-values associated with several independent variables are all moderate, but a rigorous assessment of the joint impact shows a substantial joint influence on the outcome variable. A good practice is to use a t-test to assess only one variable at a time. The f-test contrasting residual devices, however, continues to supply a rigorous assessment of the joint influence on any number of independent variables. For example, the three trimester weight gain measurements essentially reflect the total weight gained during pregnancy. To evaluate the combined influences of these three variables on the infant's log-birth weight, the contrast of two models becomes once again the basis of analysis. The full model (all 10 variables), as before, and the model with the three weight gain variables removed (seven variables) are compared. Each model produces a residual deviance, where $D_{residual} = 5.748$ (full model) and $D'_{residual} = 5.987$ (model with the three weight gain variables removed). The increase in the residual deviance is caused only by eliminating the mother's weight gained during pregnancy from consideration. An F-statistic addressing the likelihood that the difference (5.748 versus 5.987) arose by chance alone is

$$F = \frac{(D'_{residual} - D_{residual})/q}{D_{residual}/[n - (k + 1)]} = \frac{(5.987 - 5.748)/3}{0.014} = \frac{0.239/3}{0.014} = 5.744$$

where q represents the number of variables deleted. The test statistic F has an f-distribution with $q = 3$ and $n - (k + 1) = 416$ degrees of freedom when $b_8 = b_9 = b_{10} = 0$. The associated p-value is $P(D'_{residual} - D_{residual} \geq 0.239 \mid$ weight gain has no effect$) = P(F \geq 5.744 \mid$ weight gain has no effect$) = 0.001$. The small p-value provides strong evidence that one or more of the three trimester weight gain measures (wt1, wt2 and wt3) play an important role in predicting a newborn's birth weight. Following the same pattern, any subset of the independent variables can be selected and their joint influences similarly assessed with an F-statistic.

Once important coefficients are identified, the next step is to determine their relative roles in explaining the variability in the outcome variable. The regression coefficient associated with maternal height is $\hat{b}_6 = -0.0004$, and the coefficient associated with maternal prepregnancy weight is $\hat{b}_7 = 0.0024$ (Table 9.3). However, weight is not six times more important than height in predicating log-birth weight. The observed sixfold difference depends on the units of measurement. For the birth weight analysis, height is measured in centimeters and weight in kilograms. The same coefficients would have an entirely different ratio if height were measured in feet and weight in pounds. The two coefficients are not commensurate, which means they are not measured in the same units and, therefore, are not comparable (comparing "apples and oranges"). A number of methods exist to make estimated regression coefficients commensurate.

The t-statistics provide a comparison in the same units (a t-statistic is unitless). The 10 T_j-values and their ranks are given in Table 9.3. Another commensurate comparison is achieved by multiplying the jth regression coefficient by the standard deviation of the jth variable. In symbols, this commensurate coefficient (denoted $\hat{B}_j$) becomes $\hat{B}_j = \hat{b}_j S_j$. The $\hat{B}_j$-values are com-

Table 9.3. Standardized Coefficients (T_j and $\hat{B}_j$) and the Correlation Between the Dependent Variable and Each of the 10 Independent Variables (r_{yj})

Variable	$\hat{b}_j$	T_j	Rank	$\hat{B}_j^*$	Rank	r_{yj}	Rank
age	0.0021	1.90	6	1.18	6	0.08	7
parity	0.0088	1.41	8	0.91	8	0.03	9
gestation	0.0067	13.22	1	7.78	1	0.54	1
sex	-0.0342	-2.97	4	-1.71	4	-0.11	3
smoking	-0.0356	-1.70	7	-0.98	7	-0.08	6
height	-0.0004	-0.40	9	-0.25	9	0.03	8
weight	0.0024	3.82	2	2.41	2	0.24	2
weight/first	0.0040	2.06	5	1.21	5	0.10	4
weight/second	0.0073	3.21	3	1.91	3	0.10	5
weight/third	-0.0001	-0.04	10	-0.03	10	-0.02	10

*Multiplied by 100.

mensurate in the sense that they measure the change in the dependent variable for a one standard deviation increase in the independent variable. A commensurate comparison of the relative influences of height and weight becomes $\hat{B}_6 = -0.25$ versus $\hat{B}_7 = 2.41$, indicating an almost 10-fold difference in impact on the dependent variable, log-birth weight. The $\hat{B}_j$-values from the log-birth weight model are also included in Table 9.3 along with their ranks.

The ranks of the commensurate standardized coefficients T_j and $\hat{B}_j$ are not different from each other and not very different from the correlation coefficient measuring the linear association between the jth independent variable and the dependent variable (correlation$(x_j, y) = r_{yj}$—Table 9.3). In fact, if the correlations among all possible pairs of the independent variables are zero, then the rank orderings of all three measures will be the same. With data such as the birth weight data, in which the correlations among the independent variables are not large, the T_j, $\hat{B}_j$, and r_{yj} summary values show only slight differences in measuring the relative importance of the independent variables.

When the correlations among the independent variables are near zero, a regression analysis allows an approximate partitioning of the total variation into pieces reflecting the separate influences of each independent variable (T_j, $\hat{B}_j$, and r_{yj}). It is meaningful to report, for example, that gestational age *explains* a large proportion (rank 1) of the variation in birth weight and that weight gained during the third trimester has little or no impact (rank 10) since the pairwise correlations among the 10 independent variables are mostly small. However, when correlations between independent variables differ appreciably from zero, similar inferences are not possible. Standardized coefficients then no longer simply or uniquely characterize the separate roles of each independent variable. Different types of standardizing procedures give different rankings, providing no unequivocal partitioning of the total variation. If such a process existed, analyses of the relative roles of environment and heredity or race and socioeconomic status would be more enlightening.

Figure 9.4 displays the regression coefficients as slopes of a line on the same scale (commensurate). The 10 plots graphically display the same issues quantified in Table 9.3. The model dictates that the impact of each independent variable is linear. The slope of each line, as before, is an estimate of the relative change in the outcome variable per unit increase in the independent variable adjusted for the influence of the nine other variables in the model. The tick marks of the horizontal axis represent the distribution of the data associated with the estimated line. Like the standardized coefficients, the days of gestation (gest) has by far the greatest impact (steepest slope) on the log-birth weight of the infant, not surprisingly. The mother's prepregnancy weight (wt) has the next strongest influence on the outcome. The third most

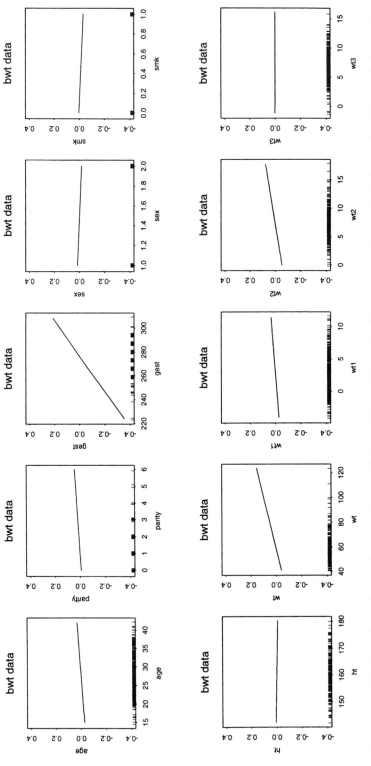

Figure 9.4. Display of standardized regression coefficients (slopes) from the linear regression analysis for each of the 10 independent variables.

important variable in predicting an infant's log-birth weight is the amount of weight gained by the mother during her second trimester (wt2). In contrast, the weight gained during her third trimester (wt3) shows essentially no impact; the slope of the line hardly differs from zero (Figure 9.4).

It is unrealistic to think that independent–dependent variable relationships are always adequately summarized by a straight line. In many situations a straight line is a useful summary, but in other situations a linear relationship is an oversimplification. Since a linear model does not restrict the form of the independent variables, other choices are available. The regression model, however, remains linear. For example, the influence of the weight gained during the first trimester can be represented as a linear or nonlinear function, and the influence of the weight gained during the second trimester can be represented as a linear or nonlinear function; however, the influence on infant birth weight is the sum of these two influences, making the birth weight model linear (additive) regardless of how the influences of the individual independent variables are measured.

Among the many ways the influence of a continuous independent variable can be modeled, one choice is to represent its impact by a polynomial expression. A polynomial expression takes on a variety of geometric shapes, depending on the defining coefficients and the number of components in the equation (*degree*). The flexibility of these polynomial representations allows the influence of each continuous independent variable to be described in a large variety of nonlinear ways.

A more general but linear birth weight model becomes

$$y_i = \log(\text{bwt}_i) = a_0 + P(\text{age}_i) + P(\text{parity}_i)$$
$$+ P(\text{gest}_i) + \cdots + P(\text{wt3}_i) + a_1\text{sex}_i + a_2\text{smk}_i + e_i \quad i = 1, 2, 3, \ldots, n = 427$$

where $P(x)$ represents a third-degree polynomial given by

$$P(x) = ax + bx^2 + cx^3.$$

The shape of the curve describing the influence of each dependent variable is determined by the polynomial coefficients a, b, and c. Selection of the polynomial degree is rather arbitrary, but a third degree polynomial is

1. not too complex,
2. sufficiently flexible to reflect a large variety of nonlinear influences,
3. linear when $b = c = 0$ (special case of nonlinearity), and
4. requires only three parameters.

The last point is particularly important since a model with too many parameters is not very useful. A rule of thumb is that the number of parameters used to define a model should be less than 10% of the number of observations. Applied to the UCSF data, a model with more than $427(0.10) \approx 43$ parameters is overspecified and will fit the observations well (the more parameters, the better the fit), but it does not provide a parsimonious summary of the relationships under study. A simple and understandable statistical structure is one of the primary reasons for postulating a mathematical model in the first place. Models, in general, involve a trade-off between simplicity (few parameters with a relatively poor fit) and complexity (many parameters with a relatively good fit), with the goal of producing a sophisticated but easily understood description of the relationships within a data set.

Polynomial representations of the independent variables introduce additional complexity into the birth weight model (27 parameters), in contrast to a linear representation (11 parameters). Polynomial expressions, however, allow a more realistic description of the relationship between each predictor and the outcome variable. This is particularly the case for a graphic display of these relationships. Figure 9.5 displays the estimated polynomial relationships associated with each of the eight continuous independent variables based on a third-degree polynomial function plotted on the same scale (commensurate). Gender and smoking exposure are binary variables consisting of only two points (as in Figure 9.4). The linear (additive) nature of the model ensures that each estimated polynomial curve is adjusted for the presence of the other variables in the regression equation. This property is sometimes expressed by stating that the influence is described as if the other independent variables were *held constant*. Geometrically, additivity guarantees that the curve representing the influences of a specific variable (x_j) is the same "shape" (i.e., $\hat{a}x_j + \hat{b}x_j^2 + \hat{c}x_j^3$) for all values of the other variables in the regression equation.

The eight estimated curves show several distinct patterns of influence on the outcome variable over the range of each independent variable. The two clearly nonlinear variables are gestation (a strongly increasing influence that weakens for the longer gestation periods) and parity (weak influence for parities 0, 1, and 2 followed by sharply negative influences for parity 4 or greater). The polynomial representation of the influence of maternal prepregnancy weight also displays a nonlinear influence on an infant's log-birth weight. Heavier mothers tend to have heavier infants except when the mothers are extremely heavy (weights > 80 kilograms). The other five continuous variables have, more or less, patterns that are rather accurately described by a straight line.

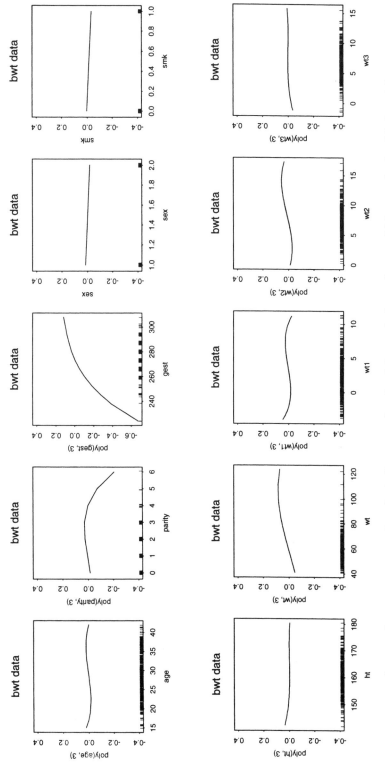

Figure 9.5. Polynomial curves representing the influences of each of the 10 independent variables on the log-birth weight measures.

CONCLUSIONS

The birth weight analysis focuses on the three trimester weight gain measures. The three estimated regression coefficients reflecting the role of maternal weight gain indicate that substantial (nonrandom) influences are likely associated with the second trimester gain (p-value < 0.001) and, to a lesser extent, with the first trimester gain (p-value $= 0.04$). No evidence of an influence from the third trimester gain is present (p-value $= 0.97$). The relative influences (standardized coefficients), as expected, follow the same pattern. The first and second trimesters are relatively important (ranks 3 and 5) and contribute about equally to the explained log-birth weight variation, while the third trimester maternal weight gain does not appear at all important (rank 10). The polynomial representations of the three weight gain patterns show no convincing evidence of a nonlinear relationship between a mother's weight gained during pregnancy and the log-birth weight of her newborn infant. For these three independent variables, a simple linear representation appears to describe the independent–dependent variable relationships adequately, making more complexity unnecessary. Therefore, in Hispanic women, the analysis clearly shows a strong and essentially multiplicative influence of the amount of weight gained during the first two trimesters, particularly the second trimester. This influence on birth weight is of the same order of magnitude as the influences of age, smoking, and parity.

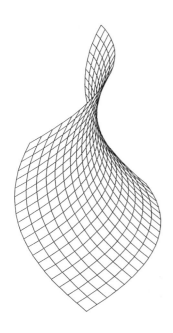

CHAPTER **10**

Linear Logistic Regression

OBJECTIVE

To describe and analyze the association between workplace exposure to noise and the risk of hypertension while accounting for several possible confounding influences, particularly salt consumption and family history of the disease.

DATA

Measures of hypertension and noise exposure were collected from 1101 women working in a textile factory in Beijing, China (only women make up the workforce). All sampled women were employed for at least five years, each at essentially the same task. Each worker was assigned to her task within the plant at "random." That is, when a current worker retired or quit (a rare event), a new worker (about age 19) was assigned to the vacated job and typically continued to do the same task until retirement. The textile factory environment was chosen because of the stability of the workforce and the spatial uniformity of each worker's exposure to noise sound pressure level (SPL). The SPL was measured as a time-weighted average. Hypertension was defined as systolic blood pressure greater than 160 mm Hg or diastolic pressure greater than 95 mm Hg. Additionally, workers taking antihypertension drugs were classified as hypertensive regardless of their blood pressure levels. This definition produced 44 hypertensive women (4.0%). Along with the measurement of each worker's noise exposure, an interview determined the worker's age, the number of years employed, her salt consumption (self-reported), and whether or not she had a family history of hypertension. In this exceptionally homogeneous cohort, one worker reported smoking, no women had more than one child, and only seven reported drinking alcohol regularly. Furthermore, all workers lived in the same industrial commune. These data constitute what is sometimes considered a *natural experiment.*

METHODS

Linear logistic models are used to estimate the risk of hypertension associated with exposure to noise while accounting for the influence of variables reflecting age, years employed, family history of the disease, and amount of salt in the diet. The risk of hypertensive disease is also explored using polynomial representations of the continuous independent variables SPL, age, and years worked.

Data type: cross-sectional (industrial hygiene measurements)
Reference: *British Medical Journal*, 1991, 48: 179–84

The variables are:

1. Hypertension: coded 1 for hypertension and 0 otherwise
2. Age: reported years
3. Years worked: reported years
4. History: coded 1 for family history and 0 otherwise
5. Salt: coded 1 for heavy use and 0 for normal or low use
6. SPL: a time-weighted average of six measurements

Part of the data file of 1101 women textile factory workers is:

```
            file name = hypertension.10.data

      hyper      age    worked   history    salt    SPL
          0    39.41    22.77         1       1     75
          0    28.12     7.63         1       1     75
          0    24.91     5.54         1       1     75
          0    40.33    21.48         0       1     75
          0    28.06     9.04         0       1     75
          0    41.17    22.82         0       1     75
          0    46.56    29.39         1       0     75
          0    45.80    29.39         1       0     75
          0    44.97    29.39         0       0     75
          0    32.97    16.38         1       0     75
          0    28.71     9.04         0       1     75
          0    36.82    16.38         0       1     75
```

0	32.48	10.52	0	1	75
0	29.43	8.56	1	0	75
0	25.69	5.77	1	1	75
–	–	–	–	–	–
–	–	–	–	–	–
–	–	–	–	–	–

DISCUSSION

A typical linear model used to predict a single outcome is defined by a sum of independent variables, each multiplied by a coefficient. The independent variables can be used exactly as measured. Frequently, however, functions of these variables are incorporated into the model, allowing considerable flexibility in the way potential influences are represented. Various forms of the outcome variable (dependent variable) are also possible. It too can be a function of the sampled observations. A special function of the outcome variable employed in conjunction with a linear model is called a *link function*. A link function creates a linear relationship between the variable or variables under study and the dependent variable. Thus, a specific postulated relationship (model) between risk factors and disease is made linear by the appropriate choice of a link function. Such a model is the logistic model. The link function is the logarithm of the odds associated with the probability of disease.

The logistic model relating k independent risk factors (denoted x_{ij}—risk factor j measured on individual i) to the probability of disease (denoted p_i) is

$$P(\text{disease} \mid x_{i1}, x_{i2}, \ldots, x_{ik}) = p_i = \frac{1}{1 + e^{-(b_0 + b_1 x_{i1} + b_2 x_{i2} + \cdots + b_k x_{ik})}}.$$

The link function $\log[p_i/(1 - p_i)]$ transforms the probability of disease into a linear model where

$$\text{log-odds} = y_i = \log[p_i/(1 - p_i)] = b_0 + b_1 x_{i1} + b_2 x_{i2} + \cdots + b_k x_{ik}.$$

In this context, the outcome variable represented by y_i is called the *logit* or *log-odds* (a.17). This equivalent but transformed model is now linear and is estimated and interpreted, in terms of the log-odds, in much the same way as all linear models.[24]

For the hypertension data, two variables are continuous (age and years worked), one is discrete (SPL), and two are binary (family history and salt consumption). A brief description of these five risk variables is presented in Table 10.1.

Table 10.1. Summary of the Five Risk Factors (Independent Variables)

Continuous data						
Variable	Symbol	Mean	Median	Std. dev.	Minimum	Maximum
sound pressure level	spl	90.8	90.0	8.83	75.0	104.0
age	age	35.5	33.9	8.40	22.0	53.0
years worked	work	16.2	16.3	9.64	5.0	38.4
Discrete data		Yes	No	Total		
salt consumption	salt	554	557	1101		
family history	history	604	497	1101		

The relationship between hypertension and SPL is summarized in Table 10.2 and Figure 10.1. Figure 10.1 shows the proportion of hypertensive women at the seven levels of SPL. The tickmarks indicate the distribution of hypertensive (top) and nonhypertensive (bottom) individuals. The tick marks are *jittered*, which means they are moved slightly from their actual values to min-

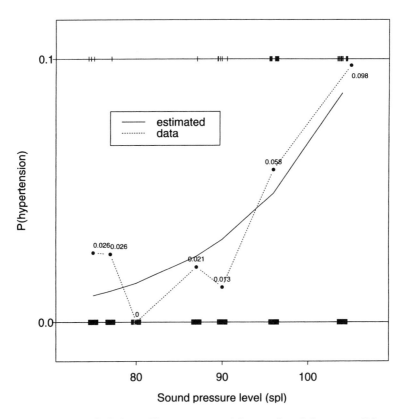

Figure 10.1. The probability of hypertension (observed and theoretical) by sound pressure levels for the Chinese textile factory workers.

imize overlap. Also included is a smooth curve estimated from a logistic relationship between the level of SPL (denoted x) and the probability of hypertension (denoted p_x). Specifically,

$$P(\text{hypertension} \mid x) = \hat{p}_x = \frac{1}{1 + e^{-(\hat{a}+\hat{b}\,x)}} = \frac{1}{1 + e^{-(-10.4+0.077\,x)}}$$

where x represents any sound pressure level. Necessarily, the model in terms of log-odds is

$$\text{log-odds}_x = \hat{a} + \hat{b}x = -10.4 + 0.077x.$$

The estimates of the parameters a and b are based on all 1101 observations in Table 10.2. Note that the model-estimated probabilities of hypertension $\hat{p}_x$ are between 0 and 1 for all levels of SPL, which is a property of the logistic model in general.

The relationship between the risk of hypertension and the five risk factors recorded for each textile factory worker summarized by an additive linear logistic model, in terms of the log-odds, is

$$\text{log-odds}_i = b_0 + b_1\text{spl}_i + b_2\text{age}_i + b_3\text{work}_i + b_4\text{history}_i + b_5\text{salt}_i$$

$i = 1, 2, 3, \ldots, 1101$. As with all regression models, the term *additive* means that the model requires each variable to influence the outcome separately (log-odds), unaffected by the levels of the other independent variables. The form of the independent variables in a logistic model is unrestricted and, to start, they are entered into the estimation process exactly as measured. The modeled relationship allows the estimation of the regression coefficients and their standard errors (Table 10.3).

A notable property of the Beijing textile factory workers is the correlation between age and years worked. Each sampled worker holds essentially the same job for her entire career. Therefore, the correlation between age and years worked is almost collinear (correlation $= 0.966$ since age $- 19 \approx$ years

Table 10.2. Frequency and Proportion of Hypertensive Women by SPL Observed in the Chinese Textile Factory Workers

SPL	75	77	80	87	90	96	104	Total
hypertensive	4	1	0	1	5	17	16	44
nonhypertensive	149	38	23	47	375	277	148	1057
total	153	39	23	48	380	294	164	1101
proportion	0.026	0.026	0.0	0.021	0.013	0.058	0.098	0.04

Table 10.3. The Estimated Regression Coefficients for the Five
Variable Logistic Model

	Coefficient	Estimate	Std. error	z-Value	p-Value
intercept	b_0	−14.718	—	—	—
SPL	b_1	0.056	0.021	2.607	0.009
age	b_2	0.150	0.075	1.999	0.046
years worked	b_3	−0.012	0.064	−0.184	0.854
family history	b_4	0.326	0.329	0.990	0.332
salt consumption	b_5	0.800	0.334	2.394	0.017

residual deviance = 306.186 with degrees of freedom = 1095

worked). Not surprisingly, almost no impact on the goodness-of-fit occurs when either of the two variables is removed from the model. For the full model (all five risk factors), the residual deviance is 306.186 and when years worked is removed, for example, the resulting residual deviance hardly changes. It is 306.219.

The high correlation between age and years worked dramatically affects the precision of the estimated regression coefficients associated with these two nearly collinear variables. The estimated standard error associated with the age coefficient $(\hat{b}_2)$ is 0.075 $(S_{\hat{b}_2})$ with years worked included in the model (Table 10.3). When years worked is not included in the model, the standard error is sharply reduced $(S'_{\hat{b}_2} = 0.025)$. The threefold decrease in variability increases the z-statistic associated with evaluating the influence of age from 1.999 to 5.582. The p-value decreases correspondingly from 0.046 to less than 0.001. However, the price paid for the increased precision is a bias in the estimate of the age/hypertension coefficient. That is, $\hat{b}_2 = 0.150$ when years worked is included in the regression model and $\hat{b}'_2 = 0.137$ when years worked is removed from the model. The difference (0.150 versus 0.137) is the confounding bias incurred by not accounting for the influence of years worked.

When the variable age is removed from the logistic model, the changes in the coefficient associated with years worked is striking. For the full model (all five variables—Table 10.3), the coefficient associated with years worked is $\hat{b}_3 = -0.012$, but when the variable age is removed, the coefficient becomes $\hat{b}'_3 = 0.113$. As with the coefficient associated with age (b_2), there is also a large decease in precision $[S_{\hat{b}_3} = 0.064$ (full model) and $S'_{\hat{b}_3} = 0.025$ (age deleted)]. This considerable difference in estimated coefficients arises from failure to account for the influence of age (−0.012 versus 0.113).

Occasionally, a statistical analysis involves a trade-off between bias and precision. The investigator, by and large, is then forced to choose between two alternatives, a biased estimate with relatively high precision or a less biased estimate with substantially lower precision. In the case of the SPL data, it is probably better to trade a decrease in precision for a less biased estimate, since SPL, not age or years worked, is the focus of the analysis, making the precision of these two regression coefficients less of a concern. The removal of bias is the primary reason age and years worked were measured and included in the model in the first place.

Figure 10.2 displays the relationship between the five risk factors and the log-odds of hypertension (Table 10.3). The jittered tick marks again show the distributions of the observations. The form of the model constrains these relationships to be linear, producing estimates of the separate impact of each variable in terms of a straight line (displayed on the same scale—commensurate).

Goodness-of-fit is always an issue with an estimated model. For a linear logistic model with continuous independent variables, a goodness-of-fit test is not a straightforward comparison of observed to estimated values. The observed outcomes are binary (hypertensive or not), and the values estimated from the logistic model are log-odds or probabilities. The observed binary data are not estimated directly by the logistic model, ensuring a lack of correspondence between the observed and expected values regardless of the fit of the model.

To produce a Pearson-like chi-square goodness-of-fit analysis, the estimated logistic model is used to create a somewhat artificial table. Once the table is constructed, observed cell frequencies are compared directly to frequencies based on model estimates. The degree of correspondence is then evaluated with a chi-square statistic in the usual way.

To create a goodness-of-fit table, first probabilities of hypertension are estimated from the logistic model using each participant's five measured risk factors, producing 1101 estimated $\hat{p}_i$-values, one for each study subject. These estimated individual probabilities $\hat{p}_i$ of hypertension are then classified into 10 categories defined by percentiles. The 10% of the individuals with the lowest estimated probabilities form the first category, the next lowest 10% form the second category, and so forth until the last category makes up the 10% of individuals with the highest probabilities. These 10 categories are called *deciles of risk*. For most data sets, the deciles of risk will not contain exactly 10% of the observations. However, the table is constructed so that each decile contains 10% or as close as possible to 10% of the data. Ten mean probabilities (denoted $\bar{p}_k$) are then calculated, one for each decile category. In symbols, for the kth decile, the mean probability of hypertension is

$$\bar{p}_k = \frac{1}{n_k} \sum \hat{p}_j \quad j = 1, 2, 3, \ldots, n_k$$

where $n_k \approx n/10$ and $k = 1, 2, 3, \ldots, 10$.

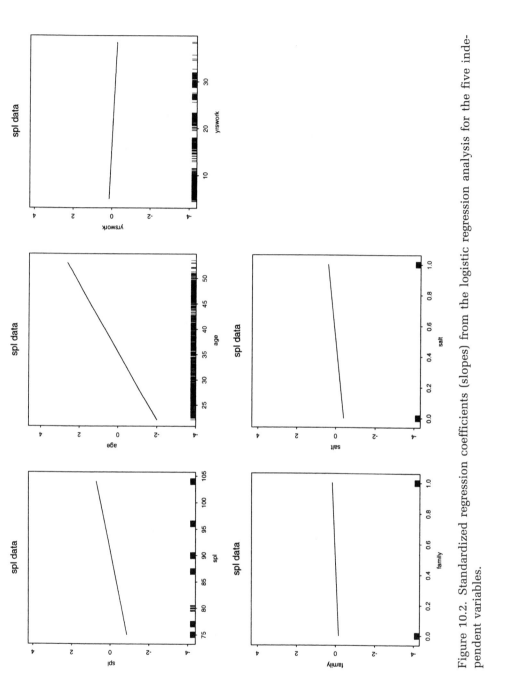

Figure 10.2. Standardized regression coefficients (slopes) from the logistic regression analysis for the five independent variables.

For the textile factory workers, these 10 estimated mean probabilities are given in Table 10.4 (column 3). Furthermore, these probabilities allow 20 model-generated expected frequencies to be calculated. For the kth decile, $n_k \bar{p}_k$ cases and $n_k(1 - \bar{p}_k)$ non-cases are expected based on the estimated model. For example, the eighth decile yields $\bar{p}_8 = 0.052$ and the expected number of cases of hypertension is $n_8 \bar{p}_8 = 0.052(110) = 5.74$, and non-cases is $n_8(1 - \bar{p}_8) = 0.948(110) = 104.26$ since $n_8 = 110$. The corresponding observed values are 5 and 105, respectively. These model-generated expected values (e_k) are compared to the observed values (o_k) tabulated into the same deciles, producing 20 comparisons (Table 10.4) reflecting the goodness-of-fit of the logistic model.

Using a Pearson chi-square analysis (a.5), the goodness-of-fit test statistic for the textile factory workers data is $X^2 = \sum (o_k - e_k)^2 / e_k = 11.780$. The observed X^2-value has a chi-square distribution with eight degrees of freedom when the model is correct. "Correct" means that the only reason the observed counts differ from the expected counts is random variation. The justification of the degrees of freedom is not simple or intuitive, and the explanation is left to more advanced descriptions of the logistic model goodness-of-fit procedure.[23] The p-value is $P(X^2 \geq 11.780 \mid \text{model is correct}) = 0.19$. A p-value in the neighborhood of 0.2 provides no strong evidence that the linear logistic model based on the additive influences of five risk factors is an adequate or inadequate description of the risk–hypertension relationship.

The implementation of the decile of risk approach to assessing the goodness-of-fit is of concern for several reasons. First, classifying a large number of estimates ($\hat{p}_i$) into 10 categories incurs some loss of information, with an associated loss in statistical efficiency. Second, the chi-square test is based on an approximation that works least well when the cell frequencies are small. Small cell frequencies are the rule, not the exception, when data are distrib-

Table 10.4. The Components of the Goodness-of-Fit Procedure for the
Textile Factory Workers' Data

Decile	n_k	Cases			Non-cases		
		$\bar{p}_k$	e_k	o_k	$1 - \bar{p}_k$	e_k	o_k
1	111	0.002	0.25	1	0.998	110.75	110
2	110	0.004	0.46	0	0.996	109.54	110
3	110	0.006	0.68	0	0.994	109.32	110
4	110	0.009	0.97	0	0.991	109.03	110
5	110	0.013	1.44	0	0.987	108.56	110
6	110	0.020	2.17	4	0.980	107.83	106
7	110	0.031	3.44	3	0.969	106.56	107
8	110	0.052	5.74	5	0.948	104.26	105
9	110	0.089	9.81	15	0.911	100.19	95
10	110	0.173	19.06	16	0.827	90.94	94

uted into deciles based on logistic model estimates. Third, small, inconsequential changes in the estimated parameters lead to small changes in the expected values but can produce substantial changes in the values observed in the table (i.e., the o_i-values). That is, slightly redefining the decile bounds can shift (sometimes consequentially) the number of observed values found in the newly defined categories. These shifts occasionally cause disproportionate changes in the contributions to the chi-square statistic, particularly when the affected categories contain small numbers of observations. Finally, the Pearson-like approach to goodness-of-fit does not produce a rigorous comparison of nested models since a simple model can produce a chi-square statistic that is smaller than that of a more complex model. If independent variables are deleted from the regression equation, the model always fits the data less well and comparison of the residual deviances always reflect this fact. However, the chi-square statistic from the decile-of-risk approach can increase when a variable or variables are deleted from the model, making a comparison between models not very intuitive. Certainly no rigorous interpretation is possible.

The primary purpose in applying a logistic model to the Chinese textile factory workers' data is to estimate the impact of SPL on the likelihood of hypertensive disease. The model based on the SPL measurements only (Table 10.2) allows estimation of this impact in terms of a regression coefficient ($\hat{b} = 0.077$). The second analysis based on the same SPL measurements but including four other possibly relevant variables (age, years worked, salt, and history) gives the estimate $\hat{b}_1 = 0.056$ (Table 10.3). The difference is the confounding bias incurred by ignoring these four relevant risk factors. It is to avoid this bias that the additional four variables were measured and included in the analysis.

Parallel to the coefficients from multivariable linear regression models in general, the coefficients from a linear logistic equation measure the amount of change in the independent variable for each unit increase in a specific dependent variable. That is, a one unit increase in the ith explanatory variable yields a b_i-unit change in the log-odds. The estimated coefficient associated with SPL is $\hat{b}_1 = 0.056$. A one unit increase in SPL then increases the log-odds an estimated 0.056 while accounting for the influence of the other four variables in the regression equation (held constant). An increase of 0.056 in terms of the log-odds translates into an increase in the odds by a factor of $e^{0.056} = 1.057$ per unit increase in SPL, also reflecting the influence of noise on the risk of hypertension. That is, the odds ratio associated with a one unit increase is $\hat{or} = 1.057$. Furthermore, for example, an increase of 20 units in SPL produces an estimated $(1.056)^{20} = 3.060$-fold increase in the odds measuring the risk of hypertension (i.e., $\hat{or}_{20} = 3.060$). For an additive model, the impact on risk measured by an odds ratio is multiplicative (a.17). This logistic model–estimated odds ratio is frequently called an *adjusted odds ratio* since it is adjusted for the other variables in the additive regression equation.

The logistic model described in Table 10.3 and Figure 10.2 dictates a linear relationship between each of the five independent variables and the log-odds associated with the risk of hypertension. No reason exists to assume that SPL, age, and years worked are so simply related to the log-odds.

A model allowing a nonlinear relationship between risk factors and a binary outcome is directly implemented. Using polynomial expressions to describe the influence of the continuous independent variables, the logistic model becomes

$$\text{log-odds}_i = a_0 + P(\text{spl}_i) + P(\text{age}_i) + P(\text{work}_i) + a_1\text{history}_i + a_2\text{salt}_i$$

and when a third-degree polynomial representation is chosen,

$$P(x) = ax + bx^2 + cx^3.$$

The nine individual estimated polynomial coefficients from this more complex but additive model are not easily interpreted but are not generally of great importance. The focus is not on each coefficient but on the entire polynomial, defined by three estimated coefficients. A three-term polynomial, then, serves as a description of the influence of the independent variable on the risk of hypertension. Using a polynomial function $P(x)$ rather than a linear term x adds flexibility to the description of the independent variable, better characterizing the relationship between each risk factor and the outcome. The patterns of influence are not constrained to be simply (perhaps simplistically) a straight line. These patterns are graphically displayed in Figure 10.3 for SPL, age, years worked, family history, and salt consumption, each adjusted for the presence of the other four variables in the regression equation. The family history and salt consumption variables consist of two points (always linear). The other three plots show separate and possibly nonlinear estimated influences on the log-odds.

Two choices exist with regard to these nonlinear descriptions of the risk factors; the relationship is essentially linear, and the apparent nonlinearity results from capitalizing on the inherently random variation of the observations or the relationship has an important nonlinear impact on risk. To compare these two possibilities formally, a model containing all three nonlinear influences (third-degree polynomials) is compared to models with a strictly linear influence assigned to each dependent variable ($P(x)$ versus x). The results are summarized in Table 10.5.

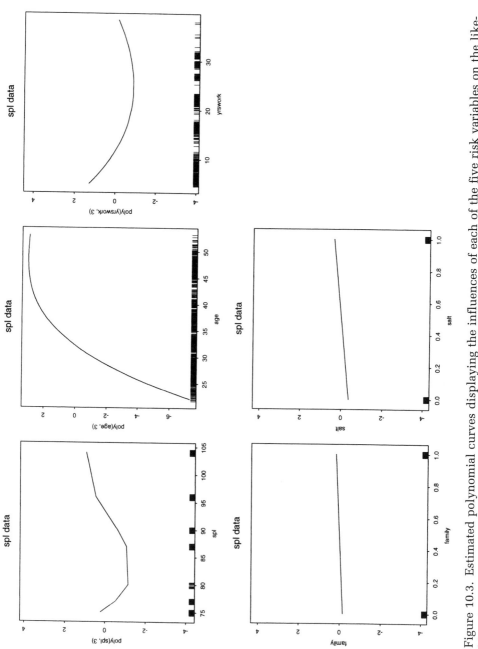

Figure 10.3. Estimated polynomial curves displaying the influences of each of the five risk variables on the likelihood of hypertension.

Table 10.5. Comparison of a Polynomial Representation to a Linear
Representation for Each Continuous Risk Factor

Model	Residual deviance	Degrees of freedom	Difference	p-Value
$P(spl) + P(age) + P(work)$*	293.175	1089	—	—
$P(work)$ replaced by $work$	294.722	1091	1.597	0.461
$P(age)$ replaced by age	298.764	1091	5.589	0.061
$P(spl)$ replaced by spl	299.641	1091	6.466	0.039

*Full five-variable model (including salt and history variables).

No convincing evidence (p-value = 0.46) of a nonlinear association with years worked emerges from the textile factory workers' data. However, some evidence exists that the risk associated with the worker's age (p-value = 0.06) increases sharply until the age of 35 or 40, then this factor has relatively little additional impact on the risk of hypertension. The representation of SPL as a nonlinear influence on the risk of hypertension also appears valuable (supported by the data—p-value = 0.04). As noise exposure increases, initially risk decreases at the lower exposure levels and then increases for SPL exposures greater than 85. The statistical analysis (Table 10.5) provides evidence that the observed pattern is not a likely result of random variation but likely represents a systematic nonlinear relationship.

Generalized Additive Model

A generalized additive model allows an unconstrained picture of the relationship between an independent variable and the outcome under study. In symbols, a generalized additive model is represented as

$$f(y_i) = a + s_1(x_{i1}) + s_2(x_{i2}) + s_3(x_{i3}) + \cdots + s_k(x_{ik})$$

where f represents a function of the dependent variable and the functions s_1, s_2, s_3, . . . s_k characterize the impact of the k independent variables. For the hypertension data, the function $f(y)$ is the logarithm of the odds associated with the probability of hypertension, and the functions s_1(spl), s_2(age) and s_3(years worked) can have any form and are estimated nonparametrically. Like the coefficients estimated as part of the previous parametric regression analysis, these estimated functions are adjusted for any confounding influences of the other variables in the additive model. The resulting estimated curves indicate the independent strength as well as the pattern of influence on the probability of hypertension associated exclusively with each risk variable.

Figure 10.4 shows five estimated functions using the hypertension data along with their approximate 95% confidence regions (dotted lines). That is, the estimated curves result from applying the model

$$\text{log-odds}_i = a_0 + s_1(\text{spl}_i) + s_2(\text{age}_i) + s_3(\text{years worked}_i) + a_1\text{history}_i + a_2\text{salt}_i$$

where the variables history and salt are binary, necessarily producing straight lines (as before). The functions s_1, s_2, and s_3 are defined by the estimation process and not by an a priori decision to use a specific parametric description. The first three plots in Figure 10.4 display the estimated functions $\hat{s}_1(\text{spl})$, $\hat{s}_2(\text{age})$, and $\hat{s}_3(\text{years worked})$. These functions are totally unconstrained since no requirements are necessary and no assumptions are made to produce the estimated curves (nonparametric estimates). The basic result is a graphic characterization of the additive relationship between each of the three continuous risk factors determined entirely from the data.

Also shown in Figure 10.4 are the associated 95% confidence bands, which help to sort out the important properties of each curve. For example, the curve estimating the adjusted influence of SPL on the risk of hypertension initially decreases and then increases as noise exposure increases. The broad confidence band for SPL where exposure is less than 85 indicates that the initial decrease, in light of random variation, is likely due to chance fluctuations but the subsequent increase is not.

The results obtained from applying a generalized additive model are not strikingly different from those obtained with the previous polynomial model (Figures 10.3 and 10.4 are similar). This similarity is not uncommon since it is rare that the adjusted relationship between a dependent and an independent variable is so complicated that a third-degree polynomial does not adequately characterize the risk factor influence. A distinct advantage of a polynomial model is that the usual regression tools apply (for example, relatively simple theory, easy estimation, and direct evaluation of goodness-of-fit measures). Nevertheless, the fact remains that the estimated response curves are flexible but constrained parametric functions.

CONCLUSIONS

A multivariable linear logistic model indicates that sound exposure is associated with the risk of hypertension. After adjusting for the possible confounding influences of worker's age, years worked, family history, and consumption of salt, an important relationship between SPL level and the risk of hypertension (p-value = 0.01) emerges from the logistic analysis. The logistic model, furthermore, adequately fits the data (p-value = 0.19), ensuring that the model-

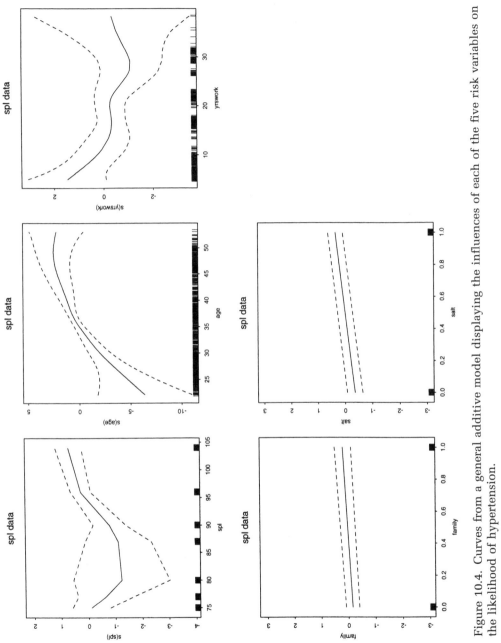

Figure 10.4. Curves from a general additive model displaying the influences of each of the five risk variables on the likelihood of hypertension.

based estimates usefully reflect risk. Additionally, a polynomial representation of the risk variables and a generalized additive model both indicate a similar but somewhat complicated and nonlinear relationship between SPL and the probability of hypertension. Low levels of exposure to noise (<85) appears to have little influence on the risk of hypertension, but higher levels of exposure (>85) produce a continuously increasing (linear) risk.

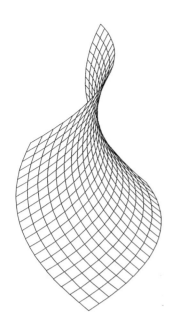

CHAPTER 11

Poisson Regression

PART I: STANDARDIZED MORTALITY RATIO

OBJECTIVE

To describe and compare the incidence of brain cancer in males and females, adjusted for the differences in the age distributions in the populations at risk.

DATA

Counts of brain cancer incidence cases and deaths were recorded as part of the Surveillance, Epidemiology, and End Results (SEER) program of the Biometry Branch of the National Cancer Institute. The SEER program acquired these incidence data from a number of surveyed areas in the United States (for example, the state of Connecticut, the city of Detroit, the state of New Mexico, and the San Francisco Bay Area). The brain cancer incidence cases and deaths were extracted from the SEER public use data for the 10 years 1985–1994 for all participating regions. Using these data, white incidence cases were selected and tabulated by gender and age (age intervals: 20 to 24 years, 25 to 29 years, 30 to 34 years, . . . , 80 to 84 years, more than 84 years). Additionally, the corresponding populations at risk were abstracted from the

SEER public use data, although the population counts originated primarily from the U.S. Census Bureau (1980 and 1990 enumerations). A total of 10,290 brain cancer incidence cases and deaths (males = 5706 and females = 4584) among 166,845,887 individuals at risk (males = 79,837,339 and females = 87,008,548) constitute the data set.

METHODS

Age-specific male and female brain cancer rates are summarized (model-free) using a standardized mortality ratio (SMR). Several other summary measures (weighted averages) of male–female differences are included. Results from a Poisson regression model employing age and gender as independent variables and the incidence rate of brain cancer as the dependent variable also describe the differences in risk between males and females while accounting for the influence of age.

Data type: incidence (cancer registry data)
Reference: SEER public use CD-ROM, U.S. National Cancer Institute

The variables are:

1. Age: as reported
2. Males cases: total number of cases reported from the SEER registry areas
3. Male population: total number of males at risk
4. Females cases: total number of cases reported from the SEER registry areas
5. Female population: total number of females at risk

The data file of 10,290 brain cancer cases tabulated into 14 five-year intervals is:

file name = brain.11.data

age	cases	males	cases	females
22.5	171	9202281	119	9049308
27.5	246	10204890	194	10265782
32.5	311	10596792	221	10817611
37.5	382	9798299	246	10071814
42.5	392	8471103	250	8797612
47.5	408	6611810	266	6825401
52.5	457	5218038	306	5489507
57.5	524	4594087	350	4984449
62.5	638	4346666	434	4929845
67.5	688	3869926	598	4705980
72.5	664	2971500	618	3937866
77.5	455	2051681	501	3096491
82.5	244	1148149	305	2111118
92.5	126	752117	176	1925764

age = midpoint of the five year age interval

DISCUSSION

Differences in the incidence of brain cancer between males and females are best identified by comparing the age-specific rates for five-year or perhaps ten-year age intervals. Comparisons of age-specific rates are essentially unaffected by the small differences in age distributions that occur between compared age-specific categories. This property is a central reason for calculating an age-specific rate. It is occasionally desirable, however, to summarize disease or mortality rates using a single value in order to compare the general risk among a series of groups equalized for differences in age distributions. A standardized mortality ratio is one such age-adjusted summary measure.[28] It is created by dividing an observed number of cases of disease or deaths by an expected number calculated from the rates of a reference population. This single statistic is designed to summarize differences in risk between populations while effectively accounting for differences in age distributions.

The data necessary to calculate the SMR to compare male and female brain cancer incidence rates are given in Table 11.1. Figure 11.1 is a plot of the age-specific rates (dotted lines).

An age-specific incidence rate* from a specific population at risk (denoted pop) for the ith age interval is the number of cases of disease $d_i^{(pop)}$ divided by the number of individuals at risk $p_i^{(pop)}$ times an arbitrary base or

$$\text{age-specific rate} = r_i^{(pop)} = \frac{d_i^{(pop)}}{p_i^{(pop)}} \times \text{base}.$$

For example, the brain cancer age-specific incidence rate in females (pop = female) for the five year age interval 60 to 64 ($i = 60$) is the number of cases $d_{60}^{(females)} = 434$ divided by the population at risk $p_{60}^{(females)} = 4,929,845$ or

$$\text{age-specific rate} = r_{60}^{(females)} = \frac{434}{4,929,845} \times 100,000 = 8.804$$

cases per 100,000 persons at risk (Table 11.1).

An expected number of cases in a specific age group is found by applying the age-specific rate from a reference population to the corresponding age-specific population count in the comparison group. A reference population

---

*The quantity called a *rate* is technically a proportion or an estimated probability, not a true rate. The differences between an estimated probability and a rate is usually unimportant in the study of human disease, particularly when ratios of rates are considered. It might also be argued that for the SEER data the rate is not a true incidence rate since deaths are also included in the count of new cases.

Table 11.1. Brain Cancer Incident Rates per 100,000 and Rate Ratios
(Male to Female)

Age	Males			Females			Ratio
	Cases	Population	Rate*	Cases	Population	Rate*	
20–24	171	9,202,281	1.9	119	9,049,308	1.3	1.413
25–29	246	10,204,890	2.4	194	10,265,782	1.9	1.276
30–34	311	10,596,792	2.9	221	10,817,611	2.0	1.437
35–39	382	9,798,299	3.9	246	10,071,814	2.4	1.596
40–44	392	8,471,103	4.6	250	8,797,612	2.8	1.628
45–49	408	6,611,810	6.2	266	6,825,401	3.9	1.583
50–54	457	5,218,038	8.8	306	5,489,507	5.6	1.571
55–59	524	4,594,087	11.4	350	4,984,449	7.0	1.624
60–64	638	4,346,666	14.7	434	4,929,845	8.8	1.667
65–69	688	3,869,926	17.8	598	4,705,980	12.7	1.399
70–74	664	2,971,500	22.3	618	3,937,866	15.7	1.424
75–79	455	2,051,681	22.2	501	3,096,491	16.2	1.371
80–84	244	1,148,149	21.3	305	2,111,118	14.4	1.471
≥85	126	752,117	16.8	176	1,925,764	9.1	1.833
total	5706	79,837,339	7.1	4584	87,008,548	5.3	1.357

*Incidence rate per 100,000 persons at risk.

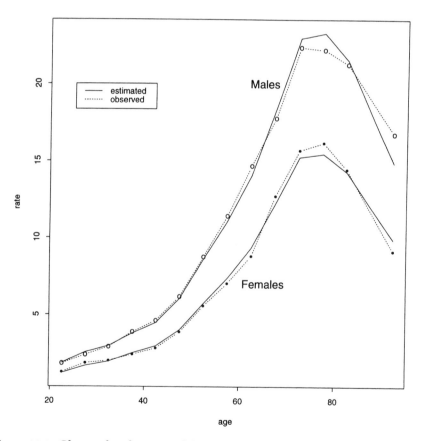

Figure 11.1. Observed and estimated (Poisson model) brain cancer incidence rates
by age for males and females.

can be an external population such as the U.S. 1970 population or an internal population such as the female population from Table 11.1 (column 6). For the brain cancer incidence data, the female population is selected as the reference group. Applying the female age-specific rates to the male age-specific population counts creates an expected number of cases in each age category (denoted e_i) as if the males had exactly the same age-specific rates observed in the female population. In symbols, the expected number of cases in the ith age category is

$$e_i = r_i^{(\text{reference})} p_i^{(\text{comparison})}$$

where $r_i^{(\text{reference})}$ represents the age-specific rate in the ith age category from the reference population (for example, the female population) and $p_i^{(\text{comparison})}$ represents the corresponding age-specific population count from the selected comparison group (for example, the male population). For example, $r_{60}^{(\text{females})} = 8.804$ cases per 100,000 at risk and $p_{60}^{(\text{males})} = 4,346,666$, so the expected number of male brain cancer cases in the age interval 60–64 is

$$e_{60} = r_{60}^{(\text{females})} p_{60}^{(\text{males})} = (0.0000880)(4,346,666) = 382.660$$

if the male rate for the age interval 60–64 was identical to the observed female age-specific rate. The observed number of cases is $d_{60}^{(\text{males})} = 6.38$.

The SMR is

$$\text{standardized mortality ratio} = \text{SMR} = \frac{\sum d_i^{(\text{comparison})}}{\sum e_i}$$

where $\sum d_i^{(\text{comparison})}$ is the total number of cases in the comparison group and $\sum e_i$ is the total number of expected cases generated using the reference population rates. Specifically, $\sum d_i^{(\text{males})} = 5706$ is the total number of male brain cancer cases ($i = 20, 25, 30, \ldots, 85$). The total expected number of brain cancer cases calculated as if the age-specific male rates were identical to those of the females is $\sum e_i = 3788.853$, giving an SMR = 5706/3788.853 = 1.506. An SMR of 1.506 indicates that the male brain cancer rate is, on average, about 1.5 times the female rate. This summary is adjusted for age distribution differences since the expected and observed numbers of deaths are derived from the same age-specific counts, namely, the male age-specific population counts (Table 11.1).

If the age-specific rates in the comparison population are almost identical to those in the reference population, then the SMR will be in the neighborhood of 1.0 regardless of differences in the respective age distributions. Values differing from 1.0 indicate differences in risk between the compared populations not associated with age.

A not so obvious property of an SMR is the requirement that the under-lying age-specific rates in the comparison population must be a constant mul-tiple of the underlying age-specific rates in the reference population for all compared ages. In terms of the brain cancer data, this requirement means that each observed age-specific ratio of male to female incidence rates (Table 11.1—last column) estimates the same underlying rate ratio for all 14 age groups. Such rate ratios are said to be *homogeneous*.[29]

For a single summary SMR to describe usefully a series of age-specific rate ratios, the rate ratios must be homogeneous. Otherwise, it would be nec-essary to summarize the differences between compared groups with more than a single value. Therefore, the brain cancer SMR of 1.506 estimates the single underlying ratio of male to female incidence rates only when the observed variability among the rate ratios is unrelated to age (homogeneous). If specific age groups exist with substantially different rate ratios, a single

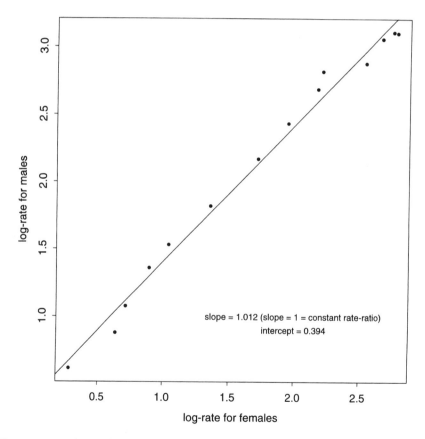

Figure 11.2. Observed brain cancer incidence rates: logarithm of the female rates plotted against the logarithm of the male rates.

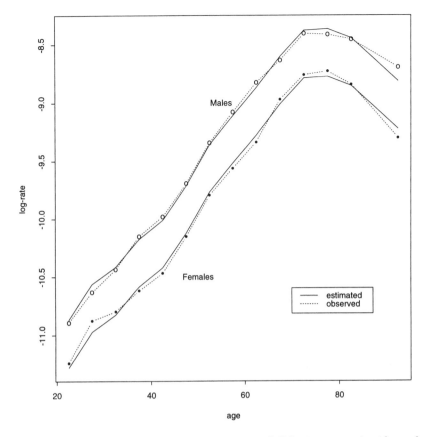

Figure 11.3. Observed and estimated (Poisson model) brain cancer incidence log-rates by age for males and females.

SMR is likely to be misleading. In general, a single value is a poor summary of heterogeneous rates, ratios, or almost any set of heterogeneous statistical measures.

The logarithms of the female brain cancer age-specific incidence rates are plotted against male age-specific log-rates in Figure 11.2. Approximately constant rate ratios yield an approximately straight line with a slope approximately equal to 1.0. In addition, for rate ratios that are nearly homogeneous with respect to age, a plot of the male and female log-rates by age will result in nearly parallel lines (Figure 11.3—dotted line). The geometry of both plots visually supports the utility of an SMR as a single summary of a common underlying difference in the risk of brain cancer between males and females.

An SMR is a traditional summary, but it is not the only way to estimate a common rate ratio. If $R_i = r_i^{(males)}/r_i^{(females)}$ represents an estimated age-specific rate ratio for the ith age group, then an estimate of the common rate ratio (denoted R) is found using a weighted average much like the weighted average described in conjunction with estimating a common odds ratio or relative risk from a series of 2 by 2 tables. A summary estimate is created by forming a weighted average of the logarithms of the rate ratios where the weights are again the reciprocal values of the estimated variances. Specifically, a weighted average of the logarithms of the rate ratios combined over k age-specific categories is

$$\overline{\log (R)} = \frac{\sum w_i \log (R_i)}{\sum w_i}$$

and

$$\text{variance of } \overline{\log (R)} = S^2_{\overline{\log (R)}} = \frac{1}{\sum w_i} \quad i = 1, 2, 3, \ldots, k$$

where $w_i = 1/S^2_{\log (R_i)}$ (a.12). An estimate of the variance of the logarithm of an estimated age-specific rate ratio is (a.10)

$$S^2_{\log (R_i)} = \frac{1}{d_i^{(\text{males})}} + \frac{1}{d_i^{(\text{females})}}.$$

For the brain cancer data, $\overline{\log (R)} = 0.408$, giving an estimate of R as $\overline{R} = e^{0.408} = 1.505$. An approximate 95% confidence interval based on $\overline{\log (R)}$ is

$$0.408 \pm 1.960(0.020) \quad \text{or} \quad (0.369, 0.448)$$

where $S_{\overline{\log (R)}} = \sqrt{1/\sum w_i} = \sqrt{1/2509.991} = 0.020$ (a.12). Following the usual pattern, an approximate 95% confidence interval for the underlying rate ratio R is

$$(e^{\text{lower bound}}, e^{\text{upper bound}}) = (e^{0.369}, e^{0.448}) = (1.447, 1.564).$$

Averaging the logarithms of the rate ratios rather than averaging the rate ratios themselves corrects (to a large extent) for the lack of symmetry typically associated with a distribution of age-specific rate ratios. In general, an approximately symmetric distribution yields summary values with distributions that are accurately approximated by a normal distribution, even for small samples of data. The normal distribution is then typically used to construct approximate statistical tests and confidence intervals (adding and subtracting a multiple of the standard error). Using log-rates also prevents meaningless negative values of the lower limit of the confidence interval for the underlying rate ratio.

A number of other approaches exist to estimate the common underlying rate ratio (SMR-like summaries). Based on the 14 observed age-specific brain cancer rate ratios $R_1, R_2, R_3, \ldots R_k$ (k = the total number of age categories = 14) given in Table 11.1 (last column), four examples are:

1. the mean estimated rate ratio $= \dfrac{1}{k}\sum R_i = 1.521$

2. the ratio of estimated mean rates $= \dfrac{\bar{R}_{\text{males}}}{\bar{R}_{\text{females}}} = \dfrac{\sum r_i^{(\text{males})}}{\sum r_i^{(\text{females})}} = 1.510$

3. the least squares estimated rate ratio $= \dfrac{\sum r_i^{(\text{females})} r_i^{(\text{males})}}{\sum [r_i^{(\text{females})}]^2} = 1.479$

4. a line based on the 14 pairs of log-rates $x_i = \log - r_i^{(\text{females})}$ and $y_i = \log - r_i^{(\text{males})}$ that allows the estimated rate ratio $= e^{\text{intercept}} = e^{0.394} = 1.483$ (Figure 11.2: intercept = 0.394 and slope = 1.012).

The estimated common rate ratios 1, 2, and 3 are different weighted averages of the age-specific rate ratios; that is,

$$\text{mean ratio} = \frac{\sum w_i R_i}{\sum w_i} = \frac{\sum w_i [r_i^{(\text{males})}/r_i^{(\text{females})}]}{\sum w_i} \quad i = 1, 2, 3, \ldots, k.$$

For case 1, the weights are $w_i = 1$; for case 2, the weights are $w_i = r_i^{(\text{females})}$; and for case 3, the weights are $w_i = [r_i^{(\text{females})}]^2$. In fact, the brain cancer SMR (1.506) is also a weighted average of rate ratios where the weights are the expected values in each age category, $w_i = e_i$.

Poisson Model

A Poisson model postulates that the collected data conform to two requirements: the logarithm of the rate (link function) is a linear function of risk factors, and the number of cases of disease or deaths recorded in each age category has at least an approximate Poisson distribution. For the brain cancer data, an additive Poisson model for an incidence rate in the ith age category is

$$\log(r_{ij}) = a + bg_j + c_1 y_{i1} + c_2 y_{i2} + c_3 y_{i3} + \cdots + c_{13} y_{i,13}$$

where g_j indicates gender (male: $g_j = 1$ and female: $g_j = 0$) and the y_{ij}-values are 13 components of a design variable representing the 14 age categories. A person's age is a known factor in the risk of brain cancer and is typically of little interest. The primary purpose of the rather complex and somewhat awkward 13-level design variable is to account for the impact of age on the risk of brain cancer so that the role of gender can be accurately assessed. The plot of the observed log-rates (Figure 11.3—dotted lines) shows two more or less parallel curves. The design variable in the Poisson model captures the shape of these two curves. The b-coefficient then measures the constant distance between the two curves.

The brain cancer data in Table 11.1 allow the estimation of the 15 model parameters (Table 11.2). Two key features to this Poisson model are as follows:

1. It provides a statistical evaluation of the conjecture that the male-to-female rate ratios are independent of age (homogeneous).
2. If the rates are homogeneous, it provides a single estimate of the influence of gender on the risk of brain cancer accounting for differences in the male/ female age distributions.

As usual, the residual deviance value reflects the goodness-of-fit. The observed residual deviance = 17.345 has an approximate chi-square distribution with 13 degrees of freedom when the model accurately represents the underlying relationships between the incidence of brain cancer and the two risk variables, age and gender. The degrees of freedom are the total number of observed age-specific rates (28) minus the number of parameters necessary to define the model (15) or $28 - 15 = 13$. The p-value associated with the goodness-of-fit is $P(X^2 \geq 17.345 \mid b = \text{constant}) = 0.18$. A probable (not extreme) residual deviance value based on millions of observations supports

Table 11.2. The Estimated Parameters from the Brain Cancer Additive Poisson Model

	Parameter	Estimate	Std. Error
intercept	a	−11.277	—
gender	b	0.409	0.020
25–29	c_1	0.304	0.076
30–34	c_2	0.451	0.073
35–39	c_3	0.692	0.071
40–44	c_4	0.856	0.071
45–49	c_5	1.154	0.070
50–54	c_6	1.507	0.069
55–59	c_7	1.758	0.068
60–64	c_8	1.999	0.066
65–69	c_9	2.266	0.065
70–74	c_{10}	2.488	0.065
75–79	c_{11}	2.502	0.067
80–84	c_{12}	2.424	0.073
≥85	c_{13}	2.054	0.082

Residual deviance = 17.345 with degrees of freedom = 13.

the usefulness of the model in representing the data, particularly the conjecture that the rate ratios are constant. Figures 11.1 and 11.3 show the geometry of the the Poisson model estimated values log $(\hat{r}_i)$ and $\hat{r}_i$ for males and females plotted for each age category (solid line). The log-rates form exactly parallel lines, as required by the additive model. Assessed visually, comparison of the plots of the observed and expected rates confirms an unimportant and nonsystematic lack of fit.

The Poisson model and estimated coefficients (Table 11.2) provide 28 estimated log-rates and, therefore, estimates of the number of cases in the 28 age categories. For example, the males ages 60–64,

$$\log[r_{60}^{(males)}] = \hat{a} + \hat{b} + \hat{c}_8 = -11.277 + 0.409 + 1.999 = -8.869.$$

The estimated age-specific male rate is then

$$r_{60}^{(males)} = e^{-8.869} = 0.000141 \quad \text{or} \quad 14.1 \text{ per } 100,000.$$

Also, for females ages 60–64,

$$\log[r_{60}^{(females)}] = \hat{a} + \hat{c}_8 = -11.277 + 1.999 = -9.278$$

and the estimated age-specific female rate is

$$r_{60}^{(females)} = e^{-9.278} = 0.000093 \quad \text{or} \quad 9.3 \text{ per } 100,000.$$

The estimated rate ratio from these model-generated estimates for the age group 60–64 is

$$\hat{R}_{60} = \frac{\hat{r}_{60}^{(males)}}{\hat{r}_{60}^{(females)}} = \frac{0.000141}{0.000093} = 1.505 = \hat{R}$$

and is necessarily the same for all age groups. The model-estimated rates are, of course, perfectly homogeneous. Using the model-derived rate estimates, the expected number of cases among males ages 60–64 is $0.000141(4,346,666) = 611.3$ (observed $= 638$) and among females it is $0.000093(4,929,845) = 460.7$ (observed $= 434$). Comparing these observed and expected numbers and the 27 other observed (o_i) and expected number of cases (e_i) for all 28 age categories creates another evaluation of the goodness-of-fit (Table 11.3). The Pearson goodness-of-fit chi-square statistic is

$$X^2 = \sum \left[\frac{(o_i - e_i)^2}{e_i} \right] = \frac{(171 - 175.4)^2}{175.4} + \cdots + \frac{(176 - 190.2)^2}{190.2} = 17.393.$$

Table 11.3. Brain Cancer Incident Rates per 100,000 and Rate Ratios
(Male to Female) Estimated from an Additive Poisson Model (b = Constant)

Age	Males			Females			Ratio
	Cases	Population	Rate*	Cases	Population	Rate*	
20–24	175.4	9,202,281	1.9	114.6	9,049,308	1.3	1.505
25–29	263.7	10,204,890	2.6	176.3	10,265,782	1.7	1.505
30–34	317.0	10,596,792	3.0	215.0	10,817,611	2.0	1.505
35–39	373.1	9,798,299	3.8	254.9	10,071,814	2.5	1.505
40–44	379.8	8,471,103	4.5	262.2	8,797,612	3.0	1.505
45–49	399.8	6,611,810	6.0	274.2	6,825,401	4.0	1.505
50–54	449.1	5,218,038	8.6	313.9	5,489,507	5.7	1.505
55–59	507.8	4,594,087	11.1	366.2	4,984,449	7.3	1.505
60–64	611.3	4,346,666	14.1	460.7	4,929,845	9.3	1.505
65–69	711.2	3,869,926	18.4	574.8	4,705,980	12.2	1.505
70–74	681.7	2,971,500	22.9	600.3	3,937,866	15.2	1.505
75–79	477.3	2,051,681	23.3	478.7	3,096,491	15.5	1.505
80–84	247.1	1,148,149	21.5	301.9	2,111,118	14.3	1.505
≥85	111.8	752,117	14.9	190.2	1,925,764	9.9	1.505
total	5706	79,837,339	7.1	4584	87,008,548	5.3	1.357

*Poisson model estimated rate per 100,000 persons at risk.

The Pearson test statistic, once again, summarizes the 28 differences between the observed (Table 11.1) and expected values (Table 11.3) and has a chi-square distribution with 13 degrees of freedom when the observed number of cases differs only by chance from the model-generated number of cases. The direct comparison gives essentially the same chi-square statistic as the residual deviance calculated from the Poisson model (17.393 versus 17.345). The two approaches to evaluating goodness-of-fit typically yield similar results, as already mentioned.

Assessing the goodness-of-fit of the additive Poisson model applied to the brain cancer rates involves primarily an evaluation of the conjecture that the rate ratio is constant. The highly flexible 13-level design variable accurately accounts for the influence of age. The additive model focuses on the parameter b because it independently measures the role of gender when, like the SMR, a single value accurately summarizes the rate ratios from all age categories (homogeneous). That is, the model dictates

$$\text{difference in logarithms of rates} = [\text{log-rate}^{(\text{males})}] - [\text{log-rate}^{(\text{females})}]$$

$$= \log [\hat{r}_i^{(\text{males})}] - \log [\hat{r}_i^{(\text{females})}]$$

$$= [\hat{a} + \hat{b} + \hat{c}_i] - [\hat{a} + \hat{c}_i]$$

$$= \hat{b} = 0.409$$

which yields, as before,

$$\hat{R} = \frac{\hat{r}_i^{(\text{males})}}{\hat{r}_i^{(\text{females})}} = e^{\hat{b}} = e^{0.409} = 1.505$$

for all 14 age categories (Table 11.3 and Figure 11.3).

For the brain cancer data, the model-based estimated summary rate ratio hardly differs from the previous nonmodel estimates. Additionally, the standard error of 0.020, which is a product of the estimation process, is also essentially the same as the value derived as part of the weighted average estimated common rate ratio ($\bar{R} = 1.505$ with variance ($\bar{R}$) = 0.020). However, the fundamental advantage of the analytic model is a formal statistical assessment of the key requirement that the age-specific rate ratio underlying the observed 14 age-specific rate ratios (Table 11.1) is constant.

PART II: ADJUSTED RATES

OBJECTIVE

To address the question: *do African-American newborn infants experience higher perinatal mortality than white infants after accounting for their generally lower birth weights?*

DATA

All African-American and white live births as well as fetal deaths reported during 1988 on the state of California birth certificates allow the comparison of perinatal mortality rates. Specifically, there were 44,356 African-American and 404,023 white infants—a total of 448,379 observations. The perinatal mortality rate is the number of deaths occurring between birth and 28 days of life plus the number of fetal deaths divided by the number of live births plus the number of fetal deaths. The perinatal rate is not a true rate but rather an estimate of the probability of a perinatal death. Birth certificates contain the mother's race/ethnicity (reported by the mother) and the infant's weight at birth (recorded in grams). The birth certificates for live births and fetal deaths were tabulated by race and classified into 100 gram birth weight categories (less than 800 grams, 801 to 900 grams, 901 to 1000 grams, . . . , 4201 to 4300 grams, and more than 4300 grams).

METHODS

Model-free techniques are used to estimate and compare perinatal mortality rates adjusted for the differences in white and black birth weight distributions. A Poisson regression model is also used to provide a similar adjustment and comparison.

Data type: vital records (birth certificates)
Reference: state of California vital records data (public data)

The variables are:

1. Weight 1: lower bound of the birth weight interval (grams)
2. Weight 2: upper bound of the birth weight interval (grams)
3. Black deaths: weight-specific counts of perinatal deaths
4. Black counts: weight-specific population counts of live births plus fetal deaths
5. Whites deaths: weight-specific counts of perinatal deaths
6. White counts: weight-specific population counts of live births plus fetal deaths

Part of the tabulated data file of 448,379 live births and fetal deaths is:

```
                 file name = perinatal.11.data
```

wt1	wt2	bdeaths	bpop	wdeaths	wpop
100	800	533	618	1585	1759
801	900	65	131	173	322
901	1000	40	122	148	337
1001	1100	30	131	134	398
1101	1200	29	137	106	381
1201	1300	21	143	103	444
1301	1400	19	143	86	427
1401	1500	19	165	108	597
1501	1600	20	167	85	560
–	–	–	–	–	–
–	–	–	–	–	–
–	–	–	–	–	–

```
        wt1 = lower bound of the weight interval
        wt2 = upper bound of the weight interval
    bdeaths = number of recorded black perinatal deaths
       bpop = number of recorded black births
    wdeaths = number of recorded white perinatal deaths
       wpop = number of recorded white births
```

DISCUSSION

The basic data, particularly the ratio of black to white perinatal mortality rates (last column), are given in Table 11.4. There are 70 race-, weight-specific categories containing the number of perinatal deaths, the number of live births plus fetal deaths (labeled "births"), and the perinatal mortality rates for white and black infants. The key issue is the role of race.[30,31] The overall perinatal mortality rate among black infants is $(520/44,356) \times 1000 = 11.723$ deaths per 1000 births, and among white infants it is $(2897/404,023) \times 1000 = 7.170$ deaths per 1000 births. However, black infants weigh less, on average, than white infants (mean values: $\bar{x}_{black} = 3143.2$ grams and $\bar{x}_{white} = 3403.4$ grams) and for all infants, lower birth weight is associated with higher mortality. The two birth weight distributions are displayed in Figure 11.4. The question, therefore, becomes: *what racial differences in perinatal mortality would be observed if the distributions of birth weights were the same for black and white infants?*

First Approach: Weight-Specific Comparisons

A direct and easily applied contrast of perinatal mortality risk essentially unaffected by differences in birth weight is accomplished by a comparison of black and white mortality rates within each birth weight category. Differences between the distributions of birth weights within a 100-gram range are small and negligible. In terms of the weight-specific rate ratios (black rate/white rate), 27 out of 35 mortality ratios are less than one (black rate < white rate). The fact that about 80% of weight-specific rates or rate ratios show black infants with lower perinatal mortality is a persuasive indication that, after equalizing birth weight differences, black infants have consistently lower mortality. In other words, when infants with essentially the same birth weights are compared, black infants, particularly those with low and extremely low birth weights, are more likely to survive. Figure 11.5 (left) displays the black and white perinatal mortality rates by birth weight. The comparisons in Table 11.4 are repeated graphically, showing that the black perinatal mortality rate (solid line) is below the white rate (dotted line) for most birth weights. A more detailed view of these differences is achieved by comparing the logarithms of the rates. Figure 11.5 (right) is a plot of the logarithms of the perinatal rates displaying a reduced range, producing a clearer picture of black and white mortality patterns. The log-rates plot identifies some instability of the estimated curves above 3600 grams, primarily due to the small number of black infants in these birth weight categories. Again, the black perinatal mortality

Table 11.4. Perinatal Deaths, Births, Rates per 1000, and Rate Ratios (Black to White) for 35 Birth Weight Categories (Grams)

Weights	White Infants			Black Infants			Ratio
	Deaths	Births	Rate	Deaths	Births	Rate	
800–901	173	322	537.27	65	131	496.18	0.924
901–1000	148	337	439.17	40	122	327.87	0.747
1001–1100	134	398	336.68	30	131	229.01	0.680
1101–1200	106	381	278.22	29	137	211.68	0.761
1201–1300	103	444	231.98	21	143	146.85	0.633
1301–1400	86	427	201.41	19	143	132.87	0.660
1401–1500	108	597	180.90	19	165	115.15	0.637
1501–1600	85	560	151.79	20	167	119.76	0.789
1601–1700	84	682	123.17	24	219	109.59	0.890
1701–1800	86	722	119.11	12	194	61.86	0.519
1801–1900	100	935	106.95	26	298	87.25	0.816
1901–2000	81	978	82.82	15	299	50.17	0.606
2001–2100	74	1,589	46.57	21	420	50.00	1.074
2101–2200	87	1,714	50.76	10	453	22.08	0.435
2201–2300	82	2,322	35.31	14	603	23.22	0.657
2301–2400	80	2,885	27.73	12	763	15.73	0.567
2401–2500	80	4,149	19.28	13	977	13.31	0.690
2501–2600	77	4,916	15.66	14	1189	11.77	0.752
2601–2700	93	7,455	12.47	10	1654	6.05	0.485
2701–2800	93	8,855	10.50	17	1796	9.47	0.901
2801–2900	100	14,197	7.04	11	2545	4.32	0.614
2901–3000	86	17,903	4.80	9	2947	3.05	0.636
3001–3100	92	19,969	4.61	12	2851	4.21	0.914
3101–3200	90	27,068	3.32	9	3557	2.53	0.761
3201–3300	96	29,107	3.30	9	3324	2.71	0.821
3301–3400	79	35,627	2.22	11	3577	3.08	1.387
3401–3500	67	32,926	2.03	1	3119	0.32	0.158
3501–3600	69	36,360	1.90	9	2952	3.05	1.607
3601–3700	58	30,612	1.89	7	2250	3.11	1.642
3701–3800	59	32,119	1.84	2	2176	0.92	0.500
3801–3900	40	24,004	1.67	3	1573	1.91	1.145
3901–4000	35	23,217	1.51	1	1348	0.74	0.492
4001–4100	30	16,232	1.85	3	909	3.30	1.786
4101–4200	19	14,233	1.33	1	735	1.36	1.019
4200–4300	17	97,81	1.74	1	489	2.04	1.177
total	2897	404,023	7.17	520	44356	11.72	1.635

rates, birth weight for birth weight, are lower than the white rates. A possible exception appears among moderately heavy infants (about 3600 grams), where the black mortality rates occasionally fluctuate above the white rates; however, this observation is based on only 18 black perinatal deaths (i.e., birth weights > 3600 grams).

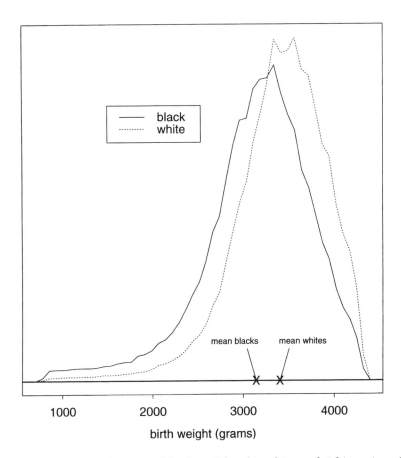

Figure 11.4. The distributions of birth weights for white and African-American newborn infants (California, 1988).

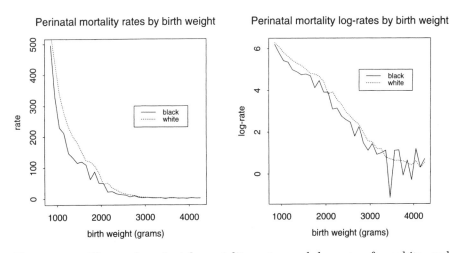

Figure 11.5. Observed perinatal mortality rates and log-rates for white and African-American newborn infants.

Second Approach: A Model-Free Summary

The 35 race-, weight-specific rate ratios do not lead to a simple or comprehensive description of the differences in black and white perinatal mortality
pattern. A weighted average of the weight-specific rate ratios, however, again
provides a single parsimonious overall summary. In addition, a measure of
the impact of the associated sampling variation on this summary is directly
estimated, leading to a statistical evaluation of the black and white differences in mortality.

Again, it is statistically advantageous to average the logarithms of the rate
ratios rather than the ratios themselves. Four specific reasons are as follows:

1. Less range (less variability) makes a graphic display clearer by increasing
   the visibility of the plot detail (Figure 11.5).
2. Log-rate ratios measure risk on an additive scale, making differences among
   rate ratios easier to describe and to manipulate statistically [i.e., ratios a/b
   become differences $\log(a) - \log(b)$].
3. The normal distribution becomes a more accurate approximation of a symmetric distribution of the log-rate ratios, especially for distributions of summary values calculated from these log-rate ratios.
4. Log-rate ratios generally have a more symmetric distribution, reducing the
   dependence of the variance on the mean, making interpretation easier.

A summary value tends to be more statistically tractable, intuitive, and inter-
pretable when the mean and the variance of its associated distribution are unrelated. For example, mean values from asymmetric distributions skewed to the
right are not readily compared since distributions with larger mean values also
have larger variances. The normal distribution has the opposite property. The
mean value is completely unrelated to the variance. Therefore, transformations
that create more symmetric (normal-like) distributions simplify the mechanics
of estimation and interpretation of analytic results.

Let the symbol $r_i^{(race)}$ denote the perinatal race-specific mortality rate from
the ith birth weight category. Then, the weight-specific rate ratio contrasting
black and white perinatal mortality rates is

$$R_i = \frac{r_i^{(black)}}{r_i^{(white)}}.$$

A weighted average (a.12) of the logarithms of the estimated rate ratios yields
a single summary of the difference in black and white perinatal mortality
risks and, as before, is

$$\overline{\text{log-}R} = \frac{\sum w_i \log(R_i)}{\sum w_i}$$

where the weights w_i are again the reciprocal of the estimated variance of $\log(R_i)$, $w_i = 1/S^2_{\log(R_i)}$. Specifically, the estimated variance of the logarithm of a perinatal rate ratio is

$$S^2_{\log(R_i)} = \frac{1}{d_i^{\text{(black)}}} + \frac{1}{d_i^{\text{(white)}}}$$

where $d_i^{\text{(race)}}$ represents the number of race-specific perinatal deaths in the ith birth weight category (a.10).

For example, for the birth weight category 2501 to 2600 grams ($i = 18$)

$$R_{18} = \frac{r_{18}^{\text{(black)}}}{r_{18}^{\text{(white)}}} = \frac{11.77}{15.66} = 0.752$$

and

$$\log(R_{18}) = \log[r_{18}^{\text{(black)}}] - \log[r_{18}^{\text{(white)}}] = \log(11.77) - \log(15.66) = -0.285.$$

An estimate of the associated variance is

$$S^2_{\log(R_{18})} = \frac{1}{d_{18}^{\text{(black)}}} + \frac{1}{d_{18}^{\text{(white)}}} = \frac{1}{14} + \frac{1}{77} = 0.084.$$

The weighted average of the logarithms of the 35 rate ratios (Table 11.4—last column) is $\overline{\text{log-}R} = -0.261$, making $\overline{R} = e^{\overline{\text{log-}R}} = e^{-0.261} = 0.770$ an estimate of the common rate ratio. That is, an estimate of the underlying ratio of black/white perinatal mortality rates is $\overline{R} = 0.770$. The black perinatal infant mortality rate is, on average, about three-quarters of the white race once it is adjusted for the generally lower birth weights experienced by African-American infants. Notice that the unadjusted black/white rate ratio is 1.635 (ratio = 11.723/7.170 = 1.635 − Table 11.1).

This single estimate of mortality risk is a useful summary only when the rate ratios from the 35 weight-specific categories are random fluctuations from the same value. Said another way, the summary rate ratio of 0.770 accurately indicates the black/white mortality differences only when race and birth weight have independent influences on the perinatal mortality risk (homogeneous rate ratios—no interaction). When a single value summarizes a series of values, there is an implicit assumption that the values summarized are each an estimate of the same quantity. The issues surrounding homogeneity and summarizing perinatal mortality rates (Part II) differ very little from those discussed in the context of contrasting male/female brain cancer incidence rates (Part I).

The estimated variance of a weighed averaged where the weights are the reciprocal of the variances of the quantities being averaged (a.12) is, once again,

$$\text{variance }(\overline{\log\text{-}R}) = \frac{1}{\sum w_i} \quad \text{and} \quad S^2_{\overline{\log\text{-}R}} = \frac{1}{427.350} = 0.00234$$

making the standard error $S_{\overline{\log R}} = \sqrt{0.00234} = 0.048$.

The approximately symmetric (approximately normal) distribution associated with the logarithm of the rate ratios allows the construction of an accurate confidence interval in the usual way. An approximate 95% confidence interval for the logarithm of the common rate ratio is

$$\overline{\log\text{-}R} \pm 1.960 S_{\overline{\log\text{-}R}} = -0.261 \pm 1.960(0.048),$$

based on the estimate $\overline{\log\text{-}R} = -0.261$, is $(-0.355, -0.166)$. Since $\overline{R} = 0.770$ is $e^{\overline{\log\text{-}R}}$, the confidence interval for the common rate ratio becomes

$$(e^{\text{lower bound}}, e^{\text{upper bound}}) = (e^{-0.355}, e^{-0.166}) = (0.701, 0.847).$$

As with all 95% confidence intervals, the probability that the interval (0.701, 0.847) contains the value estimated by $\overline{R}$ is approximately 0.95, providing a range of likely values for the underlying ratio of black to white perinatal mortality rates.

Third Approach: Poisson Regression Model

Another way to assess racial differences in perinatal mortality taking into account differences in black and white birth weight distributions is to construct a parametric model. Such a model postulates a specific relationship between mortality, birth weight, and race, making it possible to estimate, describe, and evaluate the separate influences of each component. For the California birth certificate data, a potentially useful linear model is

$$\log(r_{ij}) = a + b \text{ race}_j + P(\text{bwt}_i) \quad j = 1, 2 \quad \text{and} \quad i = 1, 2, 3, \ldots, 35$$

where $P(x) = c_1 x + c_2 x^2 + c_3 x^3 + c_4 x^4 + c_5 x^5$. The expected weight-specific perinatal mortality rate is denoted r_{ij} representing the jth race in the ith birth weight interval. The variable race is a binary indicator variable ($race_j = 1$ for black and $race_j = 0$ for white infants). A detailed description of the influence of birth weight is not a primary interest and is pragmatically represented by a rather complex function (a fifth-degree polynomial). Other functions could also represent the independent influence of infant birth weight. The polynomial expression characterizes the role of birth weight so that its influence is effectively removed, allowing a clear and focused view of the relationship between race and perinatal mortality. This strategy was used similarly to age-adjust incidence rates of brain cancer (Part I). Additionally, as in the brain cancer analysis, the number of deaths in each of the 70 race-, weight-specific categories is postulated to have a Poisson distribution. The linear model and the "Poisson assumption" make it possible to estimate the seven model coefficients and their standard errors (Table 11.5).

The Poisson model and the estimated coefficients directly yield an estimate of the log-rate $\log(r_{ij})$, which, in turn, gives an estimate of the rate r_{ij}, leading to an estimate of the number of perinatal deaths in each race-, weight-specific category. For example, the white infant log-rate ($race_j = 0$) for the weight category 2501–2600 grams ($i = 18$) is estimated by

$$\text{estimated log rate} = \log(\hat{r}_{18}^{(\text{white})}) = -3.994 - 0.290(0) + P(2550) = -4.152.$$

The estimated perinatal rate is then $\hat{r}_{18}^{(\text{white})} = e^{-4.152} \times 1000 = 15.7$ deaths per 1000 births. The number of model-estimated deaths is this rate multiplied by the number of births or $\hat{d}_{18}^{(\text{white})} = 0.0157(4916) = 77.3$. The corresponding observed quantities are $r_{18}^{(\text{white})} = (77/4916) \times 1000 = 15.7$ deaths per 1000 births (perinatal mortality rate) and $d_{18}^{(\text{white})} = 77$ perinatal deaths.

Following the typical goodness-of-fit pattern, the model-estimated number of perinatal deaths is similarly generated for all 70 race-, weight-specific categories (e_i) and compared to the corresponding numbers observed (o_i).

Table 11.5. Estimated Coefficients from the Poisson Regression Model Describing Black/White Perinatal Mortality

	Coefficient	Estimate	Std. Error
intercept	a	−3.994	—
race	b	−0.290	0.048
linear	c_1	−16.415	0.194
quadratic	c_2	1.558	0.195
cubic	c_3	2.035	0.186
quartic	c_4	0.371	0.180
quintic	c_5	−0.739	0.159

Residual deviance = 54.521 with 63 degrees of freedom.

Using a chi-square summary (a.5), the Pearson test statistic is $X^2 = \sum(o_i - e_i)^2/e_i = 56.216$ with 63 degrees of freedom. The degrees of freedom are the number of categories (counts of deaths) minus the number of parameters in the model or $70 - 7 = 63$. The p-value associated with the Pearson chi-square comparison is $P(X^2 \geq 56.216 \mid \text{model is correct}) = 0.71$. Again, "correct" means that all observed differences between observed and estimated numbers of deaths are due entirely to random fluctuations. A p-value of 0.71 indicates a rather close correspondence between the model-estimated values and the observed data, implying that the single coefficient $\hat{b}$ usefully summarizes the racial differences in black and white perinatal mortality. The Pearson chi-square statistic (56.216) is not very different from the residual deviance (54.521), which is typical for a Poisson regression analysis. As noted, these two statistics both measure lack of fit, have approximate chi-square distributions with the same degrees of freedom, and address the same issue. Not surprisingly, the graphic comparison of the observed and model-generated estimated log-rates confirms this analytic result (Figure 11.6).

The generally excellent fit of the Poisson regression model implies that the relationships within the data are accurately represented by a model with independent (additive) components measuring the race and birth weight influences on perinatal mortality risk. Specifically, the coefficient $\hat{b}$ measures a constant black/white racial difference for all birth weights (no race/birth weight interaction). In terms of the model parameters, for the ith birth weight

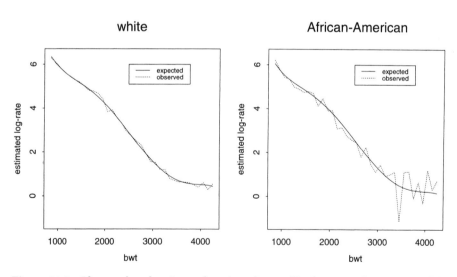

Figure 11.6. Observed and estimated perinatal mortality log-rates (Poisson model) for white and African-American newborn infants.

category, the independent influence of race measured by the estimated log-rate ratio is

$$\log{(\hat{R}_i)} = \log{(\hat{r}_i^{(\text{black})})} - \log{(\hat{r}_i^{(\text{white})})} = [\hat{a} + \hat{b}(1) + \hat{P}(\text{bwt}_i)]$$
$$- [\hat{a} + \hat{b}(0) + \hat{P}(\text{bwt}_i)] = \hat{b}.$$

Therefore, the model-estimated summary rate ratio becomes $\hat{R} = e^{\hat{b}} = e^{-0.290} = 0.749$ since $\log{(\hat{R}_i)} = \hat{b} = -0.290$ and, as before, indicates that the black perinatal rates are about 75% of the white rates for the entire range of infant birth weights.

Statistical assessment of the estimated coefficient $\hat{b}$ takes the usual two directions. Since $\hat{b}$ is subject to sampling variation, the likelihood that this estimate arose by chance alone when no racial difference in perinatal mortality exists is an important consideration. A test statistic is

$$z = \frac{\hat{b} - 0}{S_{\hat{b}}} = \frac{-0.290 - 0}{0.048} = -6.009$$

and z has an approximate standard normal distribution when $b = 0$. The estimated standard error $S_{\hat{b}} = 0.048$ is calculated as part of the estimation process (Table 11.5). The p-value associated with the estimate $\hat{b} = -0.290$ and, therefore, the approximately normally distributed z-value is $P(|\hat{b}| \geq 0.290 \mid b = 0) = P(|Z| \geq 6.009 \mid b = 0) < 0.001$. The extremely small p-value supplies clear evidence of a systematic racial difference in perinatal mortality between black and white infants independent of infant birth weight, as suspected from the weight-specific and model-free analyses.

The impact of sampling variation on the estimated summary rate ratio is also described by a confidence interval. An approximate 95% confidence interval

$$\hat{b} \pm 1.960 S_{\hat{b}} = -0.290 \pm 1.960(0.048)$$

based on the estimate $\hat{b} = -0.290$ is $(-0.384, -0.195)$. Since $\hat{R} = 0.749$ is estimated by $e^{\hat{b}} = e^{-0.290}$, the confidence interval bounds for the underlying summary rate ratio estimated by $\hat{R} = 0.749$ become

$$(e^{\text{lower bound}}, e^{\text{upper bound}}) = (e^{-0.384}, e^{-0.195}) = (0.681, 0.823).$$

Figure 11.7 (right) displays the geometry of the log-rates estimated from the model. As required by the postulated statistical structure, the curves describing the birth weight/mortality pattern by race/ethnicity group are par-

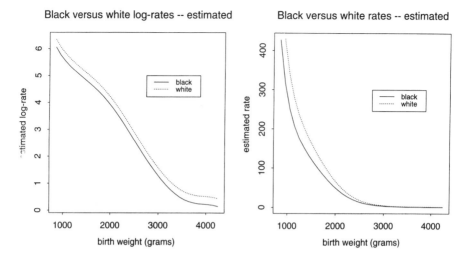

Figure 11.7. Estimated (Poisson model) perinatal mortality log-rates and rates for white and African-American newborn infants.

allel, and the constant distance between the parallel lines is $| \hat{b} | = 0.290$. Also, since $\hat{b}$ is less than zero, the estimated black perinatal mortality rates are less than the estimated white rates for all birth weights, as required by the model. Figure 11.7 (left) also shows the same estimated log-rates exponentiated, yielding model-estimated perinatal mortality rates for each birth weight. Necessarily, the black infants again have consistently lower estimated mortality over the range of birth weights.

CONCLUSIONS

Part I

A variety of estimates of the common rate ratio reflecting differences in the risk of brain cancer between males and females give almost identical values, a rate ratio in the neighborhood of 1.5. That is, the incidence rate of brain cancer is 1.5 times greater in males compared to females after adjusting for differences in age distributions. A Poisson model designed to address the same issue gives essentially the same results. Furthermore, the model allows an assessment of the homogeneity of the 14 age-specific rate ratios (p-value = 0.18), providing statistical justification for summarizing the male/female brain cancer risk with a single value.

Part II

Adjusting perinatal mortality rates for differences in birth weight distributions shows that African-American infants have lower birth weight–specific mortality than white infants. A direct comparison of 35 perinatal mortality rates within specific 100 gram birth weight categories provides substantial evidence of a lower mortality rate among African-American newborn infants. Summarizing these differences by a single rate ratio shows that the black perinatal mortality rate is, on average, 77% of the white rate, birth weight for birth weight (95% CI: 70.1%, 84.7%). As with the analysis of brain cancer incidence, a Poisson regression model addressing the same issue produces almost the same results. Again, the homogeneity of the rate ratios is a critical element in using a single summary. For the comparison of African-American and white perinatal mortality, the 35 rate ratios do no appear to differ systematically among the weight categories (p-value = 0.71).

To repeat, both analyses usefully summarize the differences in risk only when the observed rate ratios are random fluctuations from a common underlying value (no interaction between gender and age or between race and birth weight). Poisson regression analyses supply considerable evidence that this is at least approximately the case for the male/female brain cancer incidence data (Part I) and the black/white infant perinatal mortality data (Part II).

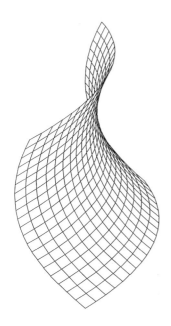

CHAPTER 12

Log-Linear Model (Poisson Model Applied to Tabular Data)

OBJECTIVE

To use case/control data to investigate the influence of vitamin use on the risk of a neural tube birth defect while accounting for possible differences associated with race/ethnicity.

DATA

The collected data are from 386 women who delivered infants or fetuses with neural tube defects (primarily anencephaly and spina bifida) ascertained by reviewing medical records from hospitals in a large number of California counties (June 1989–May 1991). Controls were randomly selected from the same areas, producing 384 singleton infants born alive without a reportable congenital anomaly. In-person interviews were conducted in English (74%) and Spanish (26%) within four or five months after delivery. Women who spoke only other languages were not included in the study. Information on race and vitamin use was obtained as part of these personal interviews. A woman was considered a vitamin user if she took single or multiple vitamin supplements in the period three months before conception and continued to take them during pregnancy (present users). Women who took vitamins only during pregnancy were classified as new users, and the remaining women were classified as nonusers. The sampled mother–infant pairs were classified by race/ethnicity (white, African-American, and Hispanic), creating a 2 by 3 by 3 table of counts (two levels of case/control status, three levels of vitamin use, and three levels of race/ethnicity).

METHODS

Poisson regression methods are applied to the tabular data, called a *log-linear model analysis* in this context. A number of log-linear models are contrasted to identify and evaluate the influences of vitamin use on the risk of a neural tube birth defect.

Data type: case/control (medical records)
Reference: *Journal of the American Medical Association*, 1996, 275(14): 1093–6

The variables are:

1. Count: the total number of observations for each status/use/race group
2. Case/control status: case coded 1 and control coded 0
3. Vitamin use: nonuse coded 1, used vitamins only during pregnancy coded 2, and present vitamin user coded 3
4. Race: coded 1 for white, 2 for African-American, and 3 for Hispanic

The tabulated data file of 770 case/control study participants is:

file name = ntds.12.data

count	status	use	race
34	1	1	1
43	0	1	1
53	1	2	1
81	0	2	1
5	1	3	1
9	0	3	1
67	1	1	2
54	0	1	2
10	1	2	2
17	0	2	2
3	1	3	2
4	0	3	2
133	1	1	3
91	0	1	3
70	1	2	3
79	0	2	3
11	1	3	3
6	0	3	3

BACKGROUND

The most frequently used definition of the independence of two events, denoted X and Y, requires the probability of the joint occurrence $P(X$ and Y occur) to equal the product $P(X$ occurs$) \times P(Y$ occurs$)$. This definition is only one of many ways to express the independence of two events. Another related expression is

$$\log (P[X \text{ and } Y \text{ occur}]) = \log (P[X \text{ occurs}]) + \log (P[Y \text{ occurs}]),$$

and the quantity

$$\delta = \log (P[X \text{ and } Y \text{ occur}]) - \log (P[X \text{ occurs}]) - \log (P[Y \text{ occurs}])$$

measures the lack of additivity between the logarithms of two probabilities, directly reflecting the lack of independence between two events. Perfect additivity of the log-probabilities is identical to exact independence ($\delta = 0$). Thus, the degree of nonadditivity between the logarithms of two probabilities is a linear measure of association ($\delta \neq 0$). Such linear measures of association are often statistically tractable tools valuable for identifying and analyzing relationships among categorical variables.

For cell frequencies within a table, a linear measure of association takes on an analogous form. For the 2 by 2 table,

	B	$\overline{B}$	Total
A	10	20	30
$\overline{A}$	20	40	60
total	30	60	90

there are various ways of demonstrating that categorical variables A and B are independent. For example, the ratio of counts $B/\overline{B}$ is the same for both levels of A ($10/20 = 20/40$). This property suggests a linear measure of association where $\log (10/20) - \log (20/40) = [\log (10) - \log (20)] - [\log (20) - \log (40)] = 0$ since A and B are independent. If A and B are not independent, then the difference between the logarithms of the ratios of the cell frequencies (B to $\overline{B}$) will not be zero, measuring the degree of association.

In general, a 2 by 2 table is denoted

	B	$\overline{B}$
A	f_{11}	f_{12}
$\overline{A}$	f_{21}	f_{22}

where f_{ij} represents the cell frequency of the joint occurrence of two specific levels of the binary variables A and B.

An additive (no interaction) log-linear model describes the logarithms of the cell frequencies f_{ij} when the categorical variables denoted A and B are independent. Specifically, for a 2 by 2 table, the additive model is

$$\log(f_{ij}) = a + b\,x_i + c\,y_j$$

where $x_i = 1$ indicates category A, $x_i = 0$ indicates category $\overline{A}$, $y_j = 1$ indicates category B, and $y_j = 0$ indicates category $\overline{B}$. In more detail, the model is

$$\log(f_{11}) = a + b + c$$
$$\log(f_{12}) = a + b$$
$$\log(f_{21}) = a + c$$
$$\log(f_{22}) = a.$$

A linear measure of association is

$$[\log(f_{11}) - \log(f_{12})] - [\log(f_{21}) - \log(f_{22})]$$

and, for the additive case,

$$[(a + b + c) - (a + b)] - [(a + c) - a] = 0$$

showing that the additive model describes the relationship between the categorical variables only when A and B are independent. An additive model requires that the difference between the differences in log-frequencies be equal, which occurs only when the ratios of the row counts are identical in each column or the column ratios are identical in each row. In other words, the column/row log-odds are equal. From the example 2 by 2 table, this measure of association is $[\log(10) - \log(20)] - [\log(20) - \log(40)] = \log(10/20) - \log(20/40) = \log(0.5) - \log(0.5) = 0$.

A nonadditive (interaction) model allows for the possibility that the row and column categorical variables A and B are associated. A nonadditive log-linear model describing the logarithms of the cell frequencies f_{ij} in a 2 by 2 table is

$$\log(f_{ij}) = a + b\,x_i + c\,y_j + d\,(x_i \times y_j)$$

where again $x_i = 1$ indicates category A, $x_i = 0$ indicates category $\overline{A}$, $y_j = 1$ indicates category B, and $y_j = 0$ indicates category $\overline{B}$. In detail, the logarithms of the cell frequencies are represented as

$$\log(f_{11}) = a + b + c + d$$
$$\log(f_{12}) = a + b$$

$$\log(f_{21}) = a + c$$

$$\log(f_{22}) = a.$$

For the nonadditive log-linear model, the previous linear measure of association is

$$[\log(f_{11}) - \log(f_{12})] - [\log(f_{21}) - \log(f_{22})]$$

but, for the nonadditive case,

$$[(a + b + c + d) - (a + b)] - [(a + c) - a] = d$$

That is, the magnitude of d reflects the difference between two log-ratios of the cell frequencies (differences in log-odds). Or

$$d = \log\left(\frac{f_{11}}{f_{12}}\right) - \log\left(\frac{f_{21}}{f_{22}}\right) = [\log(f_{11}) - \log(f_{12})] - [\log(f_{21}) - \log(f_{22})].$$

The magnitude of the quantity symbolized by d measures

1. the lack of additivity,
2. the amount of interaction,
3. the lack of independence, or
4. the amount of dependence

between the categorical variables A and B. In other words, the coefficient d from the log-linear model is the key to describing the degree of association between two binary variables in a 2 by 2 table. In short, the parameter d measures association. That is, for a difference in log-odds (a.11), as usual, $or = e^d$ where or is an odds ratio.

In general, employing a log-linear model to analyze the relationships among the categorical variables used to construct a table becomes a study of nonadditivity among the logarithms of the cell frequencies (interactions). Several textbooks provide complete descriptions of the theory and application of the log-linear model.[32,33]

DISCUSSION

Log-Linear Model—Two-Variable Case

To start, consider the relationship between maternal vitamin use and race/ethnicity (ignoring temporarily case/control status). The counts of mothers classified by vitamin use and race create a 3 by 3 table (Table 12.1).

Table 12.1. Cell Frequencies Based on the 770 Sampled Mothers Classified by Vitamin Use and Race/Ethnicity

Race	Nonuser	New User	Present User	Total
white	77	134	14	225
African-American	121	27	7	155
Hispanic	224	149	17	390
total	422	310	38	770

If vitamin use and race are unrelated, then the frequencies of these two categorical variables would be accurately described by an additive (no interaction) log-linear model where

$$\log(f_{ij}) = a + b_1 x_{1i} + b_2 x_{2i} + c_1 y_{1j} + c_2 y_{2j} \qquad i = 1, 2, 3 \quad \text{and} \quad j = 1, 2, 3.$$

The dependent variable is the logarithm of the cell frequency (again denoted f_{ij}), and the independent variables are the unordered categorical variables vitamin use and race/ethnicity. More precisely, the model components x and y represent design variables identifying the three levels of vitamin use and the three levels of race/ethnicity. Specifically, the components of the design variables are

Vitamin Use	x_{1i}	x_{2i}
nonuser	0	0
new user	1	0
present user	0	1

and

Race/Ethnicity	y_{1j}	y_{2j}
white	0	0
African-American	1	0
Hispanic	0	1

As before, perfect additivity of the logarithms of the cell frequencies occurs only when the row and column variables are perfectly independent (a.13). The additive model in complete detail is

Race	Nonuser	New User	Present User
white	$\log(f_{11}) = a$	$\log(f_{12}) = a + b_1$	$\log(f_{13}) = a + b_2$
African-American	$\log(f_{21}) = a + c_1$	$\log(f_{22}) = a + b_1 + c_1$	$\log(f_{23}) = a + b_2 + c_1$
Hispanic	$\log(f_{31}) = a + c_2$	$\log(f_{32}) = a + b_1 + c_2$	$\log(f_{33}) = a + b_2 + c_2$

The additivity is clear. The white influence adds zero, the African-American influence adds c_1, and the Hispanic influence adds c_2 to a background level represented as a. These influences are totally unaffected by the levels of vit-amin use. For example, the same coefficient (c_1) represents the influence of African-American mothers regardless of their vitamin use. Vitamin use sim-ilarly adds specific quantities (represented by 0, b_1, and b_2) to each log-cell frequency, which are totally unrelated to the levels of race/ethnicity. The additive log-linear model defines in concrete terms what is meant by the phrase "independence of vitamin use and race/ethnicity."

Based on the assumptions that vitamin use and race are independent and that each of the nine cell frequency counts has at least an approximate Pois-son distribution, the five additive model coefficients $(a, b_1, b_2, c_1, \text{and } c_2)$ and their standard errors can be estimated (Table 12.2).

The estimated logarithms of the cell frequencies, and therefore the esti-mated frequencies based on the additive Poisson model, can be directly cal-culated from the model coefficients. For example, if vitamin use and race are independent (additive), then the logarithm of the estimated number of African-Americans $(x_1 = 1 \text{ and } x_2 = 0)$ who are new users $(y_1 = 1 \text{ and } y_2 = 0)$ is esti-mated by

$$\log(\hat{f}_{22}) = \hat{a} + \hat{b}_1 + \hat{c}_1 = 4.815 - 0.308 - 0.373 = 4.134.$$

The model-estimated cell frequency becomes $\hat{f}_{22} = e^{4.134} = 62.4$. The corre-sponding observed cell frequency is $f_{22} = 27$. All nine model-estimated cell frequencies are given in Table 12.3.

The additive model dictates perfect independence. For example, the ratio of estimated nonusers to new users (1.361) is the same for the three racial categories, and the ratio of Hispanic to white estimated cell frequencies (1.733) is the same for the three kinds of vitamin use. In fact, independence of vitamin use and race/ethnicity implies that the ratio of any pair of row fre-quencies is the same for any two columns and, conversely, the ratio of any two column frequencies is the same for any two rows.

A formal comparison of the model-estimated cell frequencies (e_i) to the

Table 12.2. Estimated Coefficients and Their Standard Errors Using an Additive Log-Linear Model to Represent the Relationship Between Vitamin Use and Race/Ethnicity

Parameter	Estimate	Std. Error
a	4.815	—
b_1	−0.308	0.075
b_2	−2.407	0.169
c_1	−0.373	0.104
c_2	0.550	0.084

Residual deviance = 79.207 with degrees of freedom = 4.

Table 12.3. Estimated Cell Frequencies Based on the 770 Sampled
Mothers Classified by Vitamin Use and Race/Ethnicity
(Poisson Additive Model—Independence)

Race	Nonuser	New User	Present User	Total
white	123.3	90.6	11.1	225
African-American	84.9	62.4	7.6	155
Hispanic	213.7	157.0	19.2	390
total	422	310	38	770

observed cell frequencies (o_i) is achieved with a Pearson chi-square test statistic. The nine comparisons (Table 12.1 versus Table 12.3) yield a summary chi-square value of $X^2 = \sum(o_i - e_i)^2/e_i = 75.561$ with four degrees of freedom. The degrees of freedom are the total number of cells in the table minus the number of independent parameters needed to define the log-linear model (i.e., $3(3) - 5 = 9 - 5 = 4$). The likelihood that all nine differences occurred only because of chance variation (p-value) is $P(X^2 \geq 75.561 \mid$ use and race are independent) < 0.001. The considerable lack of correspondence between the model-generated cell frequencies and the observed values, summarized by the small p-value, indicates that the additive log-linear model is not a plausible description of the data. In other words, the data reflect a substantial association (lack of independence) between vitamin use and race/ethnicity. Figure 12.1 graphically confirms the lack of correspondence between the observed cell frequencies (left side) and the model-generated frequencies (right side). The residual deviance (79.207) calculated as part of the Poisson model analysis also has an approximate chi-square distribution with four degrees of freedom, giving essentially the same results found by comparing the nine observed and expected values (75.561).

For a two-way table, the same values estimated under the hypotheses of independence (additivity) can be calculated without a log-linear model. For example, again using the $n = 770$ sampled mothers, the number of African-Americans who are new users is estimated by

$$\hat{f}_{22} = n\,\hat{P}(\text{African-American and new user})$$

$$= n\,\hat{P}(\text{African-American}) \times \hat{P}(\text{new user})$$

$$= 770\left(\frac{310}{770}\right) \times \left(\frac{155}{770}\right) = 62.4$$

Both approaches yield the same estimated cell frequencies and, therefore, the same Pearson goodness-of-fit statistic. The log-linear model, however, generalizes in a number of directions, allowing the analysis of more complex issues arising from tables of any size or dimension.

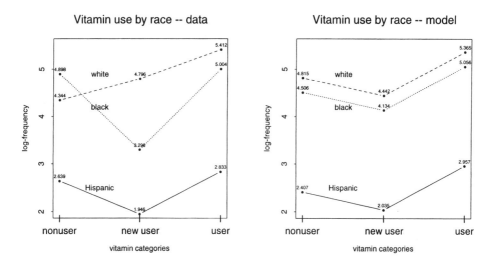

Figure 12.1. The logarithm of the cell frequencies (observed and estimated) for vitamin use categories by race/ethnicity.

Log-Linear Model—Three Variable Case

A log-linear model applies equally to the neural tube birth defects data further classified by case/control status, creating a 2 by 3 by 3 table (case/control status by vitamin use by race/ethnicity). Table 12.4 contains the 18 cell frequencies based on 770 mother–infant pairs classified by the three categorical variables.

Table 12.4. The Cell Frequencies Based on 770 Sampled Mother–Infant Pairs Classified by Case/Control Status, Maternal Vitamin Use, and Race/Ethnicity

WHITE

	Nonuser	New User	Present User	Total
case	34	53	5	92
control	43	81	9	133
total	77	134	14	225

AFRICAN-AMERICAN

	Nonuser	New User	Present User	Total
case	67	10	3	80
control	54	17	4	75
total	121	27	7	155

HISPANIC

	Nonuser	New User	Present User	Total
case	133	70	11	214
control	91	79	6	176
total	224	149	17	390

Table 12.4 makes it possible to study three pairwise relationships, particularly the relationship between case/control status and vitamin use, taking race/ethnicity into account. Race is a primary issue because the relationship between case/control status and vitamin use may differ within some or all three race/ethnicity groups. The other two less interesting pairwise relationships are case/control status and race, and vitamin use and race.

Each observed cell frequency in the three-way table is denoted f_{ijk}, where $i = 1$ or 2 (case/control status—two levels), $j = 1$, 2, or 3 (vitamin use categories—three levels), and $k = 1$, 2, or 3 (race/ethnicity classifications—three levels). A log-linear model provides an effective description of the tabular data, allowing questions concerning the categorical variables to be addressed by exploring the relationships among the logarithms of the cell frequencies ($\log[f_{ijk}]$).

Pairwise interaction terms, such as in the 2 by 2 table, remain the focus of the log-linear model since they continue to indicate the magnitude of the association between pairs of categorical variables. A log-linear model postulating three independent pairwise associations (interaction terms) is

$$\log(f_{ijk}) = x_0 + X_1 + X_2 + X_3 + (X_1 \times X_2) + (X_1 \times X_3) + (X_2 \times X_3).$$

The variables X_1, X_2, and X_3 represent design variables with one or two components representing each of the three unordered categorical variables. The design variable X_1 (case/control status) is a binary variable, while the design variables X_2 (vitamin groups) and X_3 (race/ethnicity groups) are, as before, bivariate quantities. As always, a k-level categorical variable is represented by a $(k-1)$-component design variable. The three interaction terms in the model are additive, which means that the association between any two variables is unaffected by the level of the third variable. As with the two-way table, if the cell frequencies have a Poisson distribution or at least an approximate Poisson distribution, the coefficients necessary to define the log-linear model can be estimated along with their standard errors (Table 12.5). Also, analogous to the two-way table, the measure of associations between levels of the categorical variables is the difference between the differences of the logarithms of the table frequencies. For example, the measure of association between case/control status and vitamin use (present users versus nonusers) among white mothers is

$$\log(\hat{or}) = [\log(f_{131}) - \log(f_{231})] - [\log(f_{111}) - \log(f_{211})] = [\log(5) - \log(9)]$$
$$- [\log(34) - \log(43)] = -0.588 - (-0.235) = -0.353.$$

In terms of an odds ratio, the same association (present users versus nonusers) is measured by $\hat{or} = e^{-0.353} = 0.703 = 5(43)/[34(9)]$, since -0.353 is the difference in log-odds. Similarly, the odds ratio measuring this same associa-

Table 12.5. Estimated Coefficients and Their Standard Errors Using a
Log-Linear Model to Represent the Separate (Additive) Pairwise Associations
Between Case/Control Status, Vitamin Use, and Race/Ethnicity

		Coefficient	Std. Error
intercept	x_0	3.701	—
case/control status	x_1	−0.103	0.168
vitamin use	x_{22}	0.738	0.169
	x_{23}	−1.634	0.348
race/ethnicity	x_{32}	0.326	0.182
	x_{33}	0.815	0.157
status by vitamin	$X_1 \times X_2$		
	x_1 by x_{22}	−0.436	0.158
	x_1 by x_{23}	−0.155	0.342
status by race	$X_1 \times X_3$		
	x_1 by x_{32}	0.250	0.221
	x_1 by x_{33}	0.473	0.173
vitamin by race	$X_2 \times X_3$		
	x_{22} by x_{32}	−2.027	0.257
	x_{23} by x_{32}	−1.135	0.486
	x_{22} by x_{33}	−0.911	0.180
	x_{23} by x_{33}	−0.855	0.386

Residual deviance = 2.492 with 4 degrees of freedom.

tion for African-Americans is 0.604 and for Hispanics is 1.255. These three measures of association (difference in log-odds or odds ratios) clearly differ. A critical question becomes: *do these measures of association differ systematically among the race/ethnicity groups or do they reflect random fluctuations from a common value?* The postulated log-linear model is designed to deal with this question.

The estimated coefficients in conjunction with the log-linear model produce estimated cell frequencies (denoted $\hat{f}_{ijk}$) that conform perfectly to the specified model structure. For a log-linear model based on the neural tube defects data with three additive (independent) pairwise interactions included ($X_i \times X_j$ terms), the 18 estimated cell frequencies are given in Table 12.6. For example, using the estimated coefficients (Table 12.5), the frequency of Hispanic cases whose mothers used vitamins ($\hat{f}_{133}$) is estimated by

$$\log(\hat{f}_{133}) = 3.700 - 0.103 - 1.634 + 0.815 - 0.155 + 0.473 - 0.855 = 2.242$$

and the estimated cell frequency is then $\hat{f}_{133} = e^{2.242} = 9.41$ (Table 12.6). The observed number is $f_{133} = 11$ (Table 12.4). The logarithms of the ratios of case to control cell frequencies for the three levels of vitamin use within the three race/ethnicity groups (nine log-odds values) are plotted in Figure 12.2 for the data (f_{ijk}—Table 12.1) and in Figure 12.3 for the estimated values based on the log-linear model ($\hat{f}_{ijk}$—Table 12.6).

If the fit of the pairwise model is good (say, p-value > 0.2), then little evidence exists to imply that the pairwise relationships differ among the levels of a third variable. The interactions do not interact. That is, each interaction term reflects the same degree of association between any two categorical variables for all levels of a third variable. Therefore, a single summary usefully reflects each pairwise association. For example, the model-generated cell frequencies (Table 12.6) yield estimates of the association between case/control status and vitamin use under exactly this condition. Among white mothers who are present users compared to mothers who are nonusers, then

$$\log(\hat{or}) = [\log(\hat{f}_{131}) - \log(\hat{f}_{231})] - [\log(\hat{f}_{111}) - \log(\hat{f}_{211})] = [\log(6.10)$$
$$- \log(7.90)] - [\log(36.52) - \log(40.48)] = -0.258 - (-0.103) = -0.155.$$

Furthermore, this measure of association is identical for African-American and Hispanics mothers. The estimated odds ratio measuring the association between case/control status and vitamin use is (present users versus nonusers) $\hat{or}_{white} = e^{-0.155} = 0.856 = 6.10(40.48)/[36.52(7.90)]$ and it is the same for the other two race/ethnicity groups (i.e., $\hat{or}_{black} = 3.49(56.05)/[64.95(3.51)] = 0.856$ and $\hat{or}_{hispanic} = 9.41(91.47)/[132.53(7.59)] = 0.856$).

A close fit between the model-estimated and observed cell frequencies makes the pairwise additive model a useful description of the association

Table 12.6. Estimated Number of Mother–Infant Pairs Classified by Case/Control Status, Vitamin Use, and Race/Ethnicity When All Pairwise Additive Associations are Exactly Homogeneous

WHITE	Nonuser	New User	Present User	Total
case	36.52	49.37	6.10	92
control	40.48	84.63	7.90	133
total	77	134	14	225

AFRICAN-AMERICAN	Nonuser	New User	Present User	Total
case	64.95	11.56	3.49	80
control	56.05	15.44	3.51	75
total	121	27	7	155

HISPANIC	Nonuser	New User	Present User	Total
case	132.53	72.06	9.41	214
control	91.47	76.94	7.59	176
total	224	149	17	390

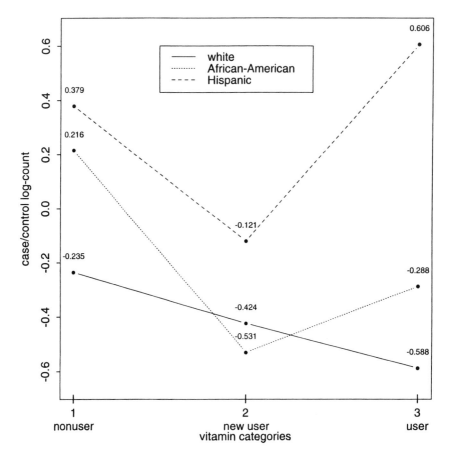

Figure 12.2. The logarithm of the ratio of the number of cases to the number of controls for three vitamin use categories by race/ethnicity.

between case/control status and vitamin use. Under these conditions, the role of vitamin use can be described by a single summary, adjusted for the influences of race. For example, the estimated odds ratio 0.856 describes the risk of being a case when present users are compared to nonusers, regardless of race/ethnicity. In other words, the measure of association is a single, summary value accounting for the influence of race/ethnicity, namely, $\log(\hat{or}) = -0.155$ or $\hat{or} = 0.856$. Such a relationship is said to be homogeneous with respect to race. The usefulness of this summary and of any other model-estimated summary of association depends on whether the pairwise additive model is an accurate representation of the relationships within the table.

Figure 12.3 displays the homogeneous pairwise relationships for the model-estimated cell frequencies (Table 12.6). The distances between the logarithms of the ratios of the case to control counts (log-odds) contrasting vitamin use categories are the same for each race (vertical axis). Geometrically, homogeneity (no interaction) generates parallel lines since the associations between pairs of variables are identical at all levels of the third variable. The geometry of the pairwise log-linear model shows three identical V-shaped case/control status and vitamin use patterns within each race/ethnicity group. Therefore, one V-shaped line equally describes the association for any one or all three of the race groups, yielding a single parsimonious summary of the impact of vitamin use on the risk of a neural tube birth defect accounting for race/ethnicity.

If the fit of the model is poor, then the relationship between each pair of the categorical variables likely differs systematically within some or all of the levels of the third variable. Misleading results generally emerge if the underlying relationships being summarized by a single value are not the same at

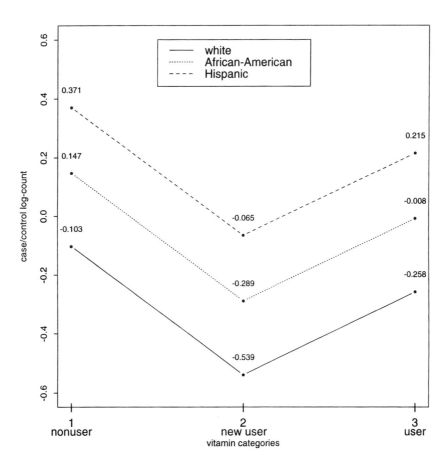

Figure 12.3. The log-ratio (Poisson model) estimated number of cases to controls for three vitamin use categories by race/ethnicity.

all levels of the third variable (not homogeneous). When a series of relationships fail to be homogeneous, an analysis of a three-way table typically becomes an analysis of a series of two-way tables. For example, if the case/control associations with vitamin use were heterogeneous with respect to race/ethnicity, then three separate analyses might be necessary, one of each race.

Comparing the estimated cell frequencies from the log-linear model (Table 12.6—e_i) and the observed data (Table 12.4—o_i), the Pearson chi-square statistic gives $X^2 = \Sigma(o_i - e_i)^2/e_i = 2.470$. Also, note the similarity to the residual deviance (2.492) produced as part of the model estimation process. As mentioned before, this similarity is typical. Both measures of goodness-of-fit have a chi-square distribution with four degrees of freedom when the model is correct. "Correct" means that the observed pairwise measures of the same association estimate the same quantity and differ only because of random variation (homogeneous). The degrees of freedom are again the total number of cells in the table minus the number of coefficients necessary to define the model, or $2(3)(3) - 14 = 18 - 14 = 4$. The p-value is $P(X^2 \geq 2.470 \mid$ homogeneous$) = 0.65$. The visual correspondence between the table values (Table 12.4 compared to Table 12.6 or Figure 12.2 compared to Figure 12.3) and the likely chi-square value provide no strong evidence of heterogeneity among the pairwise relationships within the three-way table. These relationships appear homogeneous, but this does not mean that they reflect systematic associations.

The next question becomes: *is there evidence of an association as measured by an independent pairwise interaction term* $(X_i \times X_j)$? Behaving as if the pairwise associations are homogeneous, three additional additive log-linear models are postulated. These models allow an evaluation of the strength of each independent pairwise association. The pairwise interaction terms (case/control status by vitamin use, case/control status by race, and race by vitamin use) are removed from the previous log-linear model, one at a time, creating three simpler models. For example, to evaluate the association between case/control status and vitamin use (interaction), the log-linear model becomes

$$\log(f_{ijk}) = x_0 + X_1 + X_2 + X_3 + (X_1 \times X_3) + (X_2 \times X_3)$$

where the interaction term $(X_1 \times X_2)$ reflecting the case/control by vitamin use association is removed. As before, the symbol X represents a $(k - 1)$-component design variable. The fit of this reduced model compared to the fit of the model containing all three interaction terms reflects the magnitude of the association between vitamin use and the risk of a neural tube defect.

The assessment is unaffected by race/ethnicity since this influence is treated as independent (additive) of the pairwise case/control–vitamin association.

A chi-square statistic summarizes formally the correspondence between the estimated frequencies generated by the model including all three interaction terms and the estimated frequencies generated by the model excluding one of the interaction terms. That is, the resulting residual deviances are compared and evaluated by

Summary chi-square statistic $= X^2$
$$= \text{deviance (two interaction terms included)}$$
$$- \text{deviance (all three interactions terms included)}.$$

The chi-square statistic X^2 links a significance probability to the question: *is there a systematic association between the two categorical variables that make up the deleted interaction term or are these two categorical variables unrelated (no interaction)?*

For evaluating the contribution of the case/control by vitamin use interaction ($X_1 \times X_2$) to the log-linear model, the chi-square test statistic is

$$X^2 = 10.037 - 2.470 = 7.567.$$

The test statistic X^2 has an approximate chi-square distribution with four degrees of freedom when the two models differ only because of random variation, that is, when case/control status and vitamin use are unrelated. In other words, the measured associations at all levels of race/ethnicity are not only the same (homogeneous) but equal zero (no association). The degrees of freedom are the difference between the degrees of freedom associated with each of the two compared models ($4 - 2 = 2$). The p-value is then $P(X^2 \geq 7.567 \mid$ no association) $= 0.02$. The comparison of these two models yields persuasive evidence of a systematic association between case/control status and vitamin use accounting for race/ethnicity. Geometrically, the V-shaped pattern is not likely a random deviation for a horizontal line (Figure 12.3 versus Figure 12.4).

The strength of association between the two other pairs of categorical variables is assessed the same way. All three evaluations of the independent pairwise associations from the birth defects three-way table are summarized in Table 12.7. The two-way table result that vitamin use and race are strongly related is repeated in the three-way analysis (p-value < 0.001). In addition, case/control status and vitamin use, accounting for the influence of race/ethnicity, are associated to a lesser but significant extent (p-value $= 0.02$). Also, case/control status is similarly associated with race/ethnicity (p-value $=$

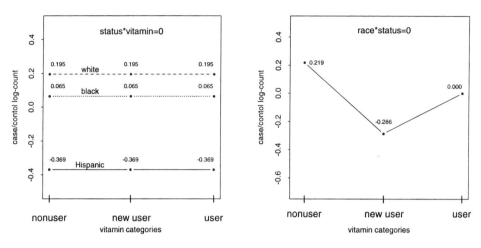

Figure 12.4. The log-ratio for two model-estimated number of cases to controls for three vitamin use categories.

0.02). The three inferences (Table 12.7) can be treated separately only when the pairwise relationships are homogeneous and the log-linear analysis provides evidence that homogeneity is a plausible assumption for the neural tube birth defects data.

Figure 12.4 (left side) displays the log-ratios of cases to controls (log-odds) for the situation where case/control status is postulated as unrelated to vitamin use ($X_1 \times X_2$ deleted from the model). The three different horizontal lines indicate an association between case/control status and race but no association between case/control status and vitamin use. Figure 12.4 (right side) displays the results from the model where case/control status is postulated to be unrelated to race/ethnicity ($X_1 \times X_3$ deleted from the model). The single nonhorizontal V-shaped line indicates an association between case/control status and vitamin use but no association between case/control status and race/ethnicity (one line, not three). Neither model is a plausible description of the neural tube defects data (Table 12.7).

Table 12.7. Tests of the Pairwise Associations from the Neural Tube Defect Case/Control Data

Deleted	Independent?	Chi-square	Degrees of Freedom	p-Value
$X_2 \times X_3$	vitamin and race	72.490	4	<0.001
$X_1 \times X_2$	case/control and vitamin	7.567	2	0.02
$X_1 \times X_3$	case/control and race	7.662	2	0.02

CONCLUSIONS

The collected case/control data provide evidence that vitamin use influences the risk of a neural tube defect while accounting for the confounding influences of race/ethnicity (white, African-American, and Hispanic). Using a log-linear model, the relationship between case/control status and vitamin use appears homogeneous among three race/ethnicity groups (p-value = 0.65). This homogeneity allows a specific and powerful single assessment of the vitamin–risk relationship adjusted for race. Accounting for race/ethnicity, the statistical evaluation of case/control status as a predictor of vitamin use produces a small significance probability (p-value = 0.02), providing substantial evidence of an association.

This analysis illustrates that the log-linear model is no more than a specific application of a Poisson model where unordered and categorical variables are represented by design variables, which is true in general.

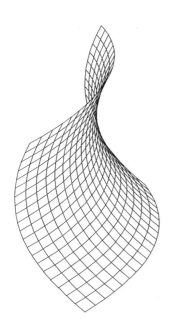

CHAPTER **13**

Survival Analysis (Cox's Proportional Hazards Model)

OBJECTIVE

To evaluate the prognostic roles in the development of acquired immune deficiency syndrome (AIDS) of two indicators of infection (CD4 lymphocyte counts and β_2-microglobulin levels) in human immunodeficiency virus (HIV)-positive men when these values are recorded at the initial HIV diagnosis.

DATA

The San Francisco Men's Health Study is based on a sample of 1034 single men ages 24 to 54 years. These men were recruited using a multistage probability sample and were followed from July 1984 to December 1987. Members of the cohort were interviewed and examined every six months. The vital status of 88.5% of these men was known. Other studies have noted an association of initial low CD4 lymphocyte counts and high β_2-microglobulin levels with a poor prognosis and increased severity of AIDS. A group of 88 HIV-positive homosexual/bisexual men were identified among the participants of the Men's Health Study. The progression time experiences of these men were analyzed to describe the role of these two measures in predicting the time from the diagnosis of HIV-positive status to the conversion to AIDS, referred to as *survival time*. By December 1987, there were 37 HIV-positive study participants and 51 participants with AIDS available for analysis.

METHODS

Under the parametric assumption of a constant hazard rate, the influence of
CD4 counts on survival time is explored. Two fundamental survival analysis
techniques are also applied—the Kaplan-Meier estimation of survival probabilities (nonparametric) and Cox's proportional hazards model (semiparametric).

Data type: prospective (follow-up survival data)
Reference: *Archives of Internal Medicine*, 1990, 150: 73–7

The variables are:

1. HIV/AIDS status: coded 1 if diagnosed with AIDS and 0 if HIV-positive (censored)
2. Survival time: time (recorded in weeks) between HIV and AIDS diagnoses
3. CD4 counts: lymphocyte counts as recorded
4. β_2-microglobulin: measured levels as recorded
5. Age: binary variable—observations 1–52 are less or equal to 30 years old and
   observations 53–88 are greater than 30 years old

Part of the data file of the 88 HIV-positive study subjects is:

```
file name = aids.13.data
```

status	time	beta	CD4
0	5	5.51	263
0	96	2.17	681
1	45	3.95	261
0	96	2.97	493
1	77	2.71	536
0	97	1.66	970
1	1	2.79	485
1	50	1.86	738
1	18	4.13	389
1	59	4.22	981
1	45	2.40	533
1	76	1.84	568
1	20	2.12	581
0	100	1.60	592
0	37	1.81	937
–	–	–	–
–	–	–	–
–	–	–	–

DISCUSSION

The analysis of the HIV-positive study participants would be relatively
straightforward if all sampled men had been observed until they developed

AIDS. For the present data, however, 51 members of the cohort were diagnosed as having AIDS during the follow-up period (3.5 years), but the other 37 at the time of analysis had not developed the disease. It is probable that these individuals subsequently developed AIDS, but for the current analysis, all that is known is that they were disease free at the end of the follow-up period. Such observations are said to be censored. Thirty-seven progression times are incomplete or censored. It is the censored nature of follow-up data that complicates the survival analysis and requires special statistical tools.[34]

The exploration of the role of CD4 counts and β_2-microglobulin levels in the prognosis of AIDS starts, like most statistical analyses, with a description of each variable (Table 13.1). Figure 13.1 displays the distributions of the CD4 counts and β_2-microglobulin levels (histograms and frequency polygons) measured at diagnosis (*baseline*). A bivariate plot of these two variables is shown in Figure 13.2 along with a summary least squares line (dashed line). Several extreme but believable values are apparent. The correlation between CD4 counts and β_2-microglobulin levels is -0.328.

The mean progression time is 63.6 weeks. This value likely underestimates the underlying survival time. The estimated standard deviation of 33.5 weeks is also likely too small. Both summaries are biased because the data contain the follow-up times of 37 men who are AIDS-free. If the analysis included observations after December 1987, these participants would add more AIDS-free time to the total observed progression time, likely increasing the estimated mean value (i.e., increasing the numerator of the mean survival time calculation) as well as the estimated variance. Adjustment that compensates for censoring allows unbiased estimates, providing a clearer understanding of the role of CD4 counts and β_2-microglobulin levels in the progression time to AIDS.

A good place to begin is with a description of the influence of the CD4 count since this count is a basic indicator of the AIDS risk. Three groups are formed based on the CD4 counts, producing strata that are less variable with respect to CD4 levels: low levels (CD4 counts < 400), moderately low levels (400 ≤ CD4 counts ≤ 900), and normal levels (CD4 counts > 900). For each group, a Kaplan-Meier estimated survival curve relates the CD4 count to the probability of a diagnosis of AIDS at any time following the initial HIV

Table 13.1. Descriptive Statistics for the Variables CD4 Lymphocyte Counts, β_2-Microglobulin Levels, and Survival Times for the Cohort of 88 Homosexual/Bisexual Men

	Mean	Median	Std. Dev.	Minimum	Maximum
cd4	657.8	641.5	260.03	49.0	1486.0
beta	2.5	2.4	0.88	0.8	5.5
progression time	63.6	67.0	33.50	1.0	102.0

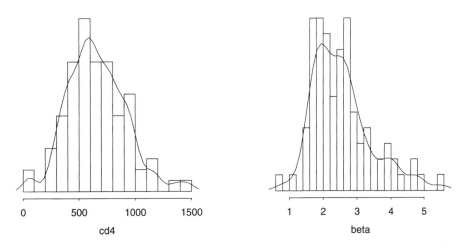

Figure 13.1. Distributions of CD4 counts and β-microglobulin levels from the sampled homosexual/bisexual HIV-positive men.

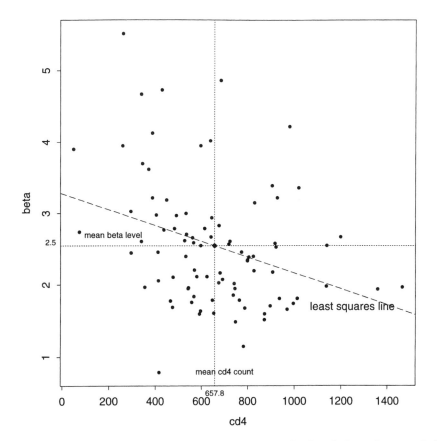

Figure 13.2. Plot of the CD4 counts and β-microglobulin levels from the sampled homosexual/bisexual HIV-positive men.

diagnosis (a.15). The probability of remaining AIDS-free (survival) beyond time t is denoted $S(t)$. In symbols, the survival function is

$$S(t) = P(\text{AIDS-free} \geq t)$$

where t is a specific time. Equivalently, the probability $S(t)$ is also interpreted as

$$S(t) = P(\text{AIDS-free during the interval } [0, t]).$$

The Kaplan-Meier process estimates $S(t)$ accounting for any censored data in an unbiased way. That is, an estimated function $\hat{S}(t)$ is constructed so that it estimates the survival probabilities that would have emerged if the data were complete (no censored individuals). Table 13.2, 13.3, and 13.4 contain estimated values of $S(t)$ for the three CD4 groups, along with estimates of the standard errors leading to 95% confidence intervals. Plots of the estimated survival curves $\hat{S}(t) = \hat{P}(\text{AIDS-free} \geq t)$ and their approximate 95% confidence intervals are displayed in Figure 13.3. Two features of the relationship between CD4 counts and the progression time to AIDS are clearly seen:

1. For the low CD4 group (CD4 counts <400) the progression time to AIDS is far more likely to be shorter than for the other two groups. The estimated $S(t)$-curve lies entirely below the moderately low and normal curves. Therefore, at any specific time the probability of being AIDS-free in this group is smaller. For example, if $t = 22$ weeks, then $S(22) = 0.51$ for individuals with CD4 counts less than 400 where $S(22) = 0.86$ for both the moderately low and normal groups. Low CD4 counts (<400) imply that about half of these individuals will progress to AIDS in less than 22 weeks but that for the other two groups only about 14% will progress to AIDS by the same time.

Table 13.2. Kaplan-Meier Survival Curve Based on 13 Homosexual/Bisexual Men with a CD4 Lymphocyte Count Less Than 400 (a.15)

Weeks	Risk	AIDS	P(AIDS-free)	Std. Error	Lower*	Upper*
0–2	13	1	0.923	0.074	0.789	1.000
2–3	12	1	0.846	0.100	0.671	1.000
3–13	10	1	0.762	0.121	0.558	1.000
13–16	9	1	0.677	0.134	0.460	0.997
16–18	8	1	0.592	0.141	0.371	0.945
18–22	7	1	0.508	0.144	0.291	0.886
22–25	5	1	0.406	0.147	0.200	0.825
25–26	4	1	0.305	0.141	0.123	0.754
26–45	3	1	0.203	0.125	0.061	0.680
45–48	2	1	0.102	0.095	0.016	0.639

*Approximate 95% confidence interval limits.

Table 13.3. Kaplan-Meier Survival Curve Based on 59 Homosexual/Bisexual Men with a CD4 Lymphocyte Count Between 400 and 900 (a.15)

Weeks	Risk	AIDS	P(AIDS-free)	Std. Error	Lower*	Upper*
0–1	59	1	0.983	0.017	0.951	1.000
1–16	58	1	0.966	0.024	0.921	1.000
16–18	57	1	0.949	0.029	0.895	1.000
18–19	56	1	0.932	0.033	0.870	0.999
19–20	55	2	0.898	0.039	0.824	0.979
20–22	53	2	0.864	0.045	0.781	0.956
22–37	51	1	0.847	0.047	0.761	0.944
37–42	50	1	0.831	0.049	0.740	0.932
42–45	49	2	0.797	0.052	0.700	0.906
45–46	47	1	0.780	0.054	0.681	0.893
46–47	46	2	0.746	0.057	0.643	0.866
47–49	44	1	0.729	0.058	0.624	0.852
49–50	42	1	0.711	0.059	0.605	0.837
50–60	40	1	0.694	0.060	0.585	0.822
60–61	39	1	0.676	0.061	0.566	0.807
61–62	38	1	0.658	0.062	0.547	0.792
62–63	37	1	0.640	0.063	0.528	0.776
63–65	36	1	0.623	0.064	0.509	0.761
65–69	35	1	0.605	0.064	0.491	0.745
69–74	33	1	0.586	0.065	0.472	0.728
74–75	32	1	0.568	0.065	0.453	0.712
75–76	31	2	0.531	0.066	0.416	0.678
76–77	29	1	0.513	0.066	0.398	0.661
77–84	27	1	0.494	0.067	0.379	0.643
84–85	26	1	0.475	0.067	0.361	0.625
85–90	25	1	0.456	0.067	0.343	0.607
90–98	17	1	0.429	0.068	0.315	0.585
98–101	10	1	0.386	0.073	0.266	0.561

*Approximate 95% confidence interval limits.

2. Only inconsequential and likely random differences appear between the moderately low and normal groups (Figure 13.3—lower right). The curves look similar and overlap, providing no convincing evidence of a systematic difference in progression times (survival) between these two CD4 groups.

Table 13.4. Kaplan-Meier Survival Curve Based on 16 Homosexual/Bisexual Men with a CD4 Lymphocyte Count Above 900 (a.15)

Weeks	Risk	AIDS	P(AIDS-free)	Std. Error	Lower*	Upper*
0–12	15	1	0.933	0.064	0.815	1.000
12–21	14	1	0.867	0.088	0.711	1.000
21–42	12	1	0.794	0.106	0.612	1.000
42–54	11	1	0.722	0.119	0.524	0.996
54–57	10	1	0.650	0.127	0.444	0.953
57–59	9	1	0.578	0.132	0.370	0.903
59–102	2	1	0.289	0.215	0.067	1.000

*Approximate 95% confidence interval limits.

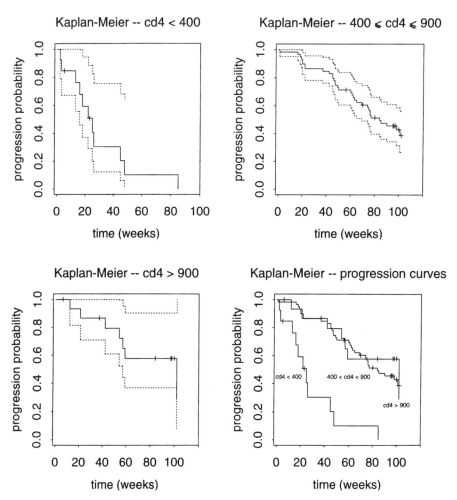

Figure 13.3. Three Kaplan-Meier survival curves displaying the progression time to AIDS with their associated 95% confidence intervals.

A Constant Hazard Function

A hazard function (denoted $\lambda(t)$) is the probability that an HIV-positive individual is diagnosed with AIDS at time t, when the individual is free of AIDS up to that time. The hazard function is related to the probability of being AIDS-free beyond time t. Specifically, the theoretical hazard function is defined as

$$\lambda(t) = \frac{dS(t)/dt}{S(t)}$$

where $S(t)$ represents a survival function.

The knowledge or assumption that the hazard function reflecting the risk of AIDS is constant considerably simplifies an analysis. The cost is the potential oversimplification of the relationship between risk and the time to AIDS (*wrong-model-bias*). When a hazard function is constant, the risk of being diagnosed as having AIDS is the same regardless of the observed follow-up time. In symbols, $\lambda(t) = \lambda$. For example, an individual who has been AIDS-free for five weeks has the same probability of developing AIDS as a person who has been AIDS-free for 50 weeks. That is, future risk does not depend on past experience when the hazard function does not depend on time.

For data sampled from a population with a constant hazard function, an estimate of the mean survival time is simply

$$\text{mean progression time to AIDS} = \bar{t} = \frac{\Sigma t_i}{d} \quad i = 1, 2, 3, \ldots, n$$

where d represents the number of complete observations (uncensored) among the total of n individuals followed and Σt_i represents the sum of all follow-up times observed, censored or not (a.16). Since the total follow-up time is likely too small (contains censored follow-up times), the sum (i.e., total person-weeks) is divided by the number of complete observations d (not $n =$ all observations in the sum) compensating for the "missing" time associated with the $n - d$ censored individuals (a.16). The estimated variance of the estimated mean survival time is $S_{\bar{t}}^2 = \bar{t}^2/d$. Both estimates depend on the number of complete observations, not the total number of individuals observed. Occasionally, follow-up data are extremely incomplete (most observations are censored). In this situation the precision of the estimated mean survival time is low because d is small, regardless of the sample size n.

When the hazard function is constant, the estimated rate of development of AIDS (estimated hazard function) is the reciprocal of the mean time to diagnosis, or

$$\text{estimated rate} = \hat{\lambda} = \frac{d}{\Sigma t_i} = \frac{1}{\bar{t}}$$

with an estimated variance of $S_{\hat{\lambda}}^2 = \hat{\lambda}^2/d$. The numerator d represents the number of diagnosed AIDS cases, and the denominator Σt_i represents the total person weeks at risk for all followed individuals. As the risk of AIDS increases, the mean time to AIDS diagnosis decreases in general. For individuals with a constant hazard function, this inverse relationship is particularly simple (i.e., rate $= \hat{\lambda} = 1/\bar{t} = 1/\text{mean}$). In addition, when the hazard function describing risk is constant, the estimated function describing the survival probabilities is then $\hat{S}(t) = e^{-\hat{\lambda}t}$. A constant hazard function causes survival time to have an exponential distribution, and vice versa.

For the three previously defined CD4 groups, the progression time to AIDS is described under the conjecture that the hazard function is constant.

Group: CD4 < 400

For those homosexual/bisexual men with a CD4 count below 400, the following describes their progression to AIDS in terms of the mean time to AIDS, the rate of AIDS, and the estimate of the progression time $S(t)$-function. From a total of $n_1 = 13$ men, complete information is available for $d_1 = 11$ individuals. The mean time to AIDS is $\bar{t}_1 = \Sigma t_i/d_i = 331/11 = 30.091$ weeks. The estimated standard error associated with this estimate is $S_{\bar{t}_1} = \bar{t}_1/\sqrt{d_1} = 30.091/\sqrt{11} = 9.073$ weeks, yielding an approximate 95% confidence interval for the value estimated by $\bar{t}_1$ as (12.308, 47.873). The estimated rate of AIDS (constant hazard rate) is $\hat{\lambda}_1 = 1/\bar{t}_1 = 1/30.091 = 0.033$, and its approximate associated 95% confidence interval is (1/47.873, 1/12.308) or (0.021, 0.081). An estimate of the progression time function follows directly as $\hat{S}_1(t) = e^{-0.033t}$ (Figure 13.4—upper left).

Group: 400 ≤ CD4 ≤ 900

For those homosexual/bisexual men with a CD4 count between 400 and 900, among the total of $n_2 = 59$ men complete information is recorded for $d_2 = 33$ individuals. The mean time to AIDS is $\bar{t}_2 = \Sigma t_i/d_2 = 4199/33 = 127.242$ weeks. The estimated standard error associated with this estimate is $S_{\bar{t}_2} = \bar{t}_2/\sqrt{d_2} = 127.242/\sqrt{33} = 22.150$ weeks, yielding an approximate 95% confidence interval for the value estimated by $\bar{t}_2$ as (83.828, 170.657). The estimated rate of AIDS (constant hazard rate) is $\hat{\lambda}_2 = 1/\bar{t}_2 = 1/127.242 = 0.008$, and its approximate associated 95% confidence interval is (1/170.657, 1/83.828) or (0.006, 0.012). An estimated progression time function follows directly as $\hat{S}_2(t) = e^{-0.008t}$ (Figure 13.4—upper right).

Group: CD4 > 900

For those homosexual/bisexual men with a CD4 count above 900, a total of $n_3 = 16$ men yielded complete information on $d_3 = 7$ individuals. The mean time to AIDS is $\bar{t}_3 = \Sigma t_i/d_3 = 1067/7 = 152.429$ weeks. The estimated standard error associated with this estimate is $S_{\bar{t}_3} = \bar{t}_3/\sqrt{d_3} = 152.429/\sqrt{7} = 57.613$ weeks, yielding an approximate 95% confidence interval for the value estimated by $\bar{t}_3$ as (39.508, 265,349). The estimated rate of AIDS (constant hazard rate) is $\hat{\lambda}_3 = 1/\bar{t}_3 = 1/152.429 = 0.007$, and its approximate associated 95% confidence interval is (1/265.349, 1/39.508) or (0.004, 0.025). An estimate of the progression time function follows directly as $\hat{S}_3(t) = e^{-0.007t}$ (Figure 13.4—lower left).

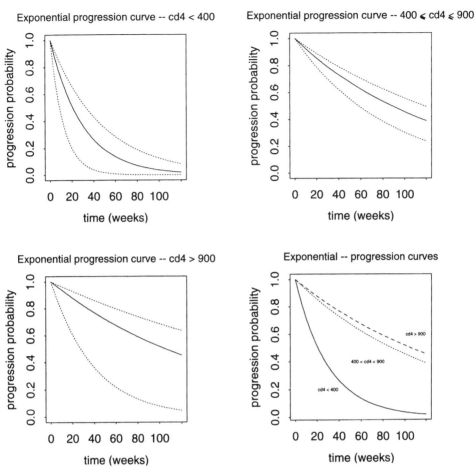

Figure 13.4. Three exponential survival curves displaying the progression time to AIDS with their associated 95% confidence intervals.

The summary values and their 95% confidence intervals are repeated in Table 13.5.

Median survival time is another summary providing a typical survival time associated with a sample of individuals. Situations arise where the median value has advantages over the mean survival time. For example, the

Table 13.5. Summary Results from Calculations Based on the Assumption of a Constant Hazard Function for the Three CD4 Groups

Group	$\bar{t}$	$S_{\bar{t}}$	Lower*	Upper*	Rate	Lower*	Upper*
CD4 < 400	30.091	9.073	12.308	47.873	0.033	0.021	0.081
400 ≤ CD4 ≤ 900	127.242	22.150	83.828	170.657	0.008	0.006	0.012
CD4 > 900	152.429	57.613	39.508	265.349	0.007	0.004	0.025

*Limits for approximate 95% confidence intervals based on the mean = $\bar{t}$ and rate = $1/\bar{t}$.

presence of outlier observations or certain patterns of censoring make the direct estimation of the mean survival time impractical. A median survival time can be estimated by interpolating between Kaplan-Meier survival probabilities. A related but simpler and frequently more effective estimate of the median is the endpoint of the interval containing the 50th percentile.[35] For the 59 individuals with CD4 counts between 400 and 900, the 50th percentile occurs in the interval 77 to 84 weeks (Table 13.3), making the estimated median value 84 weeks. That is, an estimated 50% of the individuals will convert and 50% will not convert to AIDS by 84 weeks after an HIV diagnosis. Similarly, the estimated median value for the group with CD4 counts less than 400 is 25 weeks, and for the group with CD4 counts greater than 900, the estimated median value is 102 weeks. These estimated median values require no assumptions about the statistical structure of the data. The estimation process is nonparametric, and the median accurately summarizes the survival experience whether the hazard rate is constant or not.

Another estimate of the median survival time is

$$\text{median} = \frac{1}{\lambda} \log(2) = \bar{t} \log(2).$$

This estimate is parametric and explicitly requires the hazard rate to be constant (a.16). The estimates from the Men's Health data for the three CD4 groups are $30.091\log(2) = 20.857$ weeks (CD4 < 400), $127.242\log(2) = 88.197$ weeks ($400 \leq$ CD4 ≤ 900) and $152.429\log(2) = 105.655$ weeks (CD4 < 900). Both the nonparametric and parametric approaches give roughly the same estimated median values.

If the hazard function is not at least approximately constant, then calculations based on a constant hazard function are not much use. A simple graphic approach gives some idea of whether the assumption of a constant hazard function is plausible. Note that when the hazard function is constant

$$S(t) = e^{-\lambda t}$$

and

$$\log[S(t)] = -\lambda t.$$

Then

$$\log(-\log[S(t)]) = \log(\lambda) + \log(t).$$

The last expression is a straight line function of $\log(t)$ with intercept $\log(\lambda)$ and slope 1. Therefore, if the hazard function is constant, then a plot of

$\log(-\log[S(t)])$ against $\log(t)$ randomly varies from a straight line with slope $= 1$ and intercept $= \log(\lambda)$.

Figure 13.5 shows four plots of this log-log transformed survival function for the three CD4 groups and provides a simple graphic assessment of the assumption of a constant hazard function for the Men's Health Study data. The upper left plot displays the Kaplan-Meier estimates of $S(t)$ from Tables 13.2, 13.3, and 13.4 transformed to $\log(-\log[S(t)])$ and plotted against $\log(t)$. The upper right displays the straight lines generated from the plots of the transformed $S(t)$-functions. Combining the plots (lower left) and smoothing the relationships between the transformed values of $S(t)$ and $\log(t)$ (lower right) show no strong evidence against using constant hazard functions to

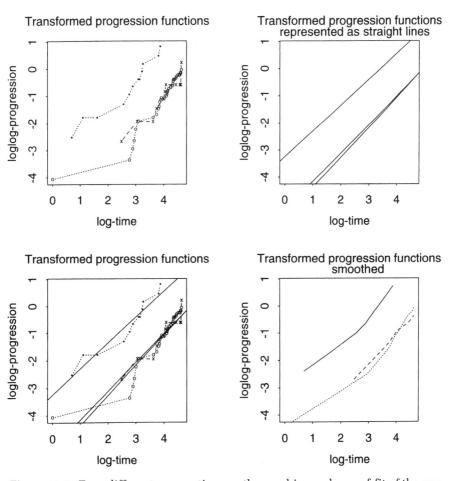

Figure 13.5. Four different perspectives on the graphic goodness-of-fit of the constant hazard assumption associated with CD4 counts.

Table 13.6. Selected Values from the Graphic Assessment
of a Constant Hazard Function

Group	Slope	Intercept	$e^{\text{intercept}} = \hat{\lambda}_i'$	$\hat{\lambda}_i$
CD4 < 400	0.952	−3.240	0.039	0.033
400 ≤ CD4 ≤ 900	1.052	−5.215	0.005	0.008
CD4 > 900	1.108	−5.478	0.004	0.007

describe the influence of CD4 counts on the progression time to AIDS within each of the three defined CD4 groups. Table 13.6 contains the key estimated values from the plots in Figure 13.5.

No formal comparison is made, but the estimated slopes (0.95, 1.05, and 1.11) do not differ substantially from a value of 1.0 (constant hazard). Each straight line appears to be an adequate if not a rather good representation of the transformed $S(t)$-function, implying that, within the CD4 groups, the risk of AIDS is meaningfully described by a constant hazard function. Since $\log(\lambda) =$ intercept, a graphic estimate of the constant hazard rates is $\hat{\lambda}' = e^{\text{intercept}}$ (Table 13.6). The hazard rates estimated graphically from the estimated lines in Figure 13.5 generally agree with the previous values based on the mean progression time (last two columns of Table 13.6), further evidence of a constant hazard rate. Figure 13.4 shows the estimated survival curves for the three CD4 groups based on a constant hazard rate (i.e., $\hat{S}(t) = e^{-\hat{\lambda}t}$). These plots are the parametric versions (based on the parameter λ) of the same survival functions estimated with the Kaplan-Meier distribution-free technique (Figure 13.3).

A Proportional Hazards Model

With a total of only 88 observations, continuing to stratify the data to evaluate the separate influences on survival from CD4 counts ($cd4$), β_2-microglobulin (beta) levels, and age (age) fails because most strata will contain too few observations to provide stable estimates. Therefore, to explore productively the joint influences of these three risk factors, a statistical model becomes the only viable alternative for analyzing their relationships to the prognosis of AIDS. A variety of models exist to explore failure time data.[36,37] One of the most popular ones is the proportional hazards model. This model (proposed by statistician D. R. Cox) relates a set of independent variables to the time an event occurs while compensating for the bias caused by any censored data.

For the Men's Health Study data, a proportional hazards model is

$$\lambda(t \mid cd4_i, \text{beta}_i, \text{age}_i) = \lambda_0(t) \times c = \lambda_0(t) \times e^{b_1 cd4_i + b_2 \text{beta}_i + b_3 \text{age}_i}.$$

The function $\lambda(t \mid cd4_i,\ beta_i,\ age_i)$ represents the hazard function at time t for the ith individual with specific levels of the three independent variables. The hazard function denoted $\lambda_0(t)$ represents a baseline or referent hazard function also at time t, and the proportionality constant c is a function of the three measured risk variables. The values for the CD4 counts (cd4) and β-microglobulin levels (beta) are represented in the model exactly as reported, while age is defined by a binary variable (age = 0 for individuals ≤ 30 and age = 1 for individuals > 30).

An alternative form of this Cox proportional hazards model is

$$\log[\lambda(t \mid cd4_i,\ beta_i,\ age_i)] = \log[\lambda_0(t)] + \log(c) = \log[\lambda_0(t)]$$
$$+ b_1 cd4_i + b_2 beta_i + b_3 age_i$$

showing that the logarithm of the hazard rate is a linear function of the risk factors and $\log[\lambda_0(t)]$ reflects an independent "background" level of risk. *Independent* in this context means that the referent hazard function does not depend on the risk factors ("constant" term in a linear model). Additionally, the impact from the risk factors is assumed not to change over time. The Cox proportional hazards model allows an assessment of the influence of the measured risk variables in much the same way as do most linear models. The additive model dictates that CD4 counts, β_2-microglobulin levels, and age have independent influences on the log-hazard function describing the risk of AIDS. The degree of influence is directly measured by the coefficients b_i associated with each variable.

A key property of the Cox model is that the b_i-coefficients are estimated without specifying the functional form of the hazard functions $\lambda(t)$ and $\lambda_0(t)$. It is, however, required that the hazard functions be proportional; that is for any two individuals denoted i and j

$$\frac{\lambda(t \mid cd4_i,\ beta_i,\ age_i)}{\lambda(t \mid cd4_j,\ beta_j,\ age_j)} = c = \text{constant with respect to time}$$

but further knowledge or conjectures are unnecessary. In other words, the Cox model requires that the ratio of hazard functions to be the same regardless of the time t considered, but it does not require the hazard function to have any additional special properties. A proportional hazards model is called *semiparametric* because the b_i-coefficients provide parametric measures of the influence of each independent variable on risk but *nonparametric* in the sense that an explicit parametric form of the hazard functions is not necessary. Frequently for survival data, the relevant hazard function is not known or is difficult to estimate, making the Cox semiparametric model particularly appealing in these situations.

A more extensive proportional hazards model describing the relationship between CD4 counts, β_2-microglobulin levels, age, and the risk of AIDS includes a series of *cross-product* terms allowing for the possibility of interactions among the independent variables. Such a nonadditive model is represented as

$$\lambda(t \mid cd4_i, beta_i, age_i) = \lambda_0(t) \times c = \lambda_0(t) \times e^q$$

where

$$q = b_1 cd4_i + b_2 beta_i + b_3 age_i + b_4(age_i \times beta_i) + b_5(age_i \times cd4_i) + b_6(beta_i \times cd4_i).$$

The algebraic relationships within the model define the interactions in the context of a proportional hazards model. For example, the influence of CD4 counts on the hazard function $\lambda(t)$ depends on three coefficients (b_1, b_5, and b_6). Rewriting the relevant part of the model gives

$$CD4 \text{ influence} = (b_1 + b_5 age_i + b_6 beta_i) \times cd4_i,$$

which defines the modeled relationship between a CD4 count and the risk of AIDS for the ith individual. The expression allows the influence of a CD4 count on the hazard function to depend on the levels of β_2-microglobulin and age ($b_5 \neq 0$ and $b_6 \neq 0$). For example, high β_2-microglobulin levels lessen the impact of the CD4 count on survival time when the b_6 coefficient is negative. Also, for older individuals, the CD4 count has an increased impact when b_5 is positive. The influence of the CD4 count is not independent of the levels of the other two variables (an interaction).

Conversely, if $b_4 = b_5 = b_6 = 0$, then the influences of the CD4 count, β_2-microglobulin level, and age on the risk of AIDS are independent (additive or no interaction). Thus, the influence of any one variable is not affected by the level of any other variable in the model. The relationship between the hazard function and the CD4 count, for example, is measured directly by the single estimated coefficient $\hat{b}_1$ for all levels of β_2-microglobulin and both levels of age. Clearly, these two models (interaction versus no interaction) describe substantially different situations. Therefore, determining whether the simpler (additive) model usefully represents the risk of AIDS is an important first step in the analysis. The choice is typically based on formally comparing the interaction model (six terms) to the no-interaction model (three terms) on the basis of differences in likelihood statistics.

The six estimated coefficients for the proportional hazards interaction model are listed in Table 13.7. The three estimated coefficients for the additive model are listed in Table 13.8. The proportional hazard model coeffi-

Table 13.7. The Six Estimated Coefficients from the Proportional
Hazards Interaction Model

Variable	Coefficient	Estimate	Std. Error
cd4	b_1	−0.0005	0.002
beta	b_2	0.886	0.515
age	b_3	−0.997	1.459
age × beta	b_4	0.071	0.348
age × cd4	b_5	0.001	0.001
beta × cd4	b_6	−0.001	0.001

$-2 \times$ log-likelihood = 383.657

cients are estimated using all 88 observations, censored and complete, but
estimated in such a way that no bias is incurred from the 37 incomplete survival times.

Log-likelihood values, calculated as part of the estimation process, reflect
the relative goodness-of-fit of each model and are key elements in comparing two analytic models (say, between model 0 and model 1). The difference
between these measures of fit is assessed directly using a chi-square distribution. The difference between two transformed likelihood statistics

$$X^2 = [-2 \times \text{log-likelihood \{model 0\}}] - [-2 \times \text{log-likelihood \{model 1\}}]$$

has an approximate chi-square distribution when model 0 is a special case
of model 1, and the two models differ only because the more general model
(model 1) better capitalizes on random variation, yielding a smaller $-2 \times$ log-
likelihood value. Usually but not necessarily, the special case is simply the
more general model with one or more of the b_i-coefficients set to zero. The
degrees of freedom associated with the chi-square distributed test statistic X^2
are the difference in the number of parameters needed to specify the two
models (for example, the number of coefficients set to zero).

For the data on progression time to AIDS, the additive model (model 0)
is a special case of the interaction model (model 1) since it is created by set-
ting three coefficients to zero ($b_4 = b_5 = b_6 = 0$). When only random variation
causes the two log-likelihood values to differ, the test statistic X^2 has an ap-

Table 13.8. The Three Estimated Coefficients from the
Proportional Hazards Additive Model

Variable	Coefficient	Estimate	Std. Error
cd4	b_1	−0.002	0.001
beta	b_2	0.405	0.158
age	b_3	−0.108	0.292

$-2 \times$ log-likelihood = 385.383

proximate chi-square distribution with $6 - 3 = 3$ degrees of freedom. Specifically, $X^2 = 385.383 - 383.657 = 1.725$ and X^2 has an approximate chi-square distribution with three degrees of freedom when no interactions are present. The significance probability (p-value) is $P(X^2 \geq 1.725 \mid b_4 = b_5 = b_6 = 0) = 0.63$. Contrasting these two log-likelihood values indicates that the interaction model likely adds unnecessary complexity to the analysis. Thus, an additive model provides a simpler representation of the important relationships and remains a useful basis for evaluating the influence of each prognostic variable on the risk of AIDS.

An assessment of the three estimated coefficients from the additive model (Table 13.8) follows a typical pattern. Since the additive model postulates independent influences, dividing each estimated coefficient by its standard error (z-statistic) serves two purposes (i.e., $z = \hat{b}/S_{\hat{b}}$). First, the z-statistics allow a separate assessment of each coefficient, providing assurance that they reflect more than a random fluctuation from zero. Second, the three z-statistics are commensurate (unitless), providing a direct comparison of the relative and independent impact of each variable on the risk of AIDS (influence on the hazard function). For the estimated coefficients associated with the variables cd4, beta, and age, the z-statistics are as follows:

CD4 counts:

$$\hat{b}_1 = -0.002 \quad \text{and} \quad z_{cd4} = \frac{-0.002 - 0}{0.00073} = -2.857 \quad (p\text{-value} = 0.004),$$

β_2-microglobulin:

$$\hat{b}_2 = 0.405 \quad \text{and} \quad z_{beta} = \frac{0.405 - 0}{0.158} = 2.559 \quad (p\text{-value} = 0.011)$$

age (≤ 30 and > 30):

$$\hat{b}_3 = -0.108 \quad \text{and} \quad z_{age} = \frac{-0.108 - 0}{0.292} = -0.370 \quad (p\text{-value} = 0.71).$$

The CD4 counts and β_2-microglobulin levels likely have important systematic and close to equivalent influences on the hazard function describing the progression time to AIDS, while an individual's age has a relatively inconsequential impact.

The same assessments can be made by comparing two log-likelihood values. For example, the log-likelihood difference resulting from removing the age variable from the proportional hazards model is

$$X^2 = [-2 \times \text{log-likelihood \{cd4, beta\}}] - [-2 \times \text{log-likelihood \{cd4, beta, age\}}]$$

and X^2 has an approximate chi-square distribution with one degree of freedom when no systematic differences exist between these two models (age has no influence—$b_4 = 0$). The specific chi-square test statistic is $X^2 = 385.521 - 385.383 = 0.137$, giving essentially the same p-value (0.71) as the value z_{age} since $(-0.370)^2 \approx 0.137$. These two approaches are usually similar ($z^2 \approx X^2$) when each coefficient is evaluated one at a time. The analogous comparison of chi-square distributed likelihood statistics, however, provides a way to statistically explore a variety of issues (single variable or combinations of variables) concerning risk, as measured by a hazard function, using a Cox proportional hazards model.

CONCLUSIONS

The analysis of the impact within three levels of CD4 counts on the probability of an HIV-positive person converting to AIDS, under the assumption that the hazard function is constant, produces three survival functions describing risk. When HIV-positive individuals have initial CD4 counts above 400, the risk of AIDS is substantially less than that of individuals with CD4 counts below 400. The estimated rates of conversion are: for CD4 < 400, the rate is 0.033 (95% CI: 0.021, 0.081); for $400 \leq$ CD4 ≤ 900, the rate is 0.008 (95% CI: 0.006, 0.012); and for CD4 > 900 the rate is 0.007 (95% CI: 0.004, 0.025). A graphic analysis supports the conjecture that the hazard functions within each of these three groups are approximately constant.

To further explore the risk of AIDS, an additive proportional hazard model is used based on three risk variables (CD4 count, β_2-microglobulin level, and age). The CD4 count continues to have a substantial influence on the risk of AIDS (p-value = 0.004), as does the level of β_2-microglobulin (p-value = 0.011), which is equally important. The inclusion of the study participant's age in the model shows little or no impact on the risk of converting to AIDS (p-value = 0.71). An evaluation of a more general proportional hazards model that allows for interactions among these risk factors indicates that a more complicated model likely differs only by chance from the additive model used in the analysis (p-value = 0.63).

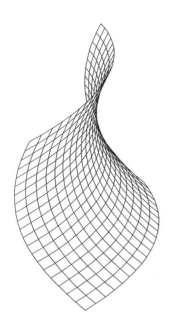

CHAPTER 14

Multivariate Comparison of Two Groups

OBJECTIVE

To explore the pattern of maternal weight change over two consecutive pregnancies, with particular focus on differences associated with the mother's parity.

DATA

Maternal weights recorded over a period including two pregnancies were abstracted from a birth records database maintained by the University of California Moffit Hospital (1980–1990). Data were collected from healthy adult white (non-Hispanic) women (age > 18) who gave birth to two consecutive single, live-born infants free of congenital anomalies. Each woman's weight was recorded prior to pregnancy (two self-reported measurements). In addition, each woman's weight was measured at or near delivery and then at about six weeks postpartum for each of the two consecutive live births (four measurements), for a total of six weight measurements on each sampled mother. Because the postpartum weights were measured at about six-weeks, six-week weight measurements were created by statistically adjusting each mother's recorded weight to estimate her weight at exactly six weeks. Maternal weight gained during pregnancy is net weight, that is, the mother's weight gain after the infant's birth weight was subtracted from the total recorded weight gained during pregnancy. Furthermore, all mothers were classified by the parity of their first recorded pregnancy, making a distinction between women whose first recorded pregnancy was their first child (nulliparous) and women whose first recorded pregnancy was parity one or higher (multiparous). Complete data for 93 white women were available to study weight change patterns.

METHODS

Means, variances, product-moment correlation coefficients, and t-tests provide univariate descriptions of six sequential weight measurements made on each mother for two parity groups. A canonical correlation analysis describes the maternal weight gain–loss association observed over two consecutive pregnancies. Multivariate comparisons are used to explore the differences in pattern of weight change between parity groups using three approaches—a canonical summary (discriminant analysis), Hotelling's T^2-test, and a multivariate analysis of variance. These analytic techniques provide different prospectives on the relationship between weight change pattern and parity but give identical statistical assessments.

Data type: longitudinal (hospital database)
Reference: Dissertation, Erica Gunderson, University of California, 1999

The variables are:

1. Parity: coded 0 for the first birth and 1 otherwise
2. Prepregnancy weight (wt1): reported maternal weight before first pregnancy
3. Delivery weight (wt2): maternal net weight at delivery of the first pregnancy
4. Postpartum weight (wt3): maternal weight six weeks after the first pregnancy
5. Prepregnancy weight (wt4): reported maternal weight before second pregnancy
6. Delivery weight (wt5): maternal net weight at delivery of the second pregnancy
7. Postpartum weight (wt6): maternal weight six weeks after the second pregnancy

Note: all maternal weight measurements are in kilograms.

Part of the data file of the 93 sampled mothers is:

file name = wtchange.14.data

parity	wt1	wt2	wt3	wt4	wt5	wt6
0	56.0	63.6	58.1	53.6	64.3	59.4
0	48.2	59.7	54.1	49.1	62.7	54.1
0	61.4	72.3	64.9	59.0	71.8	63.7
0	56.8	72.8	65.7	56.4	75.3	69.2
0	50.0	57.6	53.0	51.4	57.7	54.8
0	50.0	66.6	54.2	52.0	70.0	64.3

0	50.0	66.3	57.9	54.5	67.0	61.5
0	62.3	71.4	67.6	61.4	72.5	71.5
0	65.0	79.9	71.5	64.6	81.3	74.4
0	58.2	70.1	64.3	59.1	77.2	72.4
0	65.4	77.7	67.8	70.0	74.5	67.3
0	65.0	73.7	64.1	60.5	76.9	71.2
–	–	–	–	–	–	–
–	–	–	–	–	–	–
–	–	–	–	–	–	–

DISCUSSION

Occasionally, a deceptively subtle issue arises concerning the question of whether an observation should be treated as a dependent (outcome) variable or as an independent (predictor) variable. For example, a multivariable linear model consists of a single outcome variable and one or more predictor variables. Occasionally, it is not obvious if a variable is a predictor or an outcome variable. When symmetric variables such as the birth weights of twins are studied, the choice of dependent and independent variables is not clear and different choices yield different results. For the weight change data, the dependent variable is not a single measurement but a multivariate response consisting of six related measurements made on the same women over time. The independent variable, furthermore, is a single binary variable (parity equal to zero or parity greater than zero). The roles of these two variables in the analytic model are not based on statistical considerations but on a natural sense of the relationship between parity and weight change. Parity potentially affects weight change as an outcome, whereas the converse is not biologically very plausible. This *directionality* implies that parity is more logically the independent variable and that weight change measures are the dependent variable. Without a sense of directionality, a linear model approach is not useful analytically. When a variable consists of a number of components, it is called a *multivariate* variable. The six maternal weight measurements form a multivariate outcome variable. The statistical tools designed to explore multivariate outcomes reflect this fundamentally complex structure and are, in many cases, themselves rather complex.[37]

A summary of the 93 multivariate observations made up of six maternal weight change components is contained in Table 14.1. Quantile plots (Figure 14.1) of each of the six components of the multivariate observation show no extreme outliers and each variable appears to have an approximately normal distribution. Interest focuses not only on the multivariate response but also on differences in response associated with parity. Parity divides the sampled women into two groups—70 women whose first recorded pregnancy was their first live-born infant (coded = 0) and 23 women whose first recorded preg-

Table 14.1. Summary Statistics for the Six Weight Change Measures (Kilograms)
for 93 Women Observed Over Two Consecutive Pregnancies

Weight Change	Symbol	Mean	Median	Std. Dev.	Minimum	Maximum
prepregnancy weight	weight	59.2	59.1	10.3	40.9	106.0
gain at first pregnancy	$gain_1$	12.8	12.3	4.6	3.6	29.2
loss after first birth	$loss_1$	6.8	6.8	2.9	14.0	-0.2
intrapregnancy change	change	-4.7	-4.5	4.8	-27.5	4.6
gain at second pregnancy	$gain_2$	12.5	11.6	5.4	2.5	36.3
loss after second birth	$loss_2$	5.8	5.7	2.1	10.8	0.9

nancy was not their first live-born infant (coded = 1). The mean weight change patterns associated within these two parity groups are shown in Figure 14.2.

Measurements made on the same individual are almost always related. Recognizing this property is basic to understanding and analyzing multivariate data. For the weight gain data, like most multivariate data, accounting for the interrelationships among the six weight measurements is at the center of the analysis. For example, an issue of interest is the tendency of women to repeat their weight gain–loss patterns with consecutive pregnancies; however, weight gain and loss within a single pregnancy are related.

A starting point for exploring the interrelationships among the six weight measurements made on each of the 93 women is a correlation array. All possible correlation coefficients between pairs of weight measurements (15 correlations) are given in Table 14.2.

As a guideline to help judge the importance of an estimated correlation coefficient in light of random variation, the probability that a single correlation exceeds ± 0.206 by chance alone is 0.05 (i.e., $P(|$ a correlation $| \geq 0.206 |$ no linear association) = 0.05 for $n = 93$ pairs of observations). From this prospective, most of the correlations between pairs of the six weight change variables are not likely due strictly to random variation. Inspection of the correlation array verifies that the weight gains and losses measured within and between consecutive pregnancies are strongly related, likely in a complex way.

The correlation between the amount of weight gained during two consecutive pregnancies is 0.47 (correlation ($gain_1$, $gain_2$) = 0.47), and the similar correlation between the amount of weight lost is 0.53 (correlation ($loss_1$, $loss_2$) = 0.53). These values indicate a high degree of repetition in maternal gain–loss patterns. Weight gain and loss, however, are negatively correlated within pregnancies (correlation ($gain_1$, $loss_1$) = -0.43 and correlation ($gain_2$, $loss_2$) = -0.14, respectively). The weight gain–weight loss relationship within each pregnancy complicates the interpretation of the gain and loss pattern between pregnancies.

A canonical correlation coefficient is designed to express the degree of association between two sets of multivariate measurements with a single number

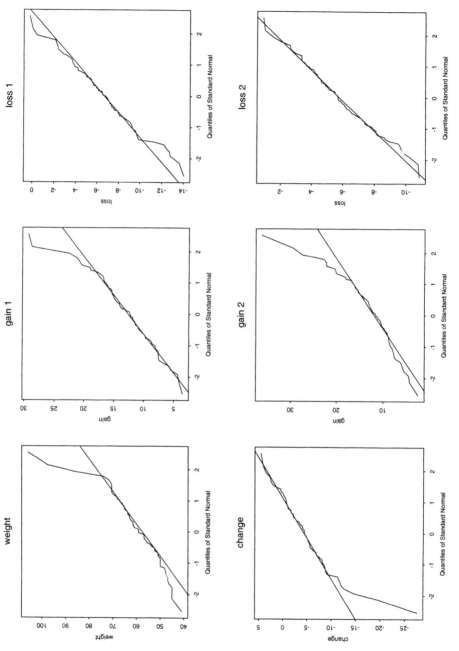

Figure 14.1. Quantile plots comparing the observed distributions of the six multivariate components to a normal distribution.

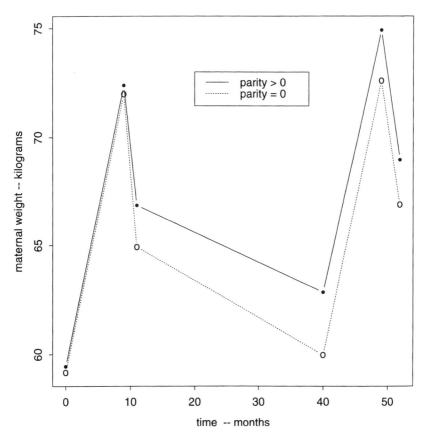

Figure 14.2. The pattern of weight change over two pregnancies by months for nulliparous and multiparous women.

Table 14.2. The Correlation Array for the Six Weight Measurements Made on 93 Women Observed Over Two Consecutive Pregnancies

	weight	gain$_1$	loss$_1$	change	gain$_2$	loss$_2$
weight	1.00	0.14	−0.18	−0.21	0.34	−0.04
gain$_1$	0.14	1.00	−0.43	−0.37	0.47	−0.32
loss$_1$	−0.18	−0.43	1.00	−0.09	−0.20	0.53
change	−0.21	−0.37	−0.09	1.00	−0.65	−0.21
gain$_2$	0.34	0.47	−0.20	−0.65	1.00	−0.14
loss$_2$	−0.04	−0.32	0.53	−0.21	−0.14	1.00

between -1 and $+1$. A canonical correlation coefficient is the usual Pearson's product-moment correlation coefficient applied to values generated by two canonical variables. For the gain–loss comparison the canonical variables are

$$x_i = a_1 \text{gain}_{1i} + a_2 \text{loss}_{1i} \quad \text{(first pregnancy canonical variable)}$$

and

$$y_i = b_1 \text{gain}_{2i} + b_2 \text{loss}_{2i} \quad \text{(second pregnancy canonical variable)}$$

for $i = 1, 2, 3, \ldots, 93$ mothers. The canonical variables x and y combine measured weight gains and losses during each pregnancy into a single summary value. Two related measurements are reduced to one summary variable per pregnancy, creating 93 pairs (x_i, y_i), one for each sampled mother. The correlation between these 93 canonical variables provides a description of the tendency of the gain–loss patterns to be repeated between two consecutive pregnancies.

A question remains; *how are the coefficients a_1, a_2, b_1, and b_2 chosen?* The mathematics of a canonical correlation analysis provides coefficients that produce the largest possible correlation between any two linear combinations of the weight gain and weight loss measurements. Other criteria exist to create other useful canonical descriptions. Maximizing the correlation is just one of several choices that produce a unique summary based on the components of a multivariate observation.

Specifically, for the weight change data, the canonical variables are

$$x_i = -0.013 \text{ gain}_{1i} + 0.022 \text{ loss}_{1i}$$

and

$$y_i = -0.010 \text{ gain}_{2i} + 0.038 \text{ loss}_{2i}$$

making the correlation between x and y the largest possible. A plot of these 93 canonical pairs (x_i, y_i) is displayed in Figure 14.3. The correlation between x and y is 0.598 (canonical correlation $= r_{xy} = 0.598$). The large canonical correlation reveals a strong tendency for women to have similar consecutive gain–loss patterns. In a totally analogous fashion, pairs of canonical variables created from any number of multivariate components provide a simpler and frequently a clearer picture of a complex multivariate relationship in terms of a single correlation coefficient.

No other linear combination of weight gain and loss has a greater correlation, making the canonical correlation unique, but, like all summary val-

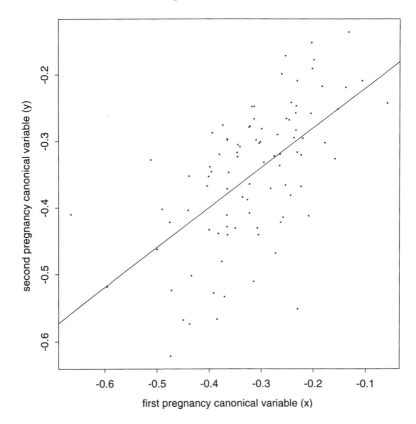

Figure 14.3. The first pregnancy canonical variate (x) plotted against the second pregnancy canonical variate (y).

ues, it is not the whole story. It is straightforward to determine which mother gained the most weight during pregnancy and which mother lost the most weight after delivery, but no single summary unequivocally combines both variables. A *linear canonical variable*, as the name suggests, reduces the complexity of a series of related measurements. The new variable is a simpler observation with worthwhile statistical properties and is frequently easier to interpret, but the observed association between weight gain and loss depends, at least to some extent, on the way the multivariate measurements are summarized.

Table 14.3 presents the estimated mean values of each of the six components of the multivariate weight change measurements for the two parity groups, contrasting the 70 nulliparous women (parity = 0) to the 23 multiparous women (parity = 1).

Pairwise comparisons among a series of related mean values are ultimately unsatisfactory because the differences result from an unknown mixture of

Table 14.3. Mean Weight Change Measurements (Kilograms) and Six Pairwise
t-Tests Comparing Nulliparous to Multiparous Women

	weight	gain$_1$	loss$_1$	change	gain$_2$	loss$_2$
parity 0	59.17	12.81	7.06	−4.95	12.63	5.71
parity 1 or more	59.45	12.94	5.53	−4.02	12.08	5.96
mean difference	0.28	0.13	−1.53	0.93	−0.55	0.26
T = t-value	0.11	0.12	−2.26	0.81	−0.42	0.50
$P\,(\mid T \mid \geq t)$*	0.91	0.91	0.03	0.42	0.67	0.62

*Two-tail p-value computed from a t-distribution with 91 degrees of freedom.

direct and indirect influences. Direct influences are a function only of the
variables compared and are completely independent of associations with other
correlated variables. Conceptually, a direct influence causes the difference that
would be observed if the comparison was perfectly balanced for all other
variables (all other relevant variables held constant). For example, the direct
difference between mean prepregnancy weights would be due strictly to differences in parity when the women compared are envisioned to be identical
in all other respects, such as age, race, height, and socioeconomic status. Conversely, indirect influences (sometimes called *confounding* influences) are due
only to the associations with other correlated variables, tending to obscure or
exaggerate the observed differences between the compared variables. For
example, the observed difference between mean prepregnancy weights (parity = 0 versus parity = 1) is influenced by other associated variables that also
differ between parity groups, such as the age of the mother. Older mothers
generally have higher parity and tend to weigh more, making age indirectly
responsible for some of the observed difference in mean prepregnancy weights
between the two parity groups (59.17 versus 59.45). To understand a multivariate relationship, it is necessary to isolate the direct influences from the
indirect influences among the components of the multivariate observation,
providing a single comprehensive assessment. Pairwise correlation coefficients (Table 14.1) and two sample t-tests (Table 14.3) do not have this property. Comparisons between both summaries reflect a mixture of direct and
indirect influences.

A Canonical Variable Approach

One approach capitalizing on all the direct information contained in the six
weight measurements depends again on constructing a canonical variable. As
before, the canonical variable is a linear combination of the components of
a multivariate observation. Represented as d_i (ith individual), a canonical
summary of the six weight change components is

$$d_i = a_1 \text{weight}_i + a_2 \text{gain}_{1i} + a_3 \text{loss}_{1i} + a_4 \text{change}_i + a_5 \text{gain}_{2i} + a_6 \text{loss}_{2i}.$$

The 93 canonical variables d_i summarize the six components of each multivariate observation by a single value. These single values lead to a simple comparison of the two mean canonical values describing the influence of parity (denoted $\bar{d}_0 - \bar{d}_1$, where $\bar{d}_0$ is the mean canonical value for the 70 women for whom parity = 0 and $\bar{d}_1$ is the mean canonical value for the 23 women for whom parity = 1). The six coefficients a_i are chosen to maximize the difference between the compared mean values relative to the estimated variance of the canonical summary d. Therefore, among all possible linear combinations of the multivariate components, comparing mean values of the linear combinations constructed from the a_i-coefficients maximizes the chances of identifying a nonrandom difference between the two parity groups when one exists. In most contexts, this specific canonical variable is called a *discriminant function*.

The a_i-coefficients are estimated as part of a linear discriminant function analysis or they are estimated as part of a linear regression analysis where the outcome variable is binary, such as parity. Specifically, for the 93 sampled women, the canonical variable is

$$d_i = 0.027\text{weight}_i + 0.127\text{gain}_{1i} + 0.462\text{loss}_{1i}$$
$$+ 0.121\text{change}_i + 0.012\text{gain}_{2i} - 0.248\text{loss}_{2i}$$

producing 93 summary values of weight change. Then, the mean values are $\bar{d}_0 = 0.676$ (parity = 0) based on $n_0 = 70$ observations and $\bar{d}_1 = -0.222$ (parity = 1) based on $n_1 = 23$ observations. The squared difference $D^2 = (\bar{d}_0 - \bar{d}_1)^2 = 0.807$ is a multivariate distance between these two parity groups. The summary D^2 is a single number that succinctly reflects the difference between the two parity groups, capitalizing on all the direct information in the multivariate weight change measurements. No other linear combination of the six weight change components gives a D^2 value greater than 0.807 (sometimes called the *Mahalonobis distance* after the statistician P. C. Mahalonobis, b. 1893).

Without a formal statistical test, it is difficult to tell whether a distance of 0.807 is likely measuring random variation or is likely due primarily to a systematic influence associated with parity on a woman's weight change pattern. Transforming the distance D^2 to have an f-distribution makes it possible to estimate the likelihood that the difference in weight change patterns between the two parity groups arose by chance alone. The transformation is

$$F = \frac{n_0 n_1 (n - k - 1)}{kn\,(n - 2)}\, D^2$$

where k = the number of multivariate components (six measurements), n_0 = the number of individuals in one group (70 women), n_1 = the number of individuals in the other group (23 women), and $n = n_1 + n_2$ is the total number of individuals sampled (93 women). As with many statistical transformations, the purpose is to create a test statistic linking the observed value to a transformed value that has a known statistical distribution, making it possible to produce a significance probability, that is, a p-value. The transformed distance $D^2 = 0.807$ becomes

$$F = \frac{70(23)(93 - 6 - 1)}{6(93)(91)}[0.676 - (-0.222)]^2 = 2.200.$$

The test statistic F has an f-distribution with $k = 6$ and $n - k - 1 = 86$ degrees of freedom when $D^2 = 0.807$ represents only a random fluctuation from zero. The p-value is then $P(D^2 \geq 0.807 \mid$ no influence of parity$) = P(F \geq 2.200 \mid$ no influence of parity$) = 0.05$. The multivariate analysis indicates "borderline" evidence of a nonrandom influence from parity on a woman's weight change pattern.

A next question is: *which components of the multivariate measurement are most influential in identifying the differences in maternal weight change pattern?* The magnitude of each a_i-coefficient making up the canonical linear combination depends on the units of measurement. When the measurement units differ, direct comparison of these coefficients has no useful interpretation. For the weight gain data, however, the six weight change measures are recorded in the same units (all six measured in kilograms). Since these variables are commensurate, a direct comparison of the coefficients indicates the relative contribution of each multivariate component to the canonical linear combination. The amounts of maternal weight loss during the first and second pregnancies ($a_3 = 0.462$ and $a_6 = -0.248$) make the most important contributions to the observed multivariate distance between the two parity groups and, perhaps somewhat surprisingly, prepregnancy weight has relatively little impact in discriminating between the two parity groups ($a_1 = 0.027$).

A Multivariate t-Test Approach

Another multivariate approach to the comparison of two groups uses the multivariate T^2-test (frequently called *Hotelling's multivariate T^2-test* after H. Hotelling (b. 1895), who developed this important technique[39]). Again, the dependent variable is the six-component weight change observation, and the two parity groups are compared. A key element of a T^2-test comparison is the variance/covariance array. This array contains all possible variances and covariances between the pairs of the components that make up the multivariate observation (denoted $\hat{v}_{ij}$ = estimated variance $(i = j)$ or covariance

$(i \neq j)$ between the ith and jth components). The six variances and 15 covariances for the weight change measurements are estimated within each parity group in the usual way and combined to give a single pooled estimate. For example,

$$\hat{v}_{23} = \hat{v}_{32} = \text{covariance}(\text{gain}_1, \text{loss}_1) = -5.76$$

$$\hat{v}_{66} = \text{variance}(\text{loss}_2) = 4.51$$

$$\hat{v}_{14} = \hat{v}_{41} = \text{covariance}(\text{weight, change}) = -10.64.$$

The entire 6 by 6 array containing all possible variances and covariances is displayed in Table 14.4. The six estimated variances are the diagonal elements $(\hat{v}_{ii})$ and the 15 estimated covariances are the off-diagonal elements $(\hat{v}_{ij} = \hat{v}_{ji})$ of the variance/covariance array.

The squared single variable (univariate) t-statistic for comparing two mean values is

$$t^2 = \frac{(\bar{x}_0 - \bar{x}_1)^2}{S^2_{\bar{x}_0 - \bar{x}_1}} = (\bar{x}_0 - \bar{x}_1) \times \frac{1}{S^2_{\bar{x}_0 - \bar{x}_1}} \times (\bar{x}_0 - \bar{x}_1).$$

Hotelling's T^2-statistic has an analogous form but in terms of matrix algebra (boldface indicates a vector or an array). The multivariate T^2-test statistic is

$$T^2 = (\bar{\mathbf{x}}_0 - \bar{\mathbf{x}}_1)' \hat{\mathbf{V}}^{-1} (\bar{\mathbf{x}}_0 - \bar{\mathbf{x}}_1).$$

For the maternal weight measurements,

$$\bar{\mathbf{x}}_i' = [\overline{\text{weight}_i}, \overline{\text{gain}_{1i}}, \overline{\text{loss}_{1i}}, \overline{\text{change}_i}, \overline{\text{gain}_{2i}}, \overline{\text{loss}_{2i}}]$$

represents a vector containing the six mean values, one vector for each parity group ($i = 0$ and 1) and $\hat{\mathbf{V}}^{-1}$ represents the inverse of the 6 by 6 estimated variance/covariance array (Table 14.4). The observed mean value vectors $\bar{\mathbf{x}}_0$

Table 14.4. The Estimated Variance/Covariance Array for
the Six Weight Change Measurements

	weight	gain$_1$	loss$_1$	change	gain$_2$	loss$_2$
weight	108.11	6.74	−5.56	−10.64	18.93	−0.89
gain$_1$	6.74	21.13	−5.76	−8.07	11.64	−3.15
loss$_1$	−5.56	−5.76	7.85	−1.57	−2.88	3.31
change	−10.64	−8.07	−1.57	22.74	−16.67	−2.05
gain$_2$	18.93	11.64	−2.88	−16.67	29.09	−1.67
loss$_2$	−0.89	−3.15	3.31	−2.05	−1.67	4.51

and $\bar{x}_1$ are the first two rows in Table 14.3, and the vector of the six differences $\bar{x}_1 - \bar{x}_0$ makes up the third row. To repeat, the two sets of six mean values are

$$\bar{x}_0 = [59.17,\ 12.81,\ 7.06,\ -4.85,\ 12.62,\ 5.71]$$

and

$$\bar{x}_1 = [59.45,\ 12.94,\ 5.53,\ -4.02,\ 12.08,\ 5.96]$$

giving

$$\bar{x}_0 - \bar{x}_1 = [0.28,\ 0.13,\ -1.53,\ -0.93,\ -0.55,\ 0.26].$$

Hotelling's T^2-statistic simultaneously contrasts all six mean differences between parity groups, taking into account the direct and indirect relationships among the multivariate components (covariances). For the 93 sampled women, the test statistic is $T^2 = 13.968$. Like the distance D^2, the value T^2 is difficult to interpret directly, but it too can be transformed to have an f-distribution where

$$F = \frac{n-k-1}{k\,(n-2)}\,T^2 = \frac{93-6-1}{6(91)}\ 13.968 = 2.200$$

allows evaluation in terms of a significance probability. Hotelling's T^2-test gives results identical to those found in the assessment of the multivariate distance between parity groups based on a canonical discriminant function (i.e., $F = 2.200$). Specifically, the p-value derived from an f-distribution to evaluate the observed T^2-value is again $P(T^2 \geq 13.968 \mid$ no influence of parity$) = P(F \geq 2.200 \mid$ no influence of parity$) = 0.05$. It is true in general that the two approaches (D^2 or T^2) are only different perspectives on the same issue and always give identical statistical results (i.e., identical p-values).

A Multivariate Analysis of Variance Approach

A third approach is a specific application of multivariate analysis of variance. In comparing two groups of multivariate measurements, the analysis of variance becomes a comparison of two variance/covariance arrays, as the name suggests. The first of these two arrays is estimated based on the conjecture that the parity groups differ systematically ($\bar{x}_0 \neq \bar{x}_1$ reflects a nonrandom difference—Table 14.3). The estimated variance/covariance array is then $\hat{\mathbf{V}}$ (Table 14.4).

A more restrictive conjecture is then made that no systematic differences exist between the two parity groups (only random variation causes the six mean weight measurements to differ between parity groups). The variance/covariance array is then calculated as if a mother's previous pregnancy history has no influence on her weight change pattern. In other words, the overall mean vector $\bar{\mathbf{x}}$ based on 93 observations (Table 14.1—column 3) estimates the common values of the six multivariate components ($\bar{\mathbf{x}}_0 \neq \bar{\mathbf{x}}_1$ reflects only random variation—Table 14.3), making no distinction between parity groups. Under this "no difference" hypothesis, a variance/covariance array (denoted $\hat{\mathbf{V}}_0$) is estimated ignoring the parity classification (Table 14.5).

When parity has an influence, this influence is likely reflected by systematic differences between the two estimated variance/covariance arrays $\hat{\mathbf{V}}$ and $\hat{\mathbf{V}}_0$. The difference between these two arrays is a direct function of the difference between the two sets of mean values $\bar{\mathbf{x}}_0$ and $\bar{\mathbf{x}}_1$. That is, if $\bar{\mathbf{x}}_0 = \bar{\mathbf{x}}_1 = \bar{\mathbf{x}}$, then $\hat{\mathbf{V}} = \mathbf{V}_0$. Otherwise, the two variance/covariance arrays differ. A single statistical criterion exists to evaluate simultaneously the magnitude of the differences between the 36 elements of these two arrays. Furthermore, this single value can be, once again, transformed to have an f-distribution linking it to a significance probability.

The impact of parity is evaluated formally by comparing the determinant of the variance/covariance array $(n - 2)\hat{\mathbf{V}}$ (parity has an influence) to the determinant of the variance/covariance array $(n - 1)\hat{\mathbf{V}}_0$ (parity has no influence). For the estimated arrays $\hat{\mathbf{V}}$ and $\hat{\mathbf{V}}_0$ (Tables 14.4 and 14.5), the test statistic is the ratio of these determinants or

$$\Lambda = \frac{\text{determinant}\,[(n - 2)\hat{\mathbf{V}}]}{\text{determinant}\,[(n - 1)\hat{\mathbf{V}}_0]} = 0.867.$$

As with the previous D^2-statistic and T^2-statistic, it is difficult to assess this criterion directly without relating the observed value to a statistical distri-

Table 14.5. Variance/Covariance Array Generated Ignoring the Parity Classification

	weight	gain_1	loss_1	change	gain_2	loss_2
weight	106.95	6.67	−5.42	−10.47	18.70	−0.89
gain_1	6.67	20.91	−5.66	−7.96	11.50	−3.12
loss_1	−5.42	−5.66	8.20	−1.29	−3.01	3.20
change	−10.47	−7.96	−1.29	22.65	−16.58	−2.07
gain_2	18.70	11.50	−3.01	−16.58	28.83	−1.63
loss_2	−0.89	−3.12	3.20	−2.07	−1.63	4.47

bution. A transformed test statistic based on Λ, like T^2 and D^2, has an f-distribution with $k = 6$ and $n - k - 1 = 86$ degrees of freedom where

$$F = \frac{n - k - 1}{k} \frac{1 - \Lambda}{\Lambda} = \frac{93 - 6 - 1}{6} \frac{1 - 0.867}{0.867} = 2.200,$$

which is identical to the previous two statistical tests. That is, the p-value is $P(\Lambda \le 0.876 \mid \text{no influence of parity}) = P(F \ge 2.200 \mid \text{no influence of parity}) = 0.05$.

One last note: if one variable is measured per observation, then these three multivariate techniques give answers identical to those obtained by applying the familiar univariate regression analysis, t-test, or analysis variance approaches.

CONCLUSIONS

A canonical correlation coefficient indicates that the pattern of weight change during and after pregnancy tends to repeat consistently between consecutive pregnancies. An observed canonical correlation of 0.598 means that a straight line rather accurately predicts the gain–loss pattern between pregnancies when summarized by a linear function.

Treating six measured weights over two pregnancies as a single multivariate response shows that parity (measured as a binary variable, no previous live births versus at least one previous live birth) likely influences the maternal weight change pattern. Three multivariate procedures give formal and identical analytic results. Specifically, the significance probability indicates that the likelihood is small that random variation is the entire reason for the observed difference in weight change pattern (p-value = 0.05), producing borderline evidence of an association.

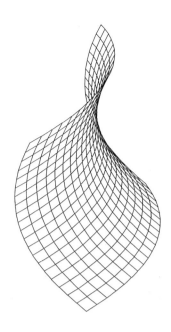

CHAPTER **15**

Smoothing
Sequential Data

OBJECTIVE

To describe the incidence and mortality patterns of Hodgkin's disease among African-Americans during the period 1973 to 1990.

DATA

A fundamental indication of the risk of disease within a population is an incidence rate (rate of new cases). A mortality rate is related to an incidence rate, and comparison reflects the survival of individuals with the disease. Using both the number of new cases of Hodgkin's disease and the number of deaths collected from 1973 to 1990 allow the calculation of annual age-adjusted incidence and mortality rates over this eight year period. The calculated rates refer to the U.S. male and female populations of African-Americans, and age adjustment was based on the U.S. 1970 age distribution. These data were collected as part of an extensive National Cancer Institute program entitled Surveillance, Epidemiology, and End Results (SEER). Incidence rates were calculated from all cases reported in the SEER areas where population-based cancer reporting systems are maintained with almost 100% completeness. The mortality data obtained from local and state vital records systems were classified by the underlying cause of death. The corresponding yearly populations at risk came from intercensus estimates based primarily on U.S. Census Bureau 1980 and 1990 enumerations. Hodgkin's disease is a complicated illness associated with a large number of epidemiologic factors. Genetic susceptibility, occupational exposures, infectious agents, environmental factors, and socioeconomic status are some of the risk factors thought to play a role in the occurrence of this disease.

METHODS

Two smoothing techniques are used to enhance the description of the secular trends in Hodgkin's disease incidence and mortality rates among African-Americans. Also, a simple linear regression analysis accurately describes the changes in mortality risk over the period 1973 to 1990.

Data type: time series (registry records)

Reference: *SEER Cancer Statistics Review*, U.S. Department of Health and Human Services, NIH Publication No. 93-2789

The variables are:

1. Year: recorded as 1973, 1974, . . . , 1990,
2. Male incidence rate: annual age-adjusted rate of new cases per 100,000 population
3. Female incidence rate: annual age-adjusted rate of new cases per 100,000 population
4. Male mortality rate: annual age-adjusted rate of deaths per 100,000 population
5. Female mortality rate: annual age-adjusted rate of deaths per 100,000 population

The tabulated data file producing 72 male and female Hodgkin's disease rates is:

name = hodgkins.15.data

year	male	female	MALE	FEMALE
1973	3.6	1.2	1.4	0.5
1974	2.4	2.1	1.2	0.6
1975	3.8	1.0	1.3	0.6
1976	3.5	1.3	1.2	0.5
1977	1.8	1.3	1.0	0.6
1978	1.8	1.1	1.0	0.4
1979	4.2	1.2	0.9	0.4
1980	2.0	1.3	1.0	0.4
1981	1.8	1.0	0.8	0.6
1982	2.7	1.7	0.7	0.5
1983	3.1	0.8	0.8	0.4
1984	2.9	1.1	1.0	0.4
1985	1.8	1.1	0.8	0.5
1986	2.5	1.6	0.7	0.4

1987	2.3	1.4	0.8	0.4
1988	1.9	1.8	0.6	0.4
1989	2.8	1.6	0.8	0.4
1990	3.0	2.5	0.7	0.3

```
  male = incidence rate among males
female = incidence rate among females
  MALE = mortality rate among males
FEMALE = mortality rate among females
```

BACKGROUND MODEL

Imagine two groups within a population, one made up of individuals who are at risk for a disease and the other made up of individuals who have the disease; N_1 individuals are at risk, and N_2 individuals have the disease. Furthermore, these two groups are at a *stable equilibrium*, which means that as new susceptible individuals enter the at-risk group, a number of susceptible individuals become ill and some of the already ill individuals die but the size of each group does not change. In symbols, over a specific time period, D_1 at-risk individuals contract the disease, D_2 individuals die, and since the population is at equilibrium, $D_1 = D_2$.

The disease incidence rate in this stable population is

$$R_1 = \frac{D_1}{P_1}$$

where D_1 new cases of disease occur among the N_1 susceptible individuals and P_1 represents the total person time accumulated among the at-risk individuals. Also, the death rate among those individuals with the disease is

$$R_2 = \frac{D_2}{P_2}$$

where D_2 deaths occurs among the N_2 ill persons and P_2 represents the total person-time accumulated among the ill individuals at risk of death. The quantity R_2 is a case fatality rate. Additionally, it is assumed that the rates R_1 and R_2 are constant with respect to time. The purpose of this model is to conceptualize the dynamics of these two important epidemiologic measures of risk (incidence and mortality rates), not to provide a statistical model in the sense of estimation and inference.[40]

This idealized equilibrium model illustrates three properties useful in understanding the relationship between disease incidence and mortality.

Property 1:

$$\text{rate in group } i = R_i = \frac{1}{\mu_i}$$

where μ_i represents the mean time to occurrence ($i = 1 = $ disease and $i = 2 = $ death). The property that a rate is the reciprocal of the mean time at risk is a direct result of a constant rate within both groups (i.e., constant hazard rate). It is a natural property that a high rate is associated with a shorter time at risk and a low rate is associated with a longer time at risk.

Property 2:

The mortality rate (denoted M) in the equilibrium population reflecting risk among all individuals (well and ill) is

$$\text{mortality rate} = M = \frac{D_2}{P_1 + P_2} = \frac{1}{\mu_1 + \mu_2}.$$

The mortality rate is simply the reciprocal of the mean time to occurrence of the disease among the disease-free individuals (μ_1) plus the mean time to death among those individuals with the disease (μ_2).

Property 3:

The ratio of the mortality rate to the incidence rate in this model population is

$$\text{mortality/incidence rate ratio} = \frac{M}{R_1} = \frac{P_1}{P_1 + P_2} = \frac{N_1}{N_1 + N_2}.$$

Not surprisingly, the incidence rate is greater than the mortality rate, or $R_1 > M$. Also, the ratio of the mortality rate to the incidence rate equals the proportion of susceptible individuals in the equilibrium population. Therefore, for populations at or close to equilibrium, the mortality to incidence rate ratio depends only on the relative population sizes N_1 and N_2.

DISCUSSION

Figure 15.1 displays annual age-adjusted incidence and mortality rates for African-Americans males and females per 100,000 persons-years at risk plotted by year of occurrence (1973 to 1990). The specific rates are given in Table 15.1. The incidence and mortality rates for males and females over the 18-year period vary considerably (Figure 15.1). This variation is primarily caused

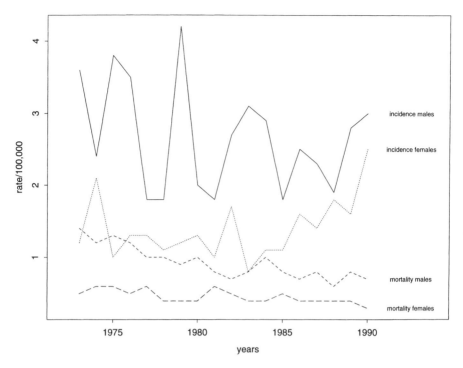

Figure 15.1. Incidence and mortality rates of Hodgkin's disease for African-American males and females (1973–1990).

by the small number of new cases and deaths occurring each year, which are highly influenced by random variation, extreme values, and a variety of biases. To identify patterns more easily and contrast the general properties of incidence and mortality risk, the rates are statistically smoothed. Smoothed rates result from trading a detailed description for a parsimonious picture, reflecting the underlying relationships between risk and year of occurrence. Two approaches are used to smooth the Hodgkin's disease rates, one simple[41] and one sophisticated.[42]

First Approach: Median/Mean Moving Average

A simple three-step process creates a smooth graphic representation of Hodgkin's disease risk over time. First, extreme values are removed; then each value is made to look more like its neighbors; and finally, new endpoints are estimated by extrapolation. Specifically, for n observed rates represented by $r_1, r_2, r_3, \ldots, r_n$, the steps are:

$$(1) \quad r_i^{(1)} = \text{median}\,(r_{i-1}, r_i, r_{i+1}) \quad \text{for } i = 2, 3, 4, \ldots, n-1$$

Table 15.1. The U.S. Incidence and Mortality Rates of Hodgkin's Disease
for the Years 1973 to 1990 for Males and Female African-Americans

Year	Incidence		Mortality	
	Male	Female	Male	Female
1973	3.6	1.2	1.4	0.5
1974	2.4	2.1	1.2	0.6
1975	3.8	1.0	1.3	0.6
1976	3.5	1.3	1.2	0.5
1977	1.8	1.3	1.0	0.6
1978	1.8	1.1	1.0	0.4
1979	4.2	1.2	0.9	0.4
1980	2.0	1.3	1.0	0.4
1981	1.8	1.0	0.8	0.6
1982	2.7	1.7	0.7	0.5
1983	3.1	0.8	0.8	0.4
1984	2.9	1.1	1.0	0.4
1985	1.8	1.1	0.8	0.5
1986	2.5	1.6	0.7	0.4
1987	2.3	1.4	0.8	0.4
1988	1.9	1.8	0.6	0.4
1989	2.8	1.6	0.8	0.4
1990	3.0	2.5	0.7	0.3

and

(2) $\quad r_i^{(2)} = w_1 r_{i-1}^{(1)} + w_2 r_i^{(1)} + w_3 r_{i+1}^{(1)} = 0.25 r_{i-1}^{(1)} + 0.50 r_i^{(1)} + 0.25 r_{i+1}^{(1)}$

$\quad$ for $\quad i = 2, 3, 4, \ldots, n - 1;$

then

(3) $\quad r_1^{(3)} = 2r_2^{(2)} - r_3^{(2)} \quad$ and $\quad r_n^{(3)} = 2r_{n-1}^{(2)} - r_{n-2}^{(2)}.$

Step 1 eliminates or minimizes the influences of extreme rates but tends to leave level spots in the smoothed curve and has no impact on consecutive sequences of three or more increasing values. Step 2 removes the flat areas and further decreases the local variability by increasing the similarity among neighboring observations. Step 2 is a special case of a general technique called a *mean moving average*. Step 3 completes the process by using the smoothed curve to estimate smoothed values for the first and last rates.

Table 15.2 illustrates the median/mean smoothing process. The median moving average (step 1) is applied to the male Hodgkin's disease incidence rates $(r_i^{(1)}$—column 2), removing extreme and possible outlier observations (for example, rates 3.8 and 4.2), producing incidence rates with less variability. The mean moving average process (step 2) further smoothes the 18

Table 15.2. The Process of Smoothing Male Hodgkin's Disease Incidence Rates

Rate	Iteration 1		Iteration 2		Iteration 3		Iteration 4	
3.6	3.6	3.62	3.62	3.74	3.74	3.83	3.83	3.90
2.4	3.6	3.60	3.60	3.60	3.60	3.60	3.60	3.60
3.8	3.6	3.58	3.58	3.46	3.46	3.37	3.37	3.30
3.5	3.5	3.09	3.09	2.94	2.94	2.89	2.89	2.87
1.8	1.8	2.12	2.12	2.29	2.29	2.38	2.38	2.44
1.8	1.8	1.93	1.98	2.06	2.06	2.14	2.14	2.20
4.2	2.0	1.98	1.98	2.01	2.04	2.07	2.10	2.13
2.0	2.0	2.00	2.00	2.04	2.04	2.10	2.10	2.16
1.8	2.0	2.17	2.17	2.25	2.25	2.29	2.29	2.32
2.7	2.7	2.62	2.62	2.57	2.57	2.54	2.54	2.52
3.1	2.9	2.83	2.78	2.73	2.72	2.67	2.67	2.63
2.9	2.9	2.78	2.78	2.72	2.72	2.67	2.67	2.64
1.8	2.5	2.57	2.57	2.58	2.58	2.58	2.58	2.58
2.5	2.5	2.47	2.47	2.49	2.49	2.51	2.51	2.53
2.3	2.3	2.34	2.44	2.45	2.49	2.50	2.51	2.53
1.9	2.3	2.44	2.44	2.52	2.52	2.58	2.58	2.62
2.8	2.8	2.76	2.76	2.78	2.78	2.80	2.80	2.81
3.0	3.0	3.08	3.08	3.04	3.04	3.01	3.01	2.99

incidence rates ($r_i^{(2)}$—column 3). Since median smoothing followed by mean smoothing does not affect the first and last observations, smoothed values are found by linear extrapolation, giving the values $r_1^{(3)}$ and $r_{18}^{(3)}$. This three-step process is applied again to the once smoothed values, and even smoother rates are produced (iteration 2—columns 4 and 5). Repeating the process several times creates a stable curve smoothly describing the incidence pattern of Hodgkin's disease among males over the 18 years (iteration 4—last column). A plot of these 18 rates and the other three similarly smoothed incidence and mortality rates are displayed in Figure 15.2.

The median/mean moving average process is a rather flexible description of a sequence of observed values. For this Hodgkin's disease application, the median moving average is based on observed rates grouped into sets of three. There is nothing special about this choice except that it yields a smooth but not too smooth pattern of Hodgkin's disease over the 18 years. Along the same lines, the choice of the mean moving average weights is equally arbitrary. The three weights ($w_1 = w_3 = 0.25$ and $w_2 = 0.5$) give a smooth representation of the incidence and mortality patterns, but other weights give equally useful smooth sequences. Smoothing techniques, in general, frequently require decisions based on subjective rather than analytic considerations.

Second Approach: Loess

A second approach to smoothing a sequence of rates involves a process called *robust locally weighted regression* (sometimes referred to as a *loess estimate*

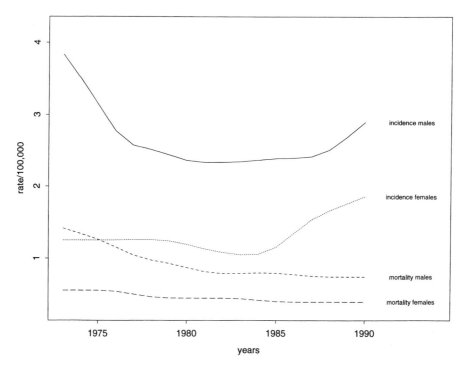

Figure 15.2. Median/mean moving average smoothed incidence and mortality rates of Hodgkin's disease for African-American males and females.

for short). Like the median/mean moving average approach, this technique provides a visually simpler picture intended to reflect the underlying pattern of Hodgkin's disease over time. Also parallel to the moving average approach, a robust locally weighted estimate combines two basic elements: minimal influence of extreme observations and reduction of local variation among neighboring observations. The implementation and some of the details of the loess smoothing process are complicated, but a general description is easily presented.

The loess smoothing process, like most smoothing processes, requires a set of weights. Here the weights are a continuous function (denoted $w(x)$) with three basic properties. For the scaled independent variable x, they are as follows:

1. $w(x) > 0$ over the range of x,
2. $w(x)$ is a smooth function of x, with its maximum value at $x = 0$, and
3. $w(-x) = w(x)$—equally distant observations are weighted equally.

The choice of a specific weight function is again somewhat arbitrary, but a popular choice is called a *tricubic function* (i.e., $w(x) = [1 - |x|^3]^3$ for $-1 \le x \le 1$).

For the Hodgkin's disease data, the polynomial expression

$$r_x = b_0 + b_1 x + b_2 x^2 + \cdots + b_k x^k$$

is used to create smooth incidence and mortality rates, using weighted least squares estimation with weights $w(x)$. The smoothed point at time x estimates the underlying rate, denoted $\hat{r}_x$. The degree of the polynomial k is small, usually as little as one or two. The process estimates a continuous function $f(x)$ from the model

$$r_x = f(x) + e$$

where, for the present data, r_x represents a Hodgkin's disease incidence or mortality rate, x represents any time of occurrence, and e represents an independent random error associated with each observation. Such a model justifies using the points in the neighborhood of a specific point as part of the estimate of that point's smoothed value. The estimated shape of the function $f(x)$ is determined entirely from the data and does not depend on any specific knowledge or assumptions. The resulting estimated rates are the first step in the loess smoothing process.

A second step is then performed in which the loess estimation process is modified. The modification is based on the size of the residual values (observed rate − estimated rate). Observations with large residual values are weighted so that they have relatively small influences; observations with small residual values, conversely, are weighted so that they have relatively large influences on the estimation of $f(x)$. Thus, the second iteration-estimated rates more strongly reflect the closely fitting values, minimizing the influences of the values that least reflect the observed/estimated pattern. This two-step process is repeated several times, yielding a stable curve relating estimated rates $\hat{r}_x$ to the time of occurrence x.

To illustrate, the robust locally weighted regression process is applied to the female Hodgkin's incidence rates, giving a smooth curve characterized by a slow decrease up to about 1985 followed by a relatively sharp increase. Figure 15.3 displays both the data and the estimated curve (upper left). As with all estimated curves, it is a good idea to inspect the residual values for outlier observations and check the normality of the error terms. Figure 15.3 contains a plot of the residual values (upper right) and a quantile-normal plot (lower left). The loess process also allows estimation of the standard errors associated with the estimated values yielding the 18 pointwise approximate 95% confidence intervals (one of each year), also displayed in Figure 15.3 (lower right). However, the basic purpose of a robust locally weighted regression estimate is a visually parsimonious description of the Hodgkin's disease incidence and mortality rates over the 18-year period (Figure 15.4).

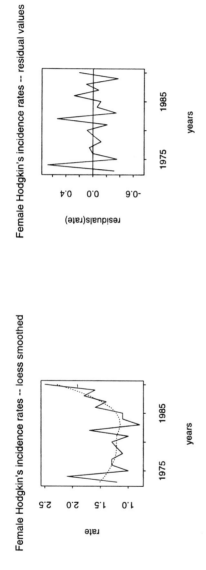

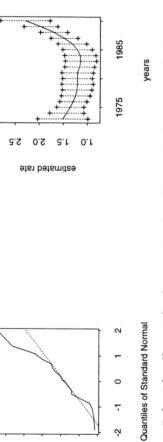

Figure 15.3. Robust locally weighted regression (loess): smoothed rates, residual values, quantile plot, and 95% confidence intervals.

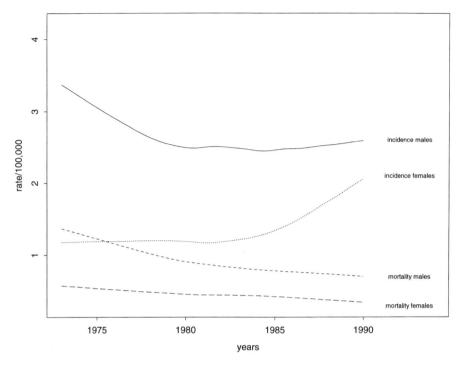

Figure 15.4. Robust locally weighted regression (loess) smoothed rates of Hodgkin's disease for African-American males and females.

CONCLUSIONS

Both moving average and loess approaches to describing incidence and mortality risk over time (years) show basically the same pattern. The smoothed incidence rates, after a 10-year period of decline in males and little change in females (1973–1982), increased over the next eight years, particularly the female rates. The smoothed mortality rates, however, continuously declined over the entire period. In fact, the decline is almost linear on the log-scale, with slopes -0.038 (male) and -0.026 (female). Therefore, the male and female mortality risk from 1973 to 1990 decreased at essentially constant rates. The males rate declined by about 4% per year and the female rate declined by about 3% per year. The clearly widening differences between incidence and mortality rates is, at least in part, because of better treatment strategies for Hodgkin's disease that have emerged in the last 20 years. In terms of the simple equilibrium model, the value of μ_2 has been extended, lowering the mortality rate M. The increase in Hodgkin's disease incidence remains unexplained.

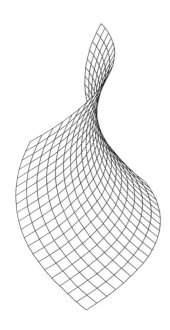

CHAPTER **16**

Nonparametric Regression Analysis

OBJECTIVE

To describe the influences on a newborn infant's birth weight of maternal prepregnancy weight and height in women who gained abnormally small amounts of weight during their pregnancies.

DATA

The Department of Obstetrics, Gynecology, and Reproductive Health at the University of California, San Francisco (UCSF) maintains a comprehensive database containing data on mothers and their newborn infants. To begin to understand the problems associated with mothers who fail to gain normal amounts of weight during pregnancy, a specific cohort of mothers and new-born infants was abstracted from this database. These women were healthy white women who gained less than 13 kilograms (25th percentile) during a term pregnancy and delivered a live-born single infant with no major congenital abnormalities. The infant's birth weight at delivery was also obtained from the UCSF database. The abstracted maternal variables, prepregnancy weight, height, smoking history, and age were self-reported during the first prenatal visit. A total 184 mother–infant pairs make up the study cohort.

METHODS

From the point of view of exploring and describing unfamiliar data, non-parametric regression methods are applied and the results primarily displayed graphically (without formal statistical testing). A parallel parametric regression analysis is also performed to provide comparable analytic results.

Data type: cross-sectional (hospital records)
Reference: *Obstetrics and Gynecology*, 1995, 86(2): 120–6

The variables are:

1. Maternal prepregnancy weight: reported in kilograms
2. Maternal height: measured in centimeters
3. Infant birth weight: measured in kilograms
4. Maternal smoking history: reported smoking coded 1 and otherwise coded 0
5. Maternal age: reported in years

Part of the data file of 184 sampled mother–infant pairs is:

```
            file name = birthweight.16.data
       wt          ht         bwt        smk        age
      52.3       167.6       2.480         0         29
      56.0       162.6       2.920         1         23
      55.5       162.6       3.800         0         33
      49.5       162.6       3.420         1         32
      52.3       162.6       3.920         0         35
      50.0       161.3       2.920         0         27
      49.2       160.0       3.350         0         23
      50.0       157.5       3.400         0         40
      84.0       160.0       4.000         0         30
      54.5       167.6       2.760         0         28
      58.2       174.0       2.800         0         22
      58.5       152.0       3.620         1         27
      75.0       176.6       3.560         0         35
      55.0       163.9       2.400         0         27
      56.8       165.1       2.100         0         22
       —           —           —           —          —
       —           —           —           —          —
       —           —           —           —          —
```

DISCUSSION

Table 16.1 contains a few descriptive statistics from the cohort of 184 UCSF mother–infant pairs. Summary values are almost always helpful; however, a more complete inspection of the properties of these variables requires more extensive statistical techniques.

Table 16.1. Summary Values for Maternal Weight, Height, Age, and Infant Birth Weight for 184 Women Who Gained Abnormally Low Amounts of Weight During Pregnancy

	Mean	Median	Std. Dev.	Minimum	Maximum
maternal weight	57.545	55.25	11.002	34.0	134.0
maternal height	163.169	162.60	8.601	110.0	190.5
maternal age	28.864	28.00	5.415	16.0	41.0
infant birth weight	3.314	3.33	0.545	0.7	4.8

Figure 16.1 is a graphic description of the 184 reported maternal prepregnancy weights. The histogram (upper left) displays the range and gives some idea of the shape of the distribution of the observed weights. A smoothed histogram (upper right) serves the same purpose and more realistically reflects the continuous nature of the maternal weight variable. As with all smoothed representations of data, a choice must be made as to how smooth a distribution to create. The smoothness is determined by selecting a bandwidth or smoothing parameter (denoted h and discussed further in the context of nonparametric regression). Increasing the bandwidth h increasingly smoothes the estimated distribution. A value of $h = 1$ yields a histogram-like estimate of the distribution. Increasing h to 20 creates a single continuous estimate of the underlying distribution of the maternal weight (lower left). A normal distribution reference band is included.[43] That is, an estimated normal distribution sampled from a population with the same mean and standard deviation as the sampled data (mean = 57.545 and standard deviation = 11.002) would likely fall within the displayed band. The estimated maternal prepregnancy weight distribution is slightly skewed to the left and more concentrated around the mean value than a normally distributed variable, producing a general lack of fit.

A smoothed estimate of a distribution is no different from most estimates. It is subject to sampling variation. Bootstrap estimates based on resampling the data and subsequent smoothing provide a visual assessment of the impact of sampling variation on the estimated distribution. Fifty such estimates ($h = 20$) are displayed in Figure 16.1 (lower right), indicating the likely range of curves expected for the estimated maternal prepregnancy weight distribution, a bootstrap-estimated *confidence band*.

The same four plots describing the maternal height variable make up Figure 16.2. Unlike the maternal prepregnancy weights, the estimated distribution of maternal heights appears to have at least an approximately normal distribution. The estimated curve is almost entirely contained within the normal distribution reference band (lower left).

Clearly, an individual's weight and height are related. For the 184 women sampled, the correlation between maternal weight and height is 0.366 ($r_{wt,ht} =$

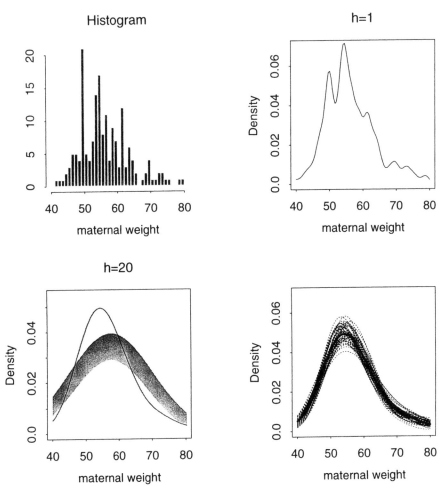

Figure 16.1. Maternal prepregnancy weight: histogram, density histogram, smoothed density plot, and a bootstrap-derived confidence region.

0.366). Since these two variables overlap in describing a woman's size, a joint distribution better characterizes the statistical properties of weight and height. Figure 16.3 is a perspective plot (sometimes called a *wire plot*) of the estimated bivariate distribution of weight and height. Like the outline of a single variable histogram, the surface of the perspective plot indicates where the data are concentrated (hills) and where the data are sparse (plains and valleys).

A less visual but more quantitative representation of the weight/height bivariate distribution is given in Figure 16.4 in terms of contours, specifically percentile contours. Each smoothed contour estimates the likelihood that a specific weight–height pair will be found within the circumscribed polygon.

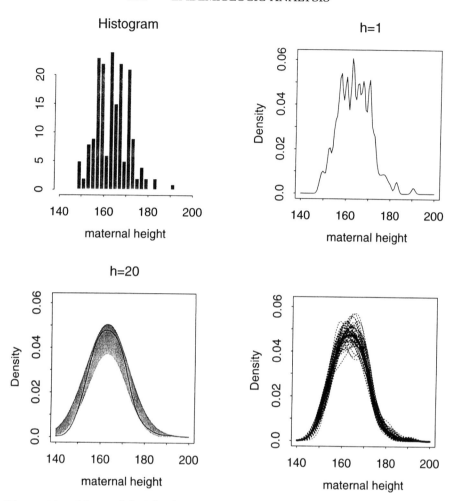

Figure 16.2. Maternal height: histogram, density histogram, smoothed density plot, and a bootstrap-derived confidence region.

For example, the median percentile (labeled 50) estimates where 50% of the weight–height pairs are likely located. Parallel to the median value associated with the distribution of a single variable, the 50th percentile contour indicates the location of the bivariate distribution. The 50th percentile contour creates a two-dimensional *interquartile range*. Additionally, the shape of the contours reflects the degree of correlation between the weight and height measurements.

Using contour polygons, differences among bivariate distributions are readily described. Figure 16.5 (left side) displays the "median contours" from the joint distributions of weight and height for mothers who smoke (dotted line) and mothers who do not smoke (solid line). The 50th percentile contours

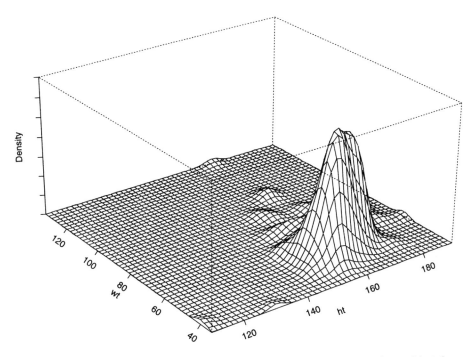

Figure 16.3. Bivariate distribution of maternal prepregnancy weight and height.

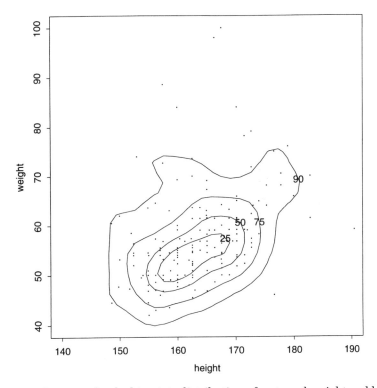

Figure 16.4. Contours for the bivariate distribution of maternal weight and height.

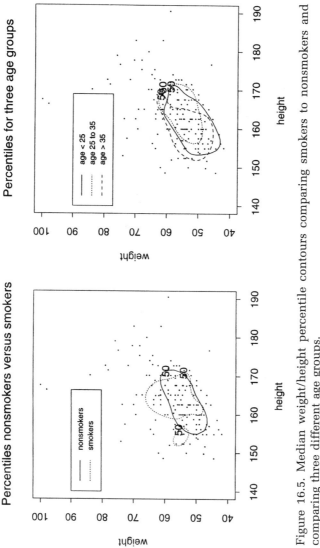

Figure 16.5. Median weight/height percentile contours comparing smokers to nonsmokers and comparing three different age groups.

have essentially the same location and size, showing little graphic evidence of systematic differences between the bivariate distributions.

Analogously, a plot of the weight/height bivariate distributions for three age categories (Figure 16.5—right side) displays the median polygons for mothers whose age is less than 25 years, for mothers whose age is between 25 and 35 years, and for mothers whose age is greater than 35 years. Again, no remarkable differences are apparent among the three 50th percentile contours, providing no indication that the weight/height distributions vary by maternal age.

Nonparametric Regression Estimation

A parametric regression analysis starts with a postulated model as the basis for describing and analyzing the relationships within a data set. A model-based approach has a number of advantages. A major issue, however, is the selection of the model (for example, linear or nonlinear and additive or non-additive). A nonparametric regression analysis does not have some of the advantages of a parametric approach. It does not, however, require the some-times difficult choice of an appropriate statistical model, providing an ideal way to explore new or unfamiliar data.

The basic structure of a nonparametric regression approach is expressed as

$$y_x = f(x) + e$$

where y_x represents a dependent variable that is a function of an independent variable x. The error term (denoted e) is assumed to have a mean = 0 and to be unrelated to x. Key to a nonparametric approach, the function $f(x)$ is not postulated from theoretical considerations but is estimated entirely from the relationships observed within the data.

A Local Mean Estimate

A local mean estimate is one way to construct an unconstrained, smooth regression curve describing the relationship between a predictor variable x and the outcome y, that is, to provide a nonparametric estimate of the function $f(x)$. A series of weights are employed, and the local mean estimate of $f(x)$ becomes

$$\hat{y}_x = \hat{f}(x) = \frac{\sum w(x_i - x \mid h) y_i}{\sum w(x_i - x \mid h)} \quad i = 1, 2, 3, \ldots, n.$$

The notation $w(x_i - x \mid h)$ represents the ith value of the n weights used to average the n observed values (denoted y_i) to estimate the dependent value

($\hat{y}_x$). The weights are used to combine all n observations into a single estimate of the function f, placing the greatest influence on the y_i-values in the neighborhood of x and relatively less weight on values of y_i as the distance $|x_i - x|$ increases. The nonparametric regression estimate is no more than a weighted average.

There are a large number of choices for the weights (denoted w) that depend on a bandwidth or smoothing parameter (again, denoted h). Such weights are chosen from generally smooth, positive, and symmetric functions peaking at zero and decreasing monotonically as the distance $|x_i - x|$ increases. Such a weighting function is also called a *kernel* function. The degree of smoothness of the estimated curve is controlled by varying the bandwidth h of the kernel function. A typical choice of a kernel function is a normal distribution with mean value x and standard deviation h.

Figure 16.6 illustrates the elements of a nonparametric local mean estimated curve (solid line) from a sample of 14 observations (circles). Any x-

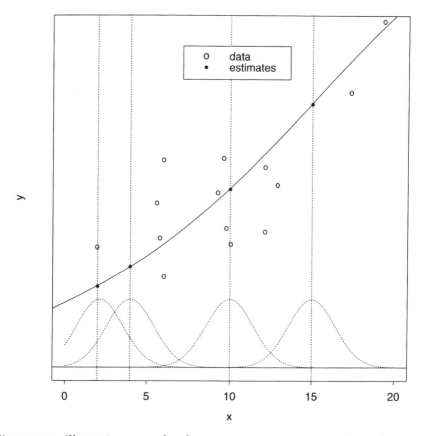

Figure 16.6. Illustrative example of a nonparametric curve constructed using a local mean estimate with a normal distribution kernel function.

value is chosen (say, x_0), and a value of the dependent variable is estimated (denoted $\hat{y}_0$—solid point) using the 14 data points (y_i) weighted by 14 heights generated at each point $x_i - x_0$ from a normal distribution with mean x_0 (kernel function—dotted lines) and variance h^2. Therefore, values of y close to x_0 receive relatively large weight and values of y farther from x_0 receive relatively less weight. The standard deviation of the normal distribution (kernel) becomes the smoothing parameter (h = bandwidth). Repeating the process over a range of x-values yields a nonparametrically estimated regression curve (solid line).

Figure 16.7 further illustrates, using the maternal weight data (x-values) to estimate a smooth curve predicting infant birth weight (y_x-values). The kernel function for the local mean estimate is a normal distribution, and four choices of a smoothing parameter are shown (standard deviations—$h = 1, 5, 10,$ and 20). When h is small, the resulting curve is locally sensitive, producing an estimated curve highly influenced by individual observations. As

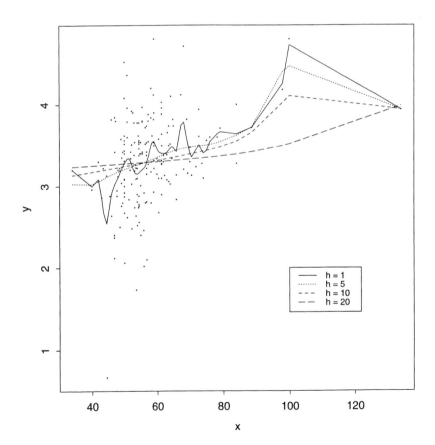

Figure 16.7. Local mean estimation of the influence of maternal prepregnancy weight on birth weight for four smoothing parameters.

h increases, neighboring maternal weights are combined, creating estimated values $\hat{y}_x$ influenced by a broader range of observations, resulting in a smoother nonparametric estimated curve.

Locally Smoothed Linear Regression

Instead of a locally smooth mean value estimate, a locally smoothed linear regression technique provides a more effectively estimated regression curve. This nonparametric approach involves minimizing a weighted least squares expression with respect to two parameters (denoted a and b) where

$$L = \sum \{y_i - [a + b(x_i - x)]\}^2 \, w\,(x_i - x \mid h) \quad i = 1, 2, 3, \ldots, n$$

produces estimates of a and b. The estimated parameter a then becomes an estimate of the dependent variable at the value x. In symbols, $\hat{a} = \hat{y}_x$ at $x_i = x$ when L is minimum. Again, a number of valuable kernel functions are available to weight the squared residual values, but the normal distribution is used in the following.

The choice of the bandwidth h is always an issue, and the results from three choices are displayed in Figure 16.8 ($h = 5, 10,$ and 20). The choice of a smoothing parameter can be based on a goodness-of-fit criterion and an optimum value selected.[43] Also, a choice can be based on nonstatistical considerations after trying a range of possibilities. A choice of $h = 10$ is illustrated in Figure 16.8 (right side) for the maternal weight data, giving an upward, nonlinear, smooth curve estimating the relationship between maternal prepregnancy weight and infant birth weight. This nonparametric estimate shows that heavier mothers tend to have heavier infants. Accompanying the local linear estimated regression curve is a 95% confidence region reflecting the impact of random variation. Note that the upper end (nonlinear part of the curve) is essentially based on five or six extremely heavy mothers. The confidence band pattern clearly indicates this uncertainty and, furthermore, indicates that infant birth weight is more or less a linear function of maternal prepregnancy weight for mothers who weigh between 40 and 80 kilograms.

The same analysis applied to the maternal height observations similarly gives an estimated curve (Figure 16.9) that predicts the pattern of infant birth weight. The chosen smoothing parameter (again, $h = 10$) yields a smooth curve indicating only slight increases in birth weight associated with increasing maternal height. The estimated curve is close to linear and, again using a 95% confidence band as a guide, shows no important relationship between a mother's height and the weight of her infant among women who gained only small amounts of weight during their pregnancy. The estimated curve is essentially a horizontal line.

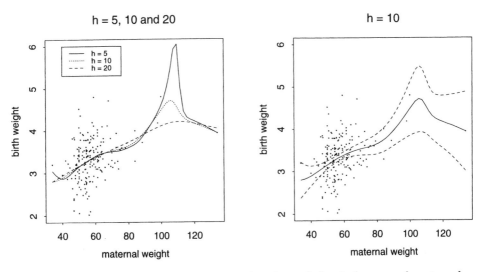

Figure 16.8. Local linear regression estimation of the influence of maternal prepregnancy weight on birth weight for three smoothing parameters.

A nonparametric estimate of a bivariate relationship is a direct extension of the single-variable local linear regression technique. Squared residual values each weighted by functions of the independent variables allow a smooth nonparametric estimate of the dependent variable y. In symbols, the quantity

$$L = \sum [y_i - (a + b_1(x_{1i} - x_1) + b_2(x_{2i} - x_2))]^2 \, w(x_{1i} - x_1 \mid h_1) w(x_{2i} - x_2 \mid h_2)$$

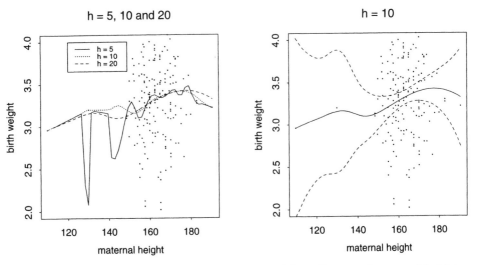

Figure 16.9. Local linear regression estimation of the influence of maternal height on birth weight for three selected smoothing parameters.

is minimized with respect to a, b_1, and b_2 where $i = 1, 2, 3, \ldots, n$. As before, the value $\hat{a}$ estimates the dependent variable ($\hat{y}$) at a selected pair of independent variables (x_1, x_2). Typical kernel functions are normal distributions with bandwidths h_1 and h_2 (standard deviations).

Using the maternal weight and height data, two plots of the nonparametric estimated regression surfaces are displayed in Figure 16.10 based on normal distribution weighting functions with two bandwidths ($h_1 = h_2 = 10$ and $h_1 = h_2 = 20$). In both cases, the estimated regression surfaces representing infant birth weight increase nonlinearly with increasing maternal weight and show little change with increasing maternal height. Additionally, the pattern of increase associated with prepregnancy weight is close to the same for all maternal heights. Necessarily, the pattern associated with maternal heights is then about the same at all maternal weights. That is, the nonparametrically estimated regression surface describes maternal weight and height as having at least approximately additive influences on the birth weight of an infant (no interaction).

Although nonparametric regression methods are most effective as data exploration tools, statistical evaluation of the impact of sampling variation is useful. Figure 16.11 shows two estimated weight and height curves with their associated reference bands. These reference bands are constructed in a fashion analogous to a confidence interval where a 95% reference band is described by

$$\hat{f}(x) \pm 1.960\sqrt{\text{variance}\,[\hat{f}(x)]}.$$

However, unlike a confidence interval, the reference band is estimated as if x was unrelated to y (null hypothesis). The reference band then describes the likely estimates of the regression curve when no association exists between

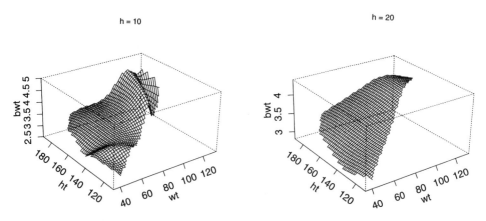

Figure 16.10. Local linear regression surfaces describing the joint influences of maternal prepregnancy weight and height on infant birth weight.

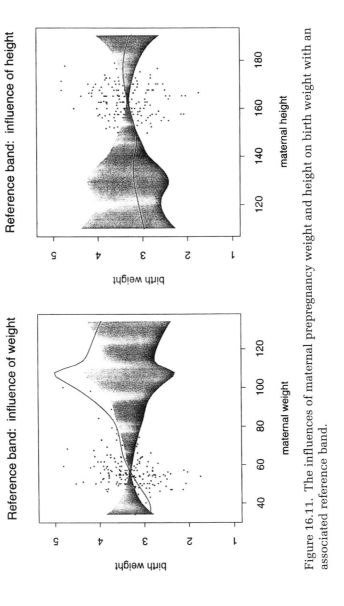

Figure 16.11. The influences of maternal prepregnancy weight and height on birth weight with an associated reference band.

independent and dependent variables, which then differ only because of random variation.

It is visually apparent (Figure 16.11) that the curve relating maternal weight to infant birth weight lies outside the "no association" generated reference band. Conversely, the curve relating maternal height to birth weight lies entirely within the reference band. These two graphic descriptions continue to indicate that maternal prepregnancy weight systematically influences the birth weight of an infant and maternal height does not.

A similar assessment of a nonparametric estimated curve is achieved with a randomization approach. A nonparametric estimate of the curve reflecting the relationship of x to y based on a random permutation of the independent variable produces an estimate of the curve as if no association exists. That is, a random permutation of the x-values guarantees that the dependent variable is unrelated to the independent variable, resulting in a nonparametric estimate influenced only by sampling variation. A collection of such curves constitutes a *randomization reference band*. Again, the variation among these curves indicates the likely range of an estimate relating the dependent x-values to the outcome y-values when no association exists.

For the maternal weight and height data, reference bands estimated from the random permutations of the 184 maternal measurements are displayed in Figure 16.12. The range of the randomization curves describes regions similar to the previously constructed "no association" reference bands. Both approaches (Figures 16.11 and 16.12) show from yet another perspective a nonlinear and likely systematic influence of maternal weight on birth weight and the absence of a relationship with maternal height among women who failed to gain normal amounts of weight during pregnancy.

Parametric Regression Analysis

Inspired by the nonparametric analysis, an additive linear parametric model with nonlinear independent variables is proposed to summarize formally the influence of maternal prepregnancy weight and height on a newborn's birth weight. That is, the form of the function $f(x_1, x_2)$ or $f(\text{wt}, \text{ht})$ is postulated rather than estimated. Specifically, the additive regression model chosen is

$$\text{bwt}_i = f(\text{wt}_i, \text{ht}_i) = b_0 + b_1\text{wt}_i + b_2\text{wt}_i^2 + b_3\text{ht}_i + b_4\text{ht}_i^2$$

where the expected birth weight (bwt_i) of an infant is a linear function of maternal prepregnancy weight (wt_i) and height (ht_i) variables. The included *squared terms* allow possible nonlinear influences from weight and height to be estimated and statistically evaluated. Least squares estimation yields estimates of the five model parameters and their standard errors (Table 16.2).

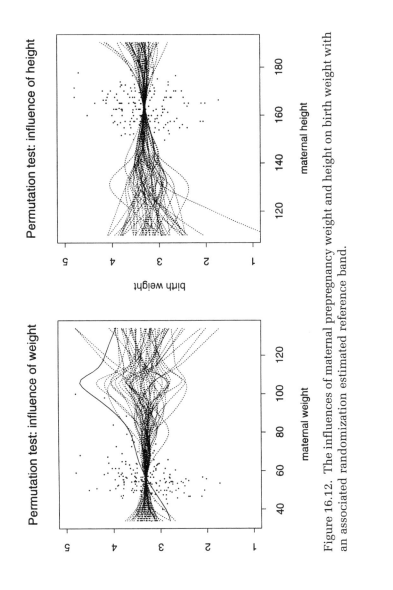

Figure 16.12. The influences of maternal prepregnancy weight and height on birth weight with an associated randomization estimated reference band.

Table 16.2. Estimates of the Model Coefficients Relating Maternal
Prepregnancy Weight and Height to Infant Birth Weight

	Coefficient	Estimate	Std. Error	t-Value
constant	b_0	1.441	—	—
weight (wt$_i$)	b_1	0.440	0.018	2.245
weight squared (wt$_i^2$)	b_2	−0.0002	0.0001	−1.332
height (ht$_i$)	b_3	0.003	0.056	0.053
height squared (ht$_i^2$)	b_4	−0.00002	0.0002	−0.850

Residual deviance = 47.399 with degrees of freedom = 179.

The parametric estimated regression surface based on the linear model
and the estimated coefficients is displayed in Figure 16.13. The additive
model dictates that the shape of the curve relating maternal prepregnancy
weight to birth weight is the same for all maternal heights; conversely, the
shape of the maternal height curve is identical for all maternal weights. This
additivity of influences is determined by the model, not the data. Similar to
the nonparametric description, increasing maternal weight is associated with
a nonlinear increasing birth weight and maternal height shows almost no
association with infant birth weight.

To display the weight and height relationships more clearly, Figure 16.14
shows separate parametric estimated regression curves and their associated

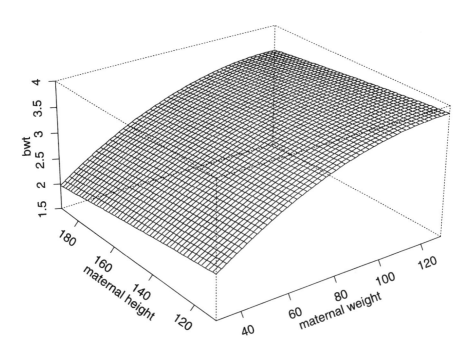

Figure 16.13. Parametric model estimated regression surface describing the joint
influences of maternal weight and height on infant birth weight.

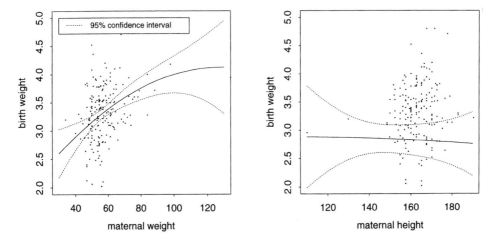

Figure 16.14. Parametric model estimated regression curves each describing the influence of maternal weight and height on infant birth weight.

95% confidence regions (dotted lines). These curves are calculated from the estimated model at the mean of the other variable. The relationship between maternal prepregnancy weight and infant birth weight (for maternal mean height = $\overline{ht}$ = 163.169) hardly differs from the corresponding nonparametric estimate (Figure 16.8—h = 20). A single model-generated curve is a particularly descriptive summary because the relationship between maternal weight and infant birth weight is identical for all maternal heights, since the curve is generated from an additive model. Figure 16.14 (right side) also clearly shows the previously observed lack of an association between maternal height (for maternal mean weight = $\overline{wt}$ = 57.545) and infant birth weight among the low weight gaining women.

To formally evaluate the independent influence of maternal prepregnancy weight, the weight variables (wt and wt^2) are deleted from the model ($b_1 = b_2 = 0$). The analysis based on the model containing only maternal height yields a residual deviance of 53.394 with 181 degrees of freedom. The residual deviance from this reduced model is compared to the value observed for the model including the weight variables (residual deviance = 47.399 with 179 degrees of freedom). The degrees of freedom in both models are the number of observations minus the number of parameters necessary to define the model (for example, n = 184 and the model requires 5 parameters, yielding $184 - 5 = 179$ degrees of freedom). The increase in the residual deviance (53.394 from 47.399) reflects the influence of maternal weight and is statistically assessed with an F-statistic or

$$F = \frac{(53.394 - 47.399)/(181 - 179)}{47.399/179} = 11.320.$$

The test statistic F has an f-distribution with 2 and 179 degrees of freedom when maternal weight is unrelated to birth weight. The p-value is then $P(F \geq 11.320 \mid b_1 = b_2 = 0) < 0.001$.

As with the nonparametric analysis, the 95% confidence region for the parametrically estimated maternal weight curve again shows that the non-linearity is primarily associated with a few extremely heavy mothers. The t-test associated with the quadratic maternal weight contribution ($\hat{b}_2$) yields little statistical evidence of an important nonlinear influence ($\hat{b}_2 = -0.0002$ and T-statistic $= -1.332$ with a p-value of 0.185). Both the confidence interval and the statistical test confirm the lack of evidence of a nonlinear association with prepregnancy weight, particularly over the range of most women's weights (40 to 80 kilograms).

Following the same pattern, the regression model has a residual deviance of 47.433 when the maternal height variables (ht and ht^2) are removed from the model ($b_3 = b_4 = 0$). The comparison of this residual deviance to the deviance produced when both weight and height variables are included in the regression equation (47.433 versus 47.399) yields an F-statistic of 0.064 with 2 and 179 degrees of freedom. The corresponding p-value is $P(F \geq 0.064 \mid b_3 = b_4 = 0) = 0.94$. As before, maternal height appears to have little if any independent influence on an infant's birth weight.

CONCLUSIONS

A nonparametric approach to assessing the influences of maternal prepregnancy weight and height shows in great detail the impact on an infant's birth weight. Using primarily graphic techniques, it is clear that heavier mothers tend to have heavier infants. This relationship is close to linear except for mothers weighing more than about 80 kilograms. For these heavier mothers, the impact on their infant's birth weight is considerably less, although this observation is based on only a few observations (i.e., large confidence intervals). Unlike maternal weight, maternal height shows no evidence of having an independent influence on an infant's birth weight. Taking these two results into account implies that the size of a mother is not an important factor in the weight of the child; rather, the mother's weight regardless of her height is a major predictor of an infant's birth weight.

A parametric linear model, designed to reflect the same relationships observed from the nonparametric approach, provides a series of formal statistical tests. That is, the linear influence of weight is substantial (p-value < 0.001), with a less important nonlinear component (p-value $= 0.18$). Parallel to the nonparametric analysis, maternal height does not appear to have an independent influence on birth weight (p-value $= 0.94$).

References*

1. W. G. Cochran, Some methods for strengthening the common χ^2 test. *Biometrics* 10:417–451, 1954.

2. B. Woolf, On estimating the relation between blood group and disease. *Ann Hum Genet* 19:251–253, 1955.

3. N. Mantel and W. Haenszel, Statistical aspects of the analysis of data from the retrospective studies of disease. *J Natl Cancer Inst* 22:719–748, 1959.

4. D. W. Hosmer and S. Lemeshow, *Applied Logistic Regression.* John Wiley and Sons, New York, 1989.

5. D. G. Kleinbaum, L. L. Kupper, and H. Morgenstern, *Epidemiologic Research.* Van Nostrand Reinhold, New York, 1982.

6. R. G. Miller, *Beyond ANOVA: Basics of Applied Statistics.* John Wiley and Sons, New York, 1986.

7. B. Efron and R. Tibshirani, *An Introduction to the Bootstrap.* Chapman & Hall, New York, 1993.

8. B. F. J. Manly, *The Design and Analysis of Research Studies.* Cambridge University Press, New York, 1992.

9. F. Galton, Regression towards mediocrity in hereditary stature. *J Anthrop Inst* 246–263, 1986.

10. C. Stern and E. R. Sherwood, *The Origin of Genetics: A Mendel Source Book.* W. H. Freedman, San Francisco, 1966.

11. R. A. Fisher, Has Mendel's work been rediscovered? *Ann Sci* 1:115–137, 1936.

12. I. Pilgrim, A solution to the too-good-to-be-true paradox and Gregor Mendel. *J Hered* 77:218–220, 1986.

---

*References frequently refer to textbooks that give a general description, which is likely more valuable for readers focused on applications. Readers who wish to pursue a topic in more detail can find references to the original papers in the cited texts.

13. F. Monaghan and A. Corcoe, Chi-square and Mendel's experiments: where is the bias? *J Hered* 76:307–309, 1985.

14. D. C. Hoaglin, F. Mosteller, and J. W. Tukey, *Understanding Robust and Exploratory Data Analysis.* John Wiley and Sons, New York, 1983.

15. S. Selvin, *Statistical Analysis of Epidemiological Data.* Oxford University Press, New York, 1996.

16. L. L. Cavalli-Sforza and W. F. Bodmer, *The Genetics of Human Populations.* W. H. Freeman, San Francisco, 1971.

17. B. Everitt, *Cluster Analysis.* John Wiley and Sons, New York, 1974.

18. R. A. Johnson and D. W. Wichern, *Applied Multivariate Statistical analysis,* 2nd ed. Prentice-Hall, Englewood Cliffs, NJ, 1988.

19. J. Fleiss, *Statistical Methods for Rates and Proportions.* John Wiley and Sons, New York, 1981.

20. L. L. Kupper, J. M. Karon, D. G. Kleinbaum, H. Morgenstern, and K. D. Lewis, Matching in epidemiologic studies: validity and efficiency considerations. *Biometrics* 37:271–291, 1981.

21. O. Miettinen, Individual matching with multiple controls in the case of all-or-none responses. *Biometrics* 25:339–355, 1969.

22. N. E. Breslow and N. E. Day, *Statistical Methods in Cancer Research.*, Vollumn 1. IARC Scientific Publication No, 82, Lyon, France, 1987.

23. J. Neter, M. K. Kunter, C. J. Nachtsheim, and W. Wasserman, *Applied Linear Regression Models,* 3rd ed. Irwin, Chicago, 1996.

24. N. R. Draper and H. Smith, *Applied Regression Analysis.* John Wiley and Sons, New York, 1966.

25. D. W. Hosmer and S. Lemeshow, *Applied Logistic Regression.* 1989. John Wiley and Sons, New York, 1989.

26. D. W. Hosmer and S. Lemeshow, A goodness-of-fit test for the multiple logistic model. *Commun Statistics* 10:1043–1069, 1980.

27. D. W. Hosmer and S. Lemeshow, Goodness-of-fit test for the multiple logistic model when the estimated probabilities are small. *Biometric J* 30:911–924, 1988.

28. N. E. Breslow and N. E. Day, *Statistical Methods in Cancer Research.*, Volumn 1. IARC Scientific Publication No, 82, Lyon, France, 1987.

29. A. S. Whittemore, Methods old and new for analyzing occupatiojal cohort data. *Am J Industrial Med* 12:233–247, 1987.

30. A. J. Wilcox and I. T. Russell, Birth weight and perinatal mortality: III. Towards a new method of analysis. *Int J Epidemiol* 15:188–196, 1986.

31. M. M. Adams, C. J. Berg, P. H. Rhodes, and B. J. McCarthy, Another look at the black–white gap in gestation-specific perinatal mortality. *Int J Epidemiol* 20:950–956, 1991.

32. Y. M. M. Bishop, S. E. Fienberg, and P. W. Holland, *Discrete Multivariate Analysis: Theory and Practice.* MIT Press, Cambridge, MA, 1975.

33. D. H. Freeman, *Applied Categorical Data Analysis.* 1987. Marcel Dekker, New York, 1987.

34. D. Collett, *Modeling Survival Data in Medical Research.* 1994. Chapman and Hall, New York, 1994.

35. R. G. Miller, *Survival Analysis.* John Wiley and Sons, New York, 1981.

36. D. G. Kleinbaum, *Survival Analysis.* 1996. Springer Verlag, New York, 1996.

37. D. R. Cox and D. Oakes, *Analysis of Survival Data.* Chapman & Hall, New York, 1984.

38. D. Morrison, *Multivariate Statistical Methods.* McGraw-Hill Book Co., New York, 1987.

39. H. Hotelling, A generalized *T* test and measure of multivariate dispersion. *Proceedings of the Second Berkeley Symposium on Mathematical Statistics*, 1951. University of California Press, Berkeley.

40. A. S. Morrison, Sequential pathogenic components of rates. *Am J Epidemiol* 109:709–718, 1979.

41. D. R. McNeil, *Interactive Data Analysis.* John Wiley and Sons, New York, 1977.

42. W. S. Cleveland, Robust locally weighted regression and smoothing scatterplots. *J Am Statist Assoc* 74:829–836, 1979.

43. A. W. Bowman and A. Azzalini, *Applied Smoothing Techniques and Data Analysis.* Clarendon Press, Oxford, 1997.

44. J. A. Rice, *Mathematical Statistics and Data Analysis.* Brooks/Cole, Monterey, CA, 1988.

45. C. J. Stone, *A Course in Probability and Statistics.* Duxbury Press, Belmont, CA, 1996.

46. N. L. Johnson, S. Kotz, and N. Balakrishnan, *Distributions in Statistics: Continuous Univariate Distributions*, Volumn 1. John Wiley and Sons, New York, 1996.

47. A. Agresti, *An Introduction to Categorical Data Analysis.* John Wiley and Sons, New York, 1996.

48. M. G. Kendall and A. Stuart, *The Advanced Theory of Statistics*, 4th ed., Volumn 1. Macmillan, New York, 1977.

49. J. Gullberg, *Mathematics: From the Birth of Numbers.* W. W. Norton, New York, 1997.

50. O. Kempthorn, *The Design and Analysis of Experiments.* John Wiley and Sons, New York, 1952.

Appendix

SOME TECHNICAL DETAILS

CONTENTS

1. INTRODUCTION

When Blase Pascal said "God is in the details," he must of been referring to statistical techniques. To understand an analytic method completely, the mathematical and statistical details are frequently important. For example, the evaluation of most statistical estimates requires, in some form, an estimate of the variance, a detail often not explained. These details are not hard to justify, but they do require a few mathematical/statistical tools. Once these tools are available, it is relatively straightforward to describe more rigorously the statistical analysis of epidemiologic data. Knowledge of the basis and mechanics of an analytic approach produces a better sense of how and why an application of a statistical technique works.

This appendix (a.1 to a.17) develops some of the relevant statistical details so that the techniques used in the 16 workshop data analyses are less mysterious. A good deal of the focus is on the variance formulas that are at the center of many statistical evaluations. However, some effort is also spent on a closer look at such techniques as the chi-square analysis, the Mantel-Haenszel-Cochran chi-square test of independence, and the Kaplan-Meier survival curve estimation.

2. VARIANCES OF SUMS

The variance of a discrete random variable X (denoted $variance\,(X)$ or σ_X^2) is defined as

$$variance\,(X) = \sigma_X^2 = \sum_{all\ x} (x - EX)^2 p_x$$

where EX is the expectation of X given by

$$expectation\ of\ X = EX = \sum_{all\ x} x p_x.$$

The symbol p_x represents the probability that the variable X takes on the specific value denoted x, or $p_x = P(X = x)$ and the sum contains all possible values of x.

The variance is a special case of the covariance defined as

$$covariance\,(X,\ Y) = \sigma_{XY} = \sum_{all\ x,y} (x - EX)(y - EY) p_{xy}$$

where $p_{xy} = P(X = x$ and $Y = y)$ is the joint probability associated with two variables X and Y. These definitions of expectation, variance, and covariance apply to discrete variables. The continuous case follows much the same pattern. The motivation and complete justification for these definitions are found in a variety of texts on elementary statistical theory.[44,45] Here the focus is on the properties of these two basic quantities and the ways these properties provide expressions for the variance of the sum of a series of observations.

If $x_1, x_2, x_3, \ldots, x_n$ represent a sample of n independent observations and each observation is transformed by multiplying or adding a constant value forming the sequence of n independent observations $ax_1 + b$, $ax_2 + b$, $ax_3 + b, \ldots, ax_n + b$ where a and b represent constants, then the expectation of the transformed variable is

$$\text{expectation of } (aX + b) = E\,(aX + b) = \sum_{\text{all } x} (ax + b)p_x = aEX + b$$

since $\sum p_x = 1$. The variance of the transformed value is

$$\text{variance } (aX + b) = \sigma^2_{aX+b} = \sum_{\text{all } x} [(ax + b) - (aEX + b)]^2 p_x$$

$$= \sum_{\text{all } x} [a\,(x - EX)]^2 p_x = a^2\sigma^2_X.$$

A special case occurs when $b = 0$; then $E\,(aX) = aEX$ and variance $(aX) = \sigma^2_{aX} = a^2\sigma^2_X$.

In general, the expectation of a sum of randomly selected observations or $E\,(\sum a_i x_i)$ is

$$E\,(a_1X_1 + a_2X_2 + a_3X_3 + \cdots + a_nX_n) = a_1E\,(X_1) + a_2E\,(X_2)$$
$$+ a_3E\,(X_3) + \cdots + a_nE\,(X_n) = \sum a_iE\,(X_i)$$

and the variance of a sum of independent observations or variance $(\sum a_i x_i)$ is

$$\text{variance } (a_1X_1 + a_2X_2 + a_3X_3 + \cdots + a_nX_n) = a_1^2 \text{ variance } (X_1)$$
$$+ a_2^2 \text{ variance } (X_2) + a_3^2 \text{ variance } (X_3) + \cdots + a_n^2 \text{ variance } (X_n)$$
$$= \sum a_i^2 \text{ variance } (X_i) \quad i = 1, 2, 3, \ldots, n$$

where all values denoted a_i are constants (nonrandom). The expectation of a sum of variables is always the sum of the individual expectations. The variance of a sum of variables is the sum of the variances only when the x_i-values are independent.

An expression for the variance of a sum of n observations that are not necessarily independent is

$$\text{variance } (a_1X_1 + a_2X_2 + a_3X_3 + \cdots + a_nX_n) = \text{variance } (\sum a_i x_i)$$

$$= \sum a_i^2 \text{ variance } (X_i) + \sum_{i \neq j} \sum a_i a_j \text{ covariance } (X_i, X_j).$$

The previous variance expression is a special case where the observations x_i are independent (i.e., covariance $(X_i, X_j) = 0$). More generally, the variance of a sum of a series of random variables is a sum of the variances and, in addition, of all possible pairwise covariances when the observations are related (i.e., covariance $(X_i, X_j) \neq 0$).

Specific Applications

VARIANCE OF A MEAN VALUE

If $x_1, x_2, x_3, \ldots, x_n$ represents a sample of n independent observations and the estimated mean value is

$$\text{mean value} = \overline{x} = \frac{1}{n} \sum x_i \quad i = 1, 2, 3, \ldots, n,$$

then

$$E(\overline{X}) = E\left(\frac{1}{n}X_1 + \frac{1}{n}X_2 + \frac{1}{n}X_3 + \cdots + \frac{1}{n}X_n\right)$$

$$= \frac{1}{n}E(X_1 + X_2 + X_3 + \cdots + X_n) = \frac{1}{n}\sum E(X_i)$$

since $a_i = 1/n$ is constant. If $E(X_i) = EX$, then $E(\overline{X}) = \frac{1}{n}(nEX) = EX$.

Additionally,

$$\text{variance}(\overline{x}) = \text{variance}\left(\frac{1}{n}\sum x_i\right) = \frac{1}{n^2}\text{variance}\left(\sum x_i\right) = \frac{1}{n^2}\sum \text{variance}(x_i).$$

Furthermore, when $\text{variance}(x_1) = \text{variance}(x_2) = \cdots = \text{variance}(x_n) = \sigma^2$, then

$$\text{variance}(\overline{x}) = \frac{1}{n^2}\sum \sigma^2 = \frac{1}{n^2}n\,\sigma^2 = \frac{1}{n}\sigma^2.$$

VARIANCE OF A DIFFERENCE

If two variables x and y are independent, then the variance of the difference $x - y$ is

$$\text{variance}(x - y) = \text{variance}[(1)x + (-1)y]$$

$$= (1)^2\text{variance}(x) + (-1)^2\text{variance}(y)$$

$$= \text{variance}(x) + \text{variance}(y).$$

Also, the variance of a sum of two independent variables is

$$\text{variance } (x + y) = \text{variance } (x) + \text{variance } (y).$$

The result that variance $(x + y) = $ variance $(x - y)$ at first may not seem intuitive but, in fact, subtraction is a special type of addition (i.e., adding a negative number). From this perspective, it is sensible that the variance of a sum and the variance of a difference of two independent variables are identical. However, when x and y are not independent, then

$$
\begin{aligned}
\text{variance } (x - y) &= \text{variance } [(1)x + (-1)y] \\
&= (1)^2\text{variance } (x) + (-1)^2\text{variance } (y) \\
&\quad + 2(1)(-1)\text{covariance } (x,y) \\
&= \text{variance } (x) + \text{variance } (y) - 2\text{covariance } (x,y)
\end{aligned}
$$

and

$$
\begin{aligned}
\text{variance } (x + y) &= \text{variance } [(1)x + (1)y] \\
&= (1)^2\text{variance } (x) + (1)^2\text{variance } (y) \\
&\quad + 2(1)(1)\text{covariance } (x,y) \\
&= \text{variance } (x) + \text{variance } (y) + 2\text{covariance } (x,y).
\end{aligned}
$$

In general, the variance of a sum of two variables x and y is

$$\text{variance } (ax \pm by) = a^2\text{variance } (x) + b^2\text{variance } (y) \pm (2ab)\text{covariance } (x, y)$$

where a and b are constants.

COMPARISON OF MEAN VALUES

An important contrast of three mean values is $\bar{x}_1 - (1/2)(\bar{x}_2 + \bar{x}_3)$ and

$$
\begin{aligned}
\text{variance } (\bar{x}_1 - (1/2)[\bar{x}_2 + \bar{x}_3]) &= \text{variance } (\bar{x}_1) + (1/4)\text{variance } (\bar{x}_2) \\
&\quad + (1/4)\text{variance } (\bar{x}_3) - 2(1/2)\text{covariance } (\bar{x}_1, \bar{x}_2) \\
&\quad - 2(1/2)\text{covariance } (\bar{x}_1, \bar{x}_3) + 2(1/4)\text{covariance } (\bar{x}_2, \bar{x}_3).
\end{aligned}
$$

If variance $(\bar{x}_1) = $ variance $(\bar{x}_2) = $ variance $(\bar{x}_3) = \sigma^2/n$, then

$$
\text{variance } (\bar{x}_1 - (1/2)[\bar{x}_2 + \bar{x}_3]) = \frac{\sigma^2}{n} + (1/4)\frac{\sigma^2}{n}
$$

$$
+ (1/4)\frac{\sigma^2}{n} - \rho\frac{\sigma^2}{n} - \rho\frac{\sigma^2}{n} + (1/2)\rho\frac{\sigma^2}{n} = 1.5\frac{\sigma^2}{n}(1 - \rho)
$$

where ρ represents the correlation coefficient measuring the linear association between all pairs (x_i, x_j) when x_1, x_2 and x_3 have the same variances and covariances.

COVARIANCE $(x, n - x)$

In general, for two variables x_1 and x_2,

variance $(x_1 + x_2)$ = variance (x_1) + variance (x_2) + 2covariance (x_1, x_2).

So, if $x_1 = x$ and $x_2 = n - x$, then

variance $(x + n - x)$ = variance (x) + variance $(n - x)$ + 2covariance $(x, n - x)$

or

$$0 = 2\text{variance } (x) + 2\text{covariance } (x, n - x).$$

Therefore,

$$\text{covariance } (x, n - x) = -\text{variance } (x).$$

Note that variance $(n - x)$ = variance (n) + $(-1)^2$variance (x) = variance (x), since n is a constant (nonrandom quantity with no variability—variance $(n) = 0$).

3. BINOMIAL PROBABILITY DISTRIBUTION

The binomial probability distribution is a centrally important discrete probability distribution, and the following defines some of its properties. A binomially distributed variable summarizes a series of variables with two outcomes. Specifically, consider a binary variable x_i (sometimes called a *Bernoulli variable*) with three properties:

1. The binary variable x_i is either 1 or 0 with probabilities p or $1 - p$, respectively.
2. Each x_i variable is statistically independent.
3. The probability p is the same for all values x_i.

The binomial variable, denoted X, is the sum of n of these binary values x_i or

$$X = x_1 + x_2 + \cdots + x_n.$$

More simply, the value X represents the count of the number of times x_i equals 1. The binary character of x_i makes the variable X an important summary for a wide range of situations with two outcomes—alive or dead, male or female, case or control, and, in general, event A or event not A.

The *binomial probability* associated with a specific outcome $X = x$ (denoted p_x) is given by

$$p_x = P(X = x) = \binom{n}{x} p^x (1 - p)^{n-x} \quad \text{where } x = 0, 1, 2, \ldots, n.$$

The term $\binom{n}{x}$ represents the number of different ways x values of 1 and $n - x$ values of 0 can occur among n values of x_i and is evaluated by, $n!/[(n - x)!x!]$. The quantity $p^x (1 - p)^{n-x}$ is the probability of a specific configuration of 1s and 0s. The product of these two quantities is the probability that x values of 1 and $n - x$ values of 0 occur in any order, making the sum $X = x$.

A direct result of applying these binomial probabilities is that the expected value of X for a series of n observations of x_i is

$$\text{expected value of } X = EX = \sum_{\text{all } x} x p_x = np$$

and the associated variance of X is

$$\text{variance } (X) = \sum_{\text{all } x} (x - EX)^2 p_x = \sigma_x^2 = np (1 - p).$$

The expectation and the variance of a binomial distributed variable also result from the application of the rules for expectations and variances of sums (a.2).

First, each binary variable x_i has an expectation and a variance. Since the probability that $x_i = 1$ is p and $x_i = 0$ is $1 - p$, the expectation and associated variance for this single binary variable are

$$EX_i = 0(1 - p) + 1p = p$$

and

$$\text{variance } (X_i) = (0 - p)^2(1 - p) + (1 - p)^2 p = p (1 - p).$$

Then, for the binomial probability distribution, the expectation (a.2) is

$$EX = E(X_1 + X_2 + X_3 + \cdots + X_n) = E(X_1) + E(X_2) + E(X_3) + \cdots + E(X_n)$$

$$= p + p + p + \cdots + p = np.$$

Since the x_i-values are required to be independent, the variance (a.2) is

$$\text{variance }(X) = \text{variance }(X_1 + X_2 + \cdots + X_n)$$
$$= \text{variance }(X_1) + \text{variance }(X_2) + \cdots + \text{variance }(X_n)$$
$$= p\,(1-p) + p\,(1-p) + \cdots + p\,(1-p) = np\,(1-p).$$

One last note: a proportion is estimated by $\hat{p} = X/n$ where X is a sum of n binary variables and

$$E\,(aX) = aEX \quad \text{so} \quad E\,(\hat{p}) = E\!\left(\frac{X}{n}\right) = \frac{1}{n}EX = \frac{1}{n}np = p$$

when X has a binomial probability distribution. Also,

$$\text{variance }(aX) = a^2\,\text{variance }(X)$$

so the variance associated with an estimated proportion is

$$\text{variance }(\hat{p}) = \text{variance}\!\left(\frac{X}{n}\right) = \frac{1}{n^2}\text{variance }(X) = \frac{1}{n^2}np\,(1-p) = \frac{p\,(1-p)}{n}.$$

4. HYPERGEOMETRIC PROBABILITY DISTRIBUTION

A hypergeometric probability distribution, like a binomial probability distribution, describes a count from a sample of observations each with two outcomes. The fundamental difference between a hypergeometric and a binomial variable (a.3) concerns the way the population is sampled. The sampling process associated with a binomial variable leaves the population unchanged (sampling with replacement—each binary event has the same probability). In the hypergeometric case, each sampled observation reduces the population size by one (sampling without replacement—each binary event has a different probability). It is sampling from a constantly changing population that produces the characteristics of a hypergeometric variable.

Formally, a hypergeometric distributed variable is made up of a series of binary observations (again denoted x_i) with two outcomes where

1. the binary variable x_i takes on the values 1 or 0,
2. each x_i value is statistically independent, and
3. the probability associated with each x_i depends only on the composition of the population at the time each observation is selected (not constant).

The hypergeometric variable X is the sum of n binary values of x_i or

$$X = x_1 + x_2 + \cdots + x_n$$

where the sample size is represented by n. Like a binomial variable, the hypergeometric variable X represents the count of the number of times x_i equals 1.

Consider a population of size N where m members have a specific binary characteristic (coded $x_i = 1$) and the rest $N - m$ do not (coded $x_i = 0$). A sample of n individuals is selected from this population. The random variable X is the count of the sampled individuals with the characteristic where each sampled observation is selected independently and without replacement. *Independently* in this context means that the probability that any individual is selected depends only on the composition of the population at the time of selection and does not depend in any way on whether the individual possesses or does not possess the characteristic. The minimum value of the hypergeometric variable X is the larger of the values 0 or $n - (N - m)$, and the maximum value of X is the smaller of the values m or n. The discrete probability associated with the variable X, called the *hypergeometric probability*, is given by

$$p_x = P\,(X = x) = \frac{\binom{m}{x}\binom{N-m}{n-x}}{\binom{N}{n}} = \frac{\binom{n}{x}\binom{N-n}{m-x}}{\binom{N}{m}}.$$

For a population size N, containing m members with the characteristic and $(N - m)$ without the characteristic, a sample of size n produces a description of the population in terms of a 2 by 2 table. The notation for a sample of size n selected from a population of size N sampled without replacement is

	With the Characteristic	Without the Characteristic	Total
sampled	x	$n - x$	n
not sampled	$m - x$	$(N - m) - (n - x)$	$N - n$
total	m	$N - m$	N

Interest is almost always focused on the number of individuals sampled with the characteristic (i.e., the value denoted x).

Using hypergeometric probabilities p_x, the expected value of the hypergeometric probability distribution is

$$\text{expected value of } X = EX = \sum_{all\ x} x p_x = n\left(\frac{m}{N}\right)$$

with the associated variance

$$\text{variance } (X) = \sigma_X^2 = \sum_{\text{all } x} (x - EX)^2 p_x = n\left(\frac{m}{N}\right)\left(1 - \frac{m}{N}\right)\left(\frac{N-n}{N-1}\right)$$

$$= \frac{nm(N-m)(N-n)}{N^2(N-1)}.$$

The term $(N-n)/(N-1)$ is called the *finite population correction factor*. This factor causes the variance of X to decrease as the proportion of the total population sampled increases (as n/N becomes closer to 1). When the population sampled consists of a finite number of observations, large sample sizes (relative to the population size) exhaust most of the observations, reducing the variability of X. Ultimately, when the entire population is sampled $(n = N)$, the variance is zero since X must always equal m for every sample $(\text{variance } (X) = 0)$.

For a small sample from a large population, the difference between sampling with and without replacement is not important. More technically, if N is much larger than n, the finite correction factor has negligible influence and the hypergeometric and binomial probability distributions become approximately equal. Not surprisingly, the expectations and variances of both probability distributions also become essentially equal $(N \gg n$ where $m/N = p)$.

5. CHI-SQUARE DISTRIBUTION: A PATTERN

A chi-square probability distribution describes the distribution of a test statistic widely used to compare observed values to values derived primarily from theoretical considerations. The complicated mathematical properties of a chi-square probability distribution are an important topic in the theory of statistics. Many applications of a chi-square distribution, however, follow a simple pattern. The pattern is:

1. When x_i represents one of m independent observations that is known or assumed to have a normal distribution, with mean $= \mu_i$ and variance $= \sigma_i^2$, then
2. $z_i = (x_i - \mu_i)/\sigma_i$ has a normal distribution with mean $= 0$ and variance $= 1$, then
3. $z_i^2 = (x_i - \mu_i)^2/\sigma_i^2$ has a chi-square distribution with one degree of freedom and
4. $\sum z_i^2 = \sum(x_i - \mu_i)^2/\sigma_i^2$ has a chi-square distribution with m degrees of freedom where m is the number of comparisons made between x_i and μ_i $(i = 1, 2, 3, \ldots, m)$; furthermore,

5. $X^2 = \sum \hat{z}_i^2 = \sum (x_i - \hat{\mu}_i)^2/\hat{\sigma}_i^2$ has a chi-square distribution with $m - b$ degrees of freedom ($i = 1, 2, 3, \ldots, m$) where b is the number of independent estimates $\hat{\mu}_i$ and $\hat{\sigma}_i^2$ used to establish the mean values μ_i and the variances σ_i^2. The value of b is not always obvious or intuitive.

The chi-square distributed value X^2 combines results from m sources of data and serves as a summary test statistic for a variety of comparisons between data and theory.

Example

The most commonly used chi-square statistics come from an expression developed by Karl Pearson around the turn of the 20th century given by

$$X^2 = \sum \left[\frac{(o_i - e_i)^2}{e_i} \right]$$

where o_i is an observed value (o for observed value) and e_i is an expected value based on theoretical considerations (e for expected value). The observed and expected values are often cell frequencies from a table.

The Pearson chi-square expression applied to tabular data is a special case of the chi-square pattern. To illustrate, consider a 2 by c table (a.14) where

	1	2	3	. . .	c
$X = 1$					
observed values	o_1	o_2	o_3	. . .	o_c
expected values	e_1	e_2	e_3	. . .	e_c
$X = 0$					
observed values	o'_1	o'_2	o'_3	. . .	o'_c
expected values	e'_1	e'_2	e'_3	. . .	e'_c

and $e_i = n_i p_i$ and $e_i' = n_i (1 - p_i)$ when p_i is postulated from theoretical considerations and $o_i = n_i \hat{p}_i$ and $o_i' = n_i (1 - \hat{p}_i)$ when $\hat{p}_i$ is calculated from the data. The index i represents a specific column of the 2 by c table. Then, the classic Pearson chi-square test statistic is

$$X^2 = \sum z_i^2 = \sum \frac{(x_i - \mu_i)^2}{\sigma_i^2} = \sum \frac{(\hat{p}_i - p_i)^2}{p_i(1 - p_i)/n_i} = \sum \left\{ \frac{(o_i - e_i)^2}{e_i} + \frac{(o_i' - e_i')^2}{e_i'} \right\}$$

from the 2 by c table ($x_i = \hat{p}_i$, $\mu_i = p_i$, $\sigma_i^2 = p_i(1 - p_i)/n_i$, and $i = 1, 2, 3, \ldots, c$). Note:

$$z_i^2 = \frac{(\hat{p}_i - p_i)^2}{p_i(1 - p_i)/n_i} = \frac{(n_i\hat{p}_i - n_ip_i)^2}{n_ip_i(1 - p_i)} = \frac{(n_i\hat{p}_i - n_ip_i)^2}{n_ip_i} + \frac{[n_i(1 - \hat{p}_i) - n_i(1 - p_i)]^2}{n_i(1 - p_i)}$$

$$= \frac{(o_i - e_i)^2}{e_i} + \frac{(o_i' - e_i')^2}{e_i'}.$$

A simple extension of this argument shows that the Pearson's special case of a chi-square statistic applies to any r by c two-way table. Therefore, in general, a Pearson chi-square summary X^2 allows observed and theoretically derived cell frequencies to be compared for all cells of a table producing a test statistic and, more importantly, a probability that all observed differences arose by chance alone (p-value). The theoretical values are derived under specific postulated conditions. These conditions determine the degrees of freedom associated with the chi-square test statistic X^2. Typically, the degrees of freedom are $(r - 1)(c - 1)$.

An Application: Woolf's Test for Homogeneity

Relationships within a series of k observed 2 by 2 tables are often characterized by a series of k estimated odds ratios, where an odds ratio $\hat{or}_i$ is calculated for each table. Woolf's procedure addresses the question of whether these odds ratios differ substantially using the test statistic

$$X_W^2 = \sum w_i [\log(\hat{or}_i) - \overline{\log(or)}]^2.$$

This chi-square statistic results from applying the previously described pattern.

The value $\log(\hat{or}_i)$ has an approximate normal distribution (i.e., $x_i = \log(or_i)$). Furthermore, each estimated log-odds ratio is assumed to estimate the same value. That is, the k estimates differ only because of random variation (homogeneous—$or_1 = or_2 = or_3 = \cdots = or_k = or$). The common value underlying the logarithms of the odds ratios is then estimated by the weighted average

$$\overline{\log(or)} = \frac{\sum w_i \log(\hat{or}_i)}{\sum w_i} \quad i = 1, 2, 3, \ldots, k$$

where the weights w_i are the reciprocal of the estimated variance of the logarithm of the odds ratio (a.11) from each 2 by 2 table. Or the weights are

$$w_i = \frac{1}{S_{\log(\hat{or}_i)}^2}.$$

Then

$$z_i = \frac{x_i - \hat{\mu}}{\hat{\sigma}_i} = \frac{\log{(\hat{or}_i)} - \overline{\log{(or)}}}{S_{\log{(\hat{or}_i)}}}$$

$$= \sqrt{w_i} \, [\log{(\hat{or}_i)} - \overline{\log{(or)}}]$$

where $\quad x_i = \log{(\hat{or}_i)}, \; \hat{\mu} = \overline{\log{(or)}}, \; \text{and} \; \hat{\sigma}_i = S_{\log{(\hat{or}_i)}}$

has an approximate standard normal distribution. Then the quantity z_i^2 has a chi-square distribution with one degree of freedom. Therefore,

$$X_W^2 = \Sigma z_i^2 = \Sigma w_i \, [\log{(\hat{or}_i)} - \overline{\log{(or)}}]^2 \quad i = 1, 2, 3, \ldots, k$$

has an approximate chi-square distribution with $k - 1$ degrees of freedom when only random differences exist among the k odds ratios.

Incidentally, when no evidence exists that the k odds ratios systematically differ (homogeneous), an estimate of the common odds ratio is

$$\text{estimated common odds ratio} = \hat{or} = e^{\overline{\log{(or)}}}.$$

6. MANTEL-HAENSZEL SUMMARY ODDS RATIO

When k odds ratios are calculated each from a series of 2 by 2 tables, it is frequently desirable to summarize all k estimates with a single value. One such approach is the Woolf weighted average estimate (a.5). Alternatively, the Mantel-Haenszel summary odds ratio also summarizes the association in a series of 2 by 2 tables denoted

table$_i$	B_1	B_2
A_1	a_i	b_i
A_2	c_i	d_i

Each table produces an estimated odds ratio. For the ith table

$$\hat{or}_i = \frac{a_i/b_i}{c_i/d_i} = \frac{a_i/c_i}{b_i/d_i} = \frac{a_i d_i}{b_i c_i}.$$

The estimated odds ratio $\hat{or}_i$ measures the association between the binary variables A and B used to construct each table (a.11).

If the odds ratios estimate the same degree of association in each of the k observed 2 by 2 tables (i.e., homogeneous—$or_1 = or_2 = or_3 = \cdots = or_k = or$), then the Mantel-Haenszel expression is a straightforward estimate of the common value. If the odds ratios are not random deviations from a common value, then a single summary is likely misleading. Woolf's procedure (a.5) is designed to evaluate the equality of a series of odds ratios.

The Mantel-Haenszel summary odds ratio based on k homogeneous tables is

$$\hat{or}_{MH} = \frac{\sum a_i d_i / n_i}{\sum b_i c_i / n_i} \quad i = 1, 2, 3, \ldots, k$$

where $n_i = a_i + b_i + c_i + d_i$ is the total number of observations contained in the ith table. The Mantel-Haenszel summary odds ratio can be viewed as a weighted average where

$$\hat{or}_{MH} = \frac{\sum w_i \hat{or}_i}{\sum w_i} = \frac{\sum (b_i c_i / n_i) \hat{or}_i}{\sum b_i c_i / n_i} = \frac{\sum a_i d_i / n_i}{\sum b_i c_i / n_i} \quad i = 1, 2, 3, \ldots, k$$

with weights $w_i = b_i c_i / n_i$. A perhaps surprising property of this summary odds ratio is that the values n_i can be small (even $n_i = 2$) and the Mantel-Haenszel summary odds ratio $\hat{or}_{MH}$ continues to estimate the common odds ratio.

Example

When the odds ratios from a series of 2 by 2 tables reflect different associations (not homogeneous), the summary odds ratio becomes a relatively meaningless average value. For example, if

table 1	B_1	B_2
A_1	50	10
A_2	10	5

then $\hat{or}_1 = 50(5)/[10(10)] = 2.5$ and if

table 2	B_1	B_2
A_1	10	5
A_2	50	10

then $\hat{or}_2 = 10(10)/[50(5)] = 0.4$.

The Mantel-Haenszel summary odds ratio is

$$\hat{or}_{MH} = \frac{50(5)/75 + 10(10)/75}{10(10)/75 + 50(5)/75} = 1.0,$$

reflecting neither $\hat{or}_1$ or $\hat{or}_2$.

Application to Matched Data

A series of matched sets are frequently described as a series of 2 by 2 tables. When a case is matched with two controls, six different 2 by 2 tables possibly occur. Using the symbol F to represent the presence and $\bar{F}$ the absence of a risk factor, these six tables become

1. one case—two controls

	F	$\bar{F}$	total
case	1	0	1
control	2	0	2
total	3	0	3

2. one case—one control

	F	$\bar{F}$	total
case	1	0	1
control	1	1	2
total	2	1	3

3. one case—no controls

	F	$\bar{F}$	total
case	1	0	1
control	0	2	2
total	1	2	3

4. no cases—two controls

	F	$\bar{F}$	total
case	0	1	1
control	2	0	2
total	2	1	3

5. no cases—one control

	F	$\bar{F}$	total
case	0	1	1
control	1	1	2
total	1	2	3

6. no cases—no controls

	F	$\bar{F}$	total
case	0	1	1
control	0	2	2
total	0	3	3

Only these six kinds of tables make up the data collected from a matched design (one case and two controls) and are summarized as follows:

Type	$a_i d_i$	$b_i c_i$	n_i	n_{ij}
1	0	0	3	n_{12}
2	1	0	3	n_{11}
3	2	0	3	n_{10}
4	0	2	3	n_{02}
5	0	1	3	n_{01}
6	0	0	3	n_{00}

where n_{ij} represents the number of identical matched sets (identical tables) and $n = n_{12} + n_{11} + n_{10} + n_{02} + n_{01} + n_{00}$ represents the total number of matched sets (tables). The Mantel-Haenszel summary odds ratio estimate is then

$$\hat{or}_m = \frac{\sum a_i d_i / n_i}{\sum b_i c_i / n_i} = \frac{0 n_{12}/3 + 1 n_{11}/3 + 2 n_{10}/3 + 0 n_{02}/3 + 0 n_{01}/3 + 0 n_{00}/3}{0 n_{12}/3 + 0 n_{11}/3 + 0 n_{10}/3 + 2 n_{02}/3 + 1 n_{01}/3 + 0 n_{00}/3}$$

$$= \frac{n_{11} + 2 n_{10}}{2 n_{02} + n_{01}}.$$

The estimated summary odds ratio $\hat{o}r_m$ (m for matched) is a direct application of the Mantel-Haenszel procedure measuring the association between case/controls status and the presence/absence of a risk factor when the sample size in each table is three ($n_i = 3$).

7. MANTEL-HAENSZEL-COCHRAN TEST FOR INDEPENDENCE

When a binary risk factor (denoted F) and a binary disease outcome (denoted D) are considered, the observations are typically displayed in a 2 by 2 table. Furthermore, if these tables are generated for each of k levels of a third categorical variable, then the ith table is again denoted as

Level i	D	$\overline{D}$	Total
F	a_i	b_i	$a_i + b_i$
$\overline{F}$	c_i	d_i	$c_i + d_i$
total	$a_i + c_i$	$b_i + d_i$	n

where F represents the risk factor present, $\overline{F}$ represents the risk factor absent, D represents the "disease" present, and $\overline{D}$ represents the "disease" absent. The cell counts a_i, b_i, c_i, and d_i ($i = 1, 2, 3, \ldots, k$) denote the frequency of the four possible joint outcomes within a specific level of a third variable (the ith level). The Mantel-Haenszel-Cochran test is used to evaluate whether the risk factor F is associated with the disease D in some or all of the 2 by 2 tables formed within each of k strata of a third variable.

A Mantel-Haenszel-Cochran evaluation of the associations within a series of tables requires each table to be independent of the other $k - 1$ tables. Additionally, each 2 by 2 table must reflect the same association; that is, all measures of association differ only because of random variation (i.e., homogeneous—no interaction). Lastly, it is convenient to treat the marginal frequencies as if they are fixed, giving the cell count a_i a hypergeometric probability distribution (a.4).

The symbol a_i represents the number of individuals with both the risk factor and the disease in a specific table. It then follows that

1. the sum of the individuals with both the risk factor and the disease ($\sum a_i$) serves as a test statistic summarizing the degree of association reflected by the k independent 2 by 2 tables;
2. the sum $\sum \hat{A}_i$ estimates the expected value of $\sum a_i$ when no association exists between risk factor and disease and is the sum of k estimates of A_i where

$$\hat{A}_i = (a_i + b_i)(a_i + c_i)/n_i;$$

3. the variance of a_i (variance (a_i)) comes from the hypergeometric distribution (a.4) and is estimated by

$$\text{variance } (a_i) = \frac{(a_i + b_i)(c_i + d_i)(a_i + c_i)(b_i + d_i)}{n_i^2(n_i - 1)}$$

and variance $(\Sigma a_i) = \Sigma \text{variance } (a_i)$ since the k tables are independent. Therefore, properties 1, 2, and 3 produce

$$z = \frac{X - EX}{\sigma_X} = \frac{\Sigma a_i - \Sigma \hat{A}_i}{\sqrt{\text{variance } (\Sigma a_i)}} = \frac{\Sigma a_i - \Sigma \hat{A}_i}{\sqrt{\Sigma \text{variance } (a_i)}}$$

and the test statistic z has an approximate normal distribution with mean = 0 and variance = 1 when the risk factor and disease are independent within all k tables. The total number of individuals with the risk factor Σa_i is contrasted to the total number expected when the risk factor is unrelated to the disease $\Sigma \hat{A}_i$. Large differences imply an association.

More typically the Mantel-Haenszel-Cochran test statistic is expressed as chi-square statistic (a.5) where

$$z^2 = X^2 = \frac{(\Sigma a_i - \Sigma \hat{A}_i)^2}{\Sigma \text{variance } (a_i)},$$

which has an approximate chi-square distribution with one degree of freedom when the risk factor (F) is unrelated to the disease (D) within all k tables.

Example

Data on smoking and low birth weight infants form four 2 by 2 tables, each displaying the relationship between smoking (F) and birth weight of less than 2500 grams (D) stratified into four race/ethnicity groups $(k = 4)$.

Birth weight	White Low	White Normal	Hispanic Low	Hispanic Normal	African-American Low	African-American Normal	Asian Low	Asian Normal
smoker	98	832	54	227	11	85	7	102
nonsmoker	169	3520	55	686	61	926	90	1936

Summary statistics are:

Race	a_i	b_i	c_i	d_i	n_i	$a_i + b_i$	$a_i + c_i$	$\hat{A}_i$	v_i^*
white	98	832	169	3520	4619	930	267	53.758	40.461
black	54	227	55	686	1022	281	109	29.970	19.431
Hispanic	11	85	61	926	1083	96	72	6.382	5.435
Asian	7	102	90	1936	2135	109	97	4.952	4.488
total	170	1246	375	7068	8859	1416	545	95.063	69.815

$^*v_i$ = variance (a_i) estimated from the hypergeometric distribution.

Summary values are:

$$\Sigma a_i = 170, \ \Sigma \hat{A}_i = 95.063, \ \Sigma a_i - \Sigma \hat{A}_i = 74.937$$

and

$$\text{variance} \ (\Sigma a_i) = \Sigma \text{variance} \ (a_i) = \Sigma v_i = 69.815$$

giving

$$X^2 = \frac{(\Sigma a_i - \Sigma \hat{A}_i)^2}{\Sigma \text{variance} \ (a_i)} = \frac{(74.937)^2}{69.815} = 80.435.$$

Then the p-value is $P(X^2 \geq 80.435 \mid \text{no association}) < 0.001$, leaving little doubt that smoking is related to the risk of a low birth weight infant. That is, the observed 170 low birth weight infants of smoking mothers is extremely unlikely to be a random deviation from the 95.063 expected when smoking and birth weight are unrelated.

Application

A sample of matched sets is no more than a series of 2 by 2 table, as already noted (a.6). Furthermore, the assessment of the association between case/control status and a risk factor is a direct application of the Mantel-Haenszel-Cochran test for independence. Data collected in matched sets of one case and two controls produce six different 2 by 2 tables. These tables and their summary values are presented in the following discussion.

Within the ith table, the values represented by a_i, $\hat{A}_i$, and v_i are the observed frequency of cases with the risk factor, the estimated number of cases when the disease and the risk factor are unrelated, and the estimated variance based on the hypergeometric distribution, respectively. The values v_i are a direct result of considering each 2 by 2 table a sample from a hypergeometric probability distribution (a.4). The symbol F again represents the presence and $\overline{F}$ the absence of the risk factor.

MATCHED DATA (1:2)

1. one case—two controls

	F	$\overline{F}$	total
case	1	0	1
control	2	0	2
total	3	0	3

n_{12} tables
$a_1 = 1$
$\hat{A}_1 = 1$
$v_1 = 0$

2. one case—one control

	F	$\overline{F}$	total
case	1	0	1
control	1	1	2
total	2	1	3

n_{11} tables
$a_2 = 1$
$\hat{A}_2 = 2/3$
$v_2 = 2/9$

3. one case—no controls

	F	$\overline{F}$	total
case	1	0	1
control	0	2	2
total	1	2	3

n_{10} tables
$a_3 = 1$
$\hat{A}_3 = 1/3$
$v_3 = 2/9$

4. no cases—two controls

	F	$\overline{F}$	total
case	0	1	1
control	2	0	2
total	2	1	3

n_{02} tables
$a_4 = 0$
$\hat{A}_4 = 2/3$
$v_4 = 2/9$

5. no cases—one control

	F	$\overline{F}$	total
case	0	1	1
control	1	1	2
total	1	2	3

n_{01} tables
$a_5 = 0$
$\hat{A}_5 = 1/3$
$v_5 = 2/9$

6. no cases—no controls

	F	$\overline{F}$	total
case	0	1	1
control	0	2	2
total	0	3	3

n_{00} tables
$a_6 = 0$
$\hat{A}_6 = 0$
$v_6 = 0$

A straightforward application of the Mantel-Haenszel-Cochran chi-square procedure using the n matched sets (i.e., all 2 by 2 tables) produce a chi-square test statistic with one degree of freedom to evaluate the association between case/control status and the presence/absence of the risk factor F in matched data.

Summary Statistics

number of matched sets $= n = n_{12} + n_{11} + n_{10} + n_{02} + n_{01} + n_{00}.$

Then

$$\Sigma a_i = n_{12} + n_{11} + n_{10},$$

$$\Sigma \hat{A}_i = (1)n_{12} + (2/3)n_{11} + (1/3)n_{10} + (2/3)n_{02} + (1/3)n_{01} + (0)n_{00},$$

$$\Sigma(a_i - \hat{A}_i) = (1/3)(n_{11} + 2n_{10} - [2n_{02} + n_{01}])$$

and

$$\Sigma \text{variance } (a_i) = n_{12}v_1 + n_{11}v_2 + n_{10}v_3 + n_{02}v_4 + n_{01}v_5 + n_{00}v_6$$
$$= (2/9) (n_{11} + n_{10} + n_{02} + n_{01})$$

giving the Mantel-Haenszel-Cochran test statistic the specific form

$$X^2 = z^2 = \frac{(\Sigma a_i - \Sigma \hat{A}_i)^2}{\Sigma \text{variance } (a_i)} = \frac{([n_{11} + 2n_{10})] - [2n_{02} + n_{01}])^2}{2(n_{11} + n_{10} + n_{02} + n_{01})}$$

which has a chi-square distribution with one degree of freedom when the risk factor is unrelated to the occurrence of the disease.

8. TAYLOR SERIES EXPANSION—POWER SERIES

A mathematical function (denoted $f(x)$) frequently can be expressed as a power series centered at a selected value[49] (denoted c) where

$$f(x) = a_0 + a_1(x - c) + a_2(x - c)^2 + a_3(x - c)^3 + a_4(x - c)^4$$
$$+ \cdots + a_k(x - c)^k + \cdots$$

which is useful when the coefficients a_i are available. In many situations, the coefficients are found by noting the following pattern:

$$f(x) = a_0 + a_1(x - c) + a_2(x - c)^2 + a_3(x - c)^3 + a_4(x - c)^4 + \cdots$$

$$f'(x) = a_1 + 2a_2(x - c) + 3a_3(x - c)^2 + 4a_4(x - c)^3 + \cdots$$

$$f''(x) = 2a_2 + 3(2)a_3(x - c) + 4(3)a_4(x - c)^2 + \cdots$$

$$f'''(x) = 3(2)a_3 + 4(3)(2)a_4(x - c) + \cdots$$

$$f''''(x) = 4(3)(2)a_4 + \cdots$$

$$\cdots$$
$$\cdots$$
$$\cdots$$

$$f^{[k]}(x) = k(k - 1)(k - 2)(k - 3) \ldots (2)a_k + \cdots = k!a_k + \cdots$$

where $f^{[k]}(x)$ denotes the kth derivate of the function $f(x)$ with respect to x. These derivatives evaluated at the selected value c are

$$f(c) = a_0$$
$$f'(c) = 1!a_1$$
$$f''(c) = 2!a_2$$
$$f'''(c) = 3!a_3$$
$$f''''(c) = 4!a_4$$
$$\cdots$$
$$\cdots$$
$$\cdots$$
$$f^{[k]}(c) = k!a_k$$

making the value of the kth coefficient in the power series

$$a_k = \frac{1}{k!}f^{[k]}(c)$$

and then

$$f(x) = f(c) + \left[\frac{1}{1!}f'(c)\right](x - c) + \left[\frac{1}{2!}f''(c)\right](x - c)^2 + \left[\frac{1}{3!}f'''(c)\right](x - c)^3 + \cdots$$

or the Taylor series expansion of the function $f(x)$ is

$$f(x) = f(c) + \sum\left[\frac{1}{k!}f^{[k]}(c)\right](x - c)^k \quad k = 1, 2, 3, \ldots$$

where $f^{[k]}(c)$ denotes the kth derivative of $f(x)$ with respect to x, evaluated at the constant value c.

Statistical Application

An observed variable denoted x frequently has known or postulated properties, but questions arise about a function of x, again denoted $f(x)$. That is, if the properties of x are known, what are the properties of $f(x)$? More specifically, if x is a random variable, what are the expectation and variance of $f(x)$ or, in symbols

$$E[f(x)] = ? \quad \text{and} \quad \text{variance } [f(x)] = ?$$

when EX and variance (x) are known? A Taylor series expansion is the key to providing approximate answers to these two questions.

To begin, only the first two terms of a Taylor series expansion are used, giving

$$f(x) \approx f(c) + f'(c)(x - c)$$

and c is selected to be the expectation of the variable x, namely, EX. Then the function $f(x)$ is approximately equal to

$$f(x) \approx f(EX) + f'(EX)(x - EX)$$

where $f'(EX)$ represents the first derivative of $f(x)$ evaluated at the constant EX.

RESULT 1

$$E[f(x)] \approx E[f(EX)] + f'(EX)E(x - EX) = f(EX)$$

since $E(x - EX) = EX - EX = 0$ and $E[f(EX)] = f(EX)$. For example, if $f(x) = e^x$, then $E[e^x] \approx e^{EX}$.

RESULT 2
Since

$$f(x) - f(EX) \approx f'(EX)(x - EX)$$

then

$$[f(x) - f(EX)]^2 \approx [f'(EX)(x - EX)]^2$$
$$E(f(x) - E[f(EX)])^2 \approx E[f'(EX)(x - EX)]^2 = [f'(EX)]^2E(x - EX)^2.$$

Because $E(x - EX)^2$ is an alternative expression of variance (x), then

$$\text{variance}[f(x)] \approx [f'(EX)]^2\text{variance}(x).$$

For example, variance $(e^x) \approx [e^{2EX}]\text{variance}(x)$ since the derivative of e^x is $de^x/dx = e^x$.

Using a truncated Taylor series expansion to approximate the expected value and the variance of a function of a random variable provides a variety of expressions for the expectation and variance of summary statistics used to analyze data.

Application

A Poisson distributed variable is sometimes transformed by taking the square root to give it a more normal-like distribution. That is, if X has a Poisson distribution with expectation $= EX = \lambda$ and the variance is variance $(x) = \lambda$, then $\sqrt{X}$ has an approximate normal distribution (if λ is not too small) with mean $= \sqrt{\lambda}$ and variance $= 1/4$.

Applying the truncated Taylor series–based approximation, the expectation of the transformed variable is

$$\text{expectation of } \sqrt{X} = E\left(\sqrt{X}\right) = \sqrt{EX} = \sqrt{\lambda}$$

and the variance is

$$\text{variance } \left(\sqrt{X}\right) = \left(-\frac{1}{2\sqrt{EX}}\right)^2 \text{variance } (X) = \frac{1}{4\lambda}\lambda = \frac{1}{4}$$

since the derivative of $\sqrt{x}$ is

$$f'(x) = \frac{d}{dx}\sqrt{x} = -\frac{1}{2\sqrt{x}}.$$

The transformed variable additionally has an approximate normal distribution because taking the square root tends to make right-skewed distributions, like the Poisson distribution, more symmetric. The details and a more rigorous justification of this transformation process are found elsewhere.[50]

9. TWO VARIANCES

Two fundamental variances are:

1. the variance of the logarithm of a variable x; then

$$\text{variance } [\log (x)] \approx \frac{1}{(EX)^2}\text{variance } (x)$$

2. the variance of a ratio of two variables x and y where $R = x/y$, then

$$\text{variance } (R) \approx \left[\frac{EX}{EY}\right]^2\left(\frac{\text{variance } (x)}{(EX)^2} + \frac{\text{variance } (y)}{(EY)^2} - 2\frac{\text{covariance } (x,\, y)}{(EX)(EY)}\right).$$

Both expressions are applications of a truncated Taylor series producing an approximate expression for the variance. These approximate variances make it possible to evaluate a number of important analytic summaries statistically. Some examples are:

variance of the estimated odds (a.9)
variance of the estimated log-odds (a.9)
variance of the estimated relative risk (a.9)
variance of the estimated rate ratio (a.10)
variance of the estimated odds ratio (a.11)
variance of the estimated survival probability (a.15).

Details

The variance of a logarithm of an observed variable x has a number of important applications. If $f(x) = \log(x)$, then

expectation of the logarithm of $f(x) = E[f(x)] = E[\log(x)] \approx \log(EX)$.

The derivative of $f(x)$ is

$$\frac{d}{dx}f(x) = \frac{d}{dx}\log(x) = \frac{1}{x}$$

making

variance of $f(x)$ = variance $[f(x)]$ = variance $[\log(x)] \approx \dfrac{1}{(EX)^2}$ variance (x).

Corollary:

$$\text{variance }(x) \approx (EX)^2 \text{variance }[\log(x)].$$

Often, quantities are transformed to have more symmetric (normal-like) distributions by using the logarithms of the values. Some examples are the odds ratio, the relative risk, and a variety of rate ratios. Then the expectation and variance of the logarithm of the transformed value becomes a necessary part of the statistical evaluation. Note: all logarithms used are natural logarithms (base $e = 2.718281828\ldots$), sometimes called *Napier logarithms* in honor of John Napier (b. 1550), who pioneered the use of logarithms.

The same Taylor series argument that produces approximate expressions for $E[f(x)]$ and variance $[f(x)]$ produces parallel expressions for a function of two variables, x and y, namely, $E[f(x, y)]$ and variance $[f(x, y)]$. That is, a truncated Taylor series applied to a bivariate function $f(x,y)$ produces (details given elsewhere[48])

$$E[f(x, y)] \approx f(EX, EY)$$

and

$$\text{variance } [f(x, y)] \approx \left[\frac{\partial f(x, y)}{\partial x}\right]^2 \text{variance }(x) + \left[\frac{\partial f(x, y)}{\partial y}\right]^2 \text{variance }(y)$$

$$+ 2\frac{\partial f(x, y)}{\partial x}\frac{\partial f(x, y)}{\partial y}\text{covariance }(x\ y)$$

where the partial derivatives are evaluated at the expectations of the variables x and y, specifically at EX and EY.

Using this expression, the approximate variance of an estimate ratio $\hat{R} = x/y$ follows. Since $f(x, y) = x/y$, the partial derivatives are

$$\frac{\partial f(x, y)}{\partial x} = \frac{\partial}{\partial x}\left[\frac{x}{y}\right] = \frac{1}{y} \quad \text{and} \quad \frac{\partial f(x, y)}{\partial y} = \frac{\partial}{\partial y}\left[\frac{x}{y}\right] = -\frac{x}{y^2}$$

and

$$\text{variance }(\hat{R}) \approx \frac{1}{(EY)^2}\text{variance }(x) + \frac{(EX)^2}{(EY)^4}\text{variance }(y)$$

$$- 2\frac{1}{(EY)}\frac{EX}{(EY)^2}\text{covariance }(x, y)$$

or, more symmetrically,

$$\text{variance }(\hat{R}) \approx \left[\frac{EX}{EY}\right]^2\left(\frac{\text{variance }(x)}{(EX)^2} + \frac{\text{variance }(y)}{(EY)^2} - 2\frac{\text{covariance }(x, y)}{(EX)(EY)}\right).$$

Application

If $X = x_1 + x_2 + x_3 + \cdots + x_n$ where x_i represents one of n independent binary variables that takes on the value 1 with probability p and the value 0 with probability $1 - p$, then an estimated proportion of the values coded equal to 1 (denoted $\hat{p}$) is

$$\hat{p} = \frac{X}{n}$$

and the estimated odds follows as

$$\hat{o} = \frac{\hat{p}}{1 - \hat{p}} = \frac{X}{n - X}.$$

The following are true when X has a binomial probability distribution (a.3) with parameters n and p:

1. $EX = np$ and $E(n - X) = n(1 - p)$,
2. variance $(X) =$ variance $(n - X) = np(1 - p)$, and
3. covariance $(X, n - X) = -$variance $(X) = -np(1 - p)$ (a.2).

Therefore, applying the Taylor series approximation gives the variance of the odds as

$$\text{variance}(\hat{o}) \approx \left[\frac{p}{1 - p}\right]^2 \left[\frac{np(1 - p)}{(np)^2} + \frac{np(1 - p)}{[n(1 - p)]^2} - 2\frac{-np(1 - p)}{(np)[n(1 - p)]}\right]$$

$$= \left[\frac{p}{1 - p}\right]^2 \frac{1}{np(1 - p)}[(1 - p)^2 + p^2 + 2p(1 - p)] = \frac{p}{n(1 - p)^3}.$$

An estimate of the variance of the estimated odds is achieved by replacing the parameter p with its corresponding estimated value $\hat{p}$ or

$$S_{\hat{o}}^2 = \frac{\hat{p}}{n(1 - \hat{p})^3} = \frac{\hat{o}}{n(1 - \hat{p})^2}.$$

Also, note that the variance of the logarithm of the odds is

$$\text{variance of the log-odds} = \text{variance}[\log(\hat{o})] \approx \frac{1}{o^2}\text{variance}(\hat{o})$$

$$= \frac{1}{np(1 - p)} = \frac{1}{np} + \frac{1}{n(1 - p)}$$

where the expectation of the estimated odds is represented by o. This variance is estimated by

$$S_{\log(\hat{o})}^2 = \frac{1}{n\hat{p}} + \frac{1}{n(1 - \hat{p})} = \frac{1}{X} + \frac{1}{n - X}$$

since $\hat{p} = X/n$.

Application

An estimate of the variance of the relative risk measure of association comes from an application of the expression for the variance of a ratio. For two binomial populations ($i = 1$ and 2) the following are true (a.3):

$$\text{expectation of an estimated proportion} = E(\hat{p}_i) = p_i$$

with associated variance

$$\text{variance}(\hat{p}_i) = \frac{p_i(1 - p_i)}{n_i}$$

where n_i represents the number of observations sampled and, as before, the estimate of p_i is denoted by $\hat{p}_i$.

The relative risk ratio is the ratio of two such independent (covariance (p_1, p_2) = 0) proportions, and the estimated relative risk (denoted $\hat{rr}$) is

$$\text{relative risk} = \hat{rr} = \frac{\hat{p}_1}{\hat{p}_2}$$

based on n_1 and n_2 observations, respectively. The expression for the variance of the ratio of two independent estimates (covariance (x, y) = 0) is

$$\text{variance}\left(\frac{X}{Y}\right) \approx \left[\frac{EX}{EY}\right]^2 \left(\frac{\text{variance}(x)}{(EX)^2} + \frac{\text{variance}(y)}{(EY)^2}\right).$$

Specifically, for the estimated relative risk where $X = p_1$ and $Y = p_2$,

$$\text{variance}(\hat{rr}) \approx \left[\frac{p_1}{p_2}\right]^2 \left(\frac{p_1(1 - p_1)/n_1}{(p_1)^2} + \frac{p_2(1 - p_2)/n_2}{(p_2)^2}\right)$$

$$= \left[\frac{p_1}{p_2}\right]^2 \left(\frac{1 - p_1}{n_1 p_1} + \frac{1 - p_2}{n_2 p_2}\right).$$

Substituting the estimate $\hat{p}_i$ for the population parameters p_i gives an estimate of the variance of the relative risk as

$$S_{\hat{rr}}^2 = \left[\frac{\hat{p}_1}{\hat{p}_2}\right]^2 \left(\frac{1 - \hat{p}_1}{n_1 \hat{p}_1} + \frac{1 - \hat{p}_2}{n_2 \hat{p}_2}\right) = [\hat{rr}]^2 \left(\frac{1 - \hat{p}_1}{n_1 \hat{p}_1} + \frac{1 - \hat{p}_2}{n_2 \hat{p}_2}\right).$$

Since variance $[\log (x)] = $ variance $(x)/(EX)^2$, the estimated variance of the logarithm of the estimated relative risk is

$$S^2_{\log (\hat{r})} = \frac{1 - \hat{p}_1}{n_1 \hat{p}_1} + \frac{1 - \hat{p}_2}{n_2 \hat{p}_2}.$$

10. RATE RATIO

To compare two rates, a ratio is commonly used. If X represents the number of events observed from one group (X has a binomial probability distribution (a.3) with parameters n_1 and p_1 making $EX = n_1 p_1$ and variance $(X) = n_1 p_1 (1 - p_1)$—group 1) and Y represents the number of events observed in an independent (covariance = 0) second group (Y has a binomial probability distribution with parameters n_2 and p_2 making $EY = n_2 p_2$ and variance $(Y) = n_2 p_2 (1 - p_2)$—group 2), then the estimated rate in the first group is $\hat{p}_1 = X/n_1$ and the estimated rate in the second group is $\hat{p}_2 = Y/n_2$. Here no distinction is made between a ratio of rates and a ratio of proportions, which is only approximately true. However, when the probability of disease or death is small (usually the case), a proportion multiplied by a constant value approximately equals a rate, making the ratio of two rates essentially equal to a ratio of the two proportions. That is, proportion $\approx \delta \times$ rate where δ is the length of the rate-interval, frequently $\delta = 1$ or 5 years.

The rate ratio $R = p_1/p_2$ is estimated by

$$\text{estimated rate ratio} = f[x, y] = \hat{R} = \frac{\hat{p}_1}{\hat{p}_2} = \frac{X/n_1}{Y/n_2}.$$

Using the expression for the variance of a ratio (a.9) gives

$$\text{variance}\left(\frac{X}{Y}\right) \approx \left[\frac{\partial f}{\partial x}\right]^2 n_1 p_1 (1 - p_1) + \left[\frac{\partial f}{\partial y}\right]^2 n_2 p_2 (1 - p_2)$$

$$+ 2 \frac{\partial f}{\partial x} \frac{\partial f}{\partial y} \text{covariance } (X, Y)$$

and analogous to the variance of the relative risk measure (a.9), the variance of $\hat{R}$ is approximately

$$\text{variance } (\hat{R}) \approx \text{variance}\left(\frac{X/n_1}{Y/n_2}\right) = \left[\frac{p_1}{p_2}\right]^2 \left(\frac{n_1 p_1 (1 - p_1)}{(n_1 p_1)^2} + \frac{n_2 p_2 (1 - p_2)}{(n_2 p_2)^2}\right)$$

$$= R^2 \left(\frac{1 - p_1}{n_1 p_1} + \frac{1 - p_2}{n_2 p_2}\right).$$

For disease and mortality data, the quantity $1 - p_i \approx 1$ where p_i is the probability of disease or death (almost always a small proportion). Furthermore, the quantity $n_i p_i$ is estimated by d_i, the number of cases of disease or deaths in the ith group ($i = 1, 2$). For the ratio of disease or mortality rates, the estimated variance of an estimated rate ratio $\hat{R}$ then becomes

$$S_{\hat{R}}^2 = \hat{R}^2 \left(\frac{1}{d_1} + \frac{1}{d_2} \right)$$

where $\hat{R}$ is the estimated rate in group 1 divided by the estimated rate in group 2. Also, since the estimated variance of the logarithm of a variable is

$$S_{\log(x)}^2 = \frac{1}{(EX)^2} S_X^2,$$

the estimated variance of the logarithm of the estimated rate ratio ($x = \hat{R}$) is

$$S_{\log(\hat{R})}^2 = \frac{1}{\hat{R}^2} \hat{R}^2 \left(\frac{1}{d_1} + \frac{1}{d_2} \right) = \frac{1}{d_1} + \frac{1}{d_2}$$

where d_1 and d_2 represent the number of cases of disease or deaths in groups 1 and 2, respectively.

11. ODDS RATIO

The odds ratio, as the name implies, is the ratio of two odds. The odds are themselves a ratio and arise typically from two different sets of independent observations. Consider the variable X_1, which results from counting a series of events among n_1 independent binary outcomes. Additionally, consider another variable X_2, which also results from a count of a series of events among n_2 independent binary variables. More specifically, the count X_1 has an binomial probability distribution (a.3) with parameters n_1 and p_1, and the count X_2 has an independent binomial probability distribution with parameters n_2 and p_2 (i.e., covariance $(X_1, X_2) = 0$).

The estimated odds associated with X_1 are $\hat{o}_1 = \hat{p}_1/(1 - \hat{p}_1)$, and the estimated odds associated with X_2 are $\hat{o}_2 = \hat{p}_2/(1 - \hat{p}_2)$. Therefore, the odds ratio is estimated by

$$\hat{or} = \frac{\hat{o}_1}{\hat{o}_2} = \frac{\hat{p}_1/(1 - \hat{p}_1)}{\hat{p}_2/(1 - \hat{p}_2)}.$$

An odds ratio of 1.0 means that the odds are identical for both binomial distributions and indicates that $p_1 = p_2$.

An expression for the variance of the estimated odds ratio derives from first considering the logarithm of the estimated odds ratio where

$$\log{(\hat{or})} = \log\left(\frac{\hat{o}_1}{\hat{o}_2}\right) = \log{(\hat{o}_1)} - \log{(\hat{o}_2)}.$$

The logarithm of the odds ratio is the difference between two independent log-odds values and the variance (a.2 and a.9) is then

$$\text{variance} [\log{(\hat{or})}] = \text{variance} (\log{[\hat{o}_1]}) + \text{variance} (\log{[\hat{o}_2]})$$

$$= \frac{1}{n_1 p_1 (1 - p_1)} + \frac{1}{n_2 p_2 (1 - p_2)}$$

$$= \frac{1}{n_1 p_1} + \frac{1}{n_1 (1 - p_1)} + \frac{1}{n_2 p_2} + \frac{1}{n_2 (1 - p_2)}$$

making the variance of the estimated odds ratio.

$$\text{variance} (\hat{or}) = (or)^2 \text{variance} [\log{(\hat{or})}].$$

The odds ratio is typically estimated from data summarized in a 2 by 2 table. Specifically, for the binary variables represented by A and B such a table is

	B_1	B_2	Total
A_1	a	b	n_1
A_2	c	d	n_2
total	m_1	m_2	n

where $\hat{p}_1 = a/n_1$ and $\hat{p}_2 = c/n_2$. The odds of B_1 versus B_2 associated with A_1 are estimated by $\hat{o}_1 = \hat{p}_1/(1 - \hat{p}_1) = a/b$, and the odds of B_1 versus B_2 associated with A_2 are estimated by $\hat{o}_2 = \hat{p}_2/(1 - \hat{p}_2) = c/d$ given an estimated odds ratio of

$$\hat{or} = \frac{\hat{o}_1}{\hat{o}_2} = \frac{a/b}{c/d} = \frac{ad}{bc}$$

contrasting the probability of the occurrence of B under conditions A_1 and A_2.

A natural estimate of the variance of the logarithm of the estimated odds ratio is

$$S^2_{\log(\hat{or})} = \frac{1}{n_1 \hat{p}_1} + \frac{1}{n_1(1 - \hat{p}_1)} + \frac{1}{n_2 \hat{p}_2} + \frac{1}{n_2(1 - \hat{p}_2)}$$

or, more simply,

$$S^2_{\log(\hat{or})} = \frac{1}{a} + \frac{1}{b} + \frac{1}{c} + \frac{1}{d}.$$

Additionally, an estimate of the variance of the estimated odds ratio becomes (a.9)

$$S^2_{\hat{or}} = (\hat{or})^2 \left[\frac{1}{a} + \frac{1}{b} + \frac{1}{c} + \frac{1}{d} \right].$$

Specifically, such a 2 by 2 table and odds ratio arise when n_1 individuals with a risk factor $(A_1 = F)$ are observed over time where a individuals with the disease $(B_1 = D)$ and b individuals without the disease $(B_2 = \bar{D})$ are recorded (i.e., $\hat{o}_1 = a/b$). Similarly, among n_2 individuals without the risk factor $(A_2 = \bar{F})$, c individuals with and d individuals without the disease are observed (i.e., $\hat{o}_2 = c/d$). Or $\hat{p}_1 = a/n_1$ and $\hat{p}_2 = c/n_1$ estimate

p_1 = P(disease among individuals with the risk factor present) = $P(D \mid F)$

p_2 = P(disease among individuals with the risk factor absent) = $P(D \mid \bar{F})$.

The estimated odds ratio is

$$\hat{or} = \frac{\hat{o}_1}{\hat{o}_2} = \frac{a/b}{c/d} = \frac{ad}{bc}.$$

An odds ratio also measures association when m_1 cases of disease are observed where a cases have the risk factor and c cases do not (i.e., $\hat{o}_1 = a/c$) and m_2 non-cases (controls) are observed where b individuals have the risk factor and d individuals do not (i.e., $\hat{o}_2 = b/d$). Then $\hat{p}_1 = a/m_1$ and $\hat{p}_2 = b/m_2$ estimate

p_1 = P(risk factor among individuals with the disease present) = $P(F \mid D)$

p_2 = P(risk factor among individuals with the disease absent) = $P(F \mid \bar{D})$.

In this case/control situation, the estimated odds ratio is, as before,

$$\hat{or} = \frac{\hat{o}_1}{\hat{o}_2} = \frac{a/c}{b/d} = \frac{ad}{bc}$$

and the estimated variance is also unchanged.

12. WEIGHTED AVERAGE

An often important summary of a series of observations or estimates is frequently achieved using a weighted average. An average is most effectively applied to values that arise from different and independent sources but estimate the same quantity. Specifically, if $\hat{g}_1$, $\hat{g}_2$, $\hat{g}_3$, . . . , $\hat{g}_k$ represent k independent estimates of the same quantity, then a weighted average of these values estimates the common value. Furthermore, the precision of this estimate, as usual, is characterized by the variance or estimated variance of the estimated value.

A weighted average of the estimates of g_i, each estimated from one of k independent sources, is

$$\overline{G} = \frac{\sum w_i \hat{g}_i}{\sum w_i} \quad i = 1, 2, 3, \ldots, k$$

producing a summary estimate of the common value G.
    The variance of $\overline{G}$ (a.2) is

$$\text{variance} (\overline{G}) = \text{variance} \left[\frac{\sum w_i \hat{g}_i}{\sum w_i} \right] = \frac{1}{(\sum w_i)^2} \text{variance} (\sum w_i \hat{g}_i)$$

$$= \frac{1}{(\sum w_i)^2} \sum w_i^2 \text{variance} (\hat{g}_i)$$

as long as the estimates $\hat{g}_i$ are independent (for example, come from entirely unrelated sources). If the weights chosen equal the reciprocal of the variance of $\hat{g}_i$ ($w_i = 1/\text{variance} (\hat{g})$), then

$$\text{variance} (\overline{G}) = \frac{1}{(\sum w_i)^2} \sum w_i = \frac{1}{\sum w_i}.$$

Although a large number of useful choices exist for the weights w_i, choosing the reciprocal of the variance of the estimated values $\hat{g}_i$ has a distinct justification and some statistical advantages.[48] Weighting by the reciprocal of the variance gives greater weight to estimates with small variances (high precision) and gives lesser weight to estimates with large variances (low precision).

Example

If $x_1, x_2, x_3, \ldots, x_n$ are independently sampled values from the same population, then each value estimates the same mean (μ) and has the same associated variance (σ^2). Thus a weighted average estimate is the usual mean value or

$$\overline{G} = \frac{\sum w_i x_i}{\sum w_i} = \frac{\sum x_i}{n} = \overline{x}$$

where reciprocal variance weights $w_i = 1/\sigma^2$ are constant. The value $\overline{G} = \overline{x}$ is an estimate of the population parameter $G = \mu$. The variance of $\overline{G}$ is then

$$\text{variance } (\overline{G}) = \text{variance } (\overline{x}) = \frac{1}{\sum w_i} = \frac{\sigma^2}{n}.$$

And the estimated variance of $\overline{G}$ follows where

$$S_{\overline{G}}^2 = S_{\overline{x}}^2 = \frac{S^2}{n}$$

when S^2 is the estimate of the variance common to the sampled values (σ^2).

Example

In the analysis of spatial data, it is frequently postulated that individuals living in a series of k geographic areas have the same probability (rate) of death, denoted p. If each area has a population of size n_i in which d_i deaths occurred, then an area specific mortality rate (ith area) is

$$\hat{r}_i = \frac{d_i}{n_i}.$$

If the observed number of deaths is assumed to be proportional to the population size (i.e., $E(d_i) = n_i p$) plus random variation, then

$$\text{variance } (\hat{r}_i) = \frac{1}{n_i^2} \text{variance } (d_i) = \frac{1}{n_i^2} n_i p = \frac{p}{n_i}$$

where p is the common probability of death among the areas considered. An overall estimated mortality rate (denoted $\hat{M}$) found by a weighted average is

$$\hat{M} = \frac{\Sigma w_i \hat{r}_i}{\Sigma w_i} = \frac{\Sigma (n_i/p)\hat{r}_i}{\Sigma (n_i/p)} = \frac{\Sigma (n_i/p \cdot d_i/n_i)}{\Sigma (n_i/p)} = \frac{\Sigma d_i}{\Sigma n_i} = \frac{D}{N}$$

when

$$\text{weights} = w_i = \frac{1}{\text{variance } (\hat{r}_i)} = \frac{n_i}{p} \quad i = 1, 2, 3, \ldots, k$$

where $D = \Sigma d_i$ represents the total number of deaths and $N = \Sigma n_i$ the total number of observed individuals. The variance of the overall estimated (weighted average) mortality rate $\hat{M}$ is

$$\text{variance } (\hat{M}) = \frac{1}{\Sigma w_i} = \frac{1}{\Sigma (n_i/p)} = \frac{p}{N}$$

and is estimated by

$$S_{\hat{M}}^2 = \frac{D}{N^2} = \frac{\hat{M}}{N}$$

since $D = \hat{M} N$.

13. ADDITIVE MODEL FOR A TWO-WAY CLASSIFICATION

Critical to summarizing and understanding the relationships between two categorical variables based on data contained in a two-way table is a decision—to proceed as if interactions exist or as if they do not exist. This issue translates into the question: *is an additive model a good representation of the tabular data?*

An additive (no interaction) model for a two-way classification of a set of observations is

$$y_{ij} = a + r_i + c_j + e_{ij}$$

where measurement y_{ij} represents the value contained in the (*i*th, *j*th)-cell of a two-way table. The parameter a represents a constant value (background level), r_i is the influence of the ith level of the row category (denoted A_i), and c_j is the influence of the jth column category (denoted B_j). The error term e_{ij} incorporates a stochastic element ("noise") into the model.

The value y_{ij} represents a continuous quantity subject to the influence of two categorical variables represented by A and B. Three examples are:

r_{ij}: a rate,
$log\,(R_{ij})$: a logarithm of a ratio, and
$log\,(f_{ij})$: a logarithm of a frequency.

The notation produces the following r by c two-way table (r = total number of rows and c = total number of columns) with a total of $n = rc$ measured values of y_{ij}:

	B_1	B_2	B_3	. . .	B_c	Mean
A_1	y_{11}	y_{12}	y_{13}	. . .	y_{1c}	$\bar{y}_{1.}$
A_2	y_{21}	y_{22}	y_{23}	. . .	y_{2c}	$\bar{y}_{2.}$
A_3	y_{31}	y_{32}	y_{33}	. . .	y_{3c}	$\bar{y}_{3.}$
. . .	. . .	. . .	. . .	. . .	. . .	. . .
. . .	. . .	. . .	. . .	. . .	. . .	. . .
. . .	. . .	. . .	. . .	. . .	. . .	. . .
A_r	y_{r1}	y_{r2}	y_{r3}	. . .	y_{rc}	$\bar{y}_{r.}$
mean	$\bar{y}_{.1}$	$\bar{y}_{.2}$	$\bar{y}_{.3}$	. . .	$\bar{y}_{.c}$	$\bar{y}$

and for the additive model

$$\bar{y} = \frac{1}{n}\sum\sum y_{ij} \quad \text{estimates } a \qquad i = 1, 2, 3, \ldots, r \quad \text{and} \quad j = 1, 2, 3, \ldots, c.$$

$$\bar{y}_{i.} = \frac{1}{c}\sum y_{ij} \quad \text{estimates } a + r_i \qquad j = 1, 2, 3, \ldots, c$$

$$\bar{y}_{.j} = \frac{1}{r}\sum y_{ij} \quad \text{estimates } a + c_j \qquad i = 1, 2, 3, \ldots, r$$

where $\sum r_i = \sum c_j = \sum_i e_{ij} = \sum_j e_{ij} = 0$. Therefore, estimates of the four components of an additive model are

$$\hat{a} = \bar{y}, \quad \hat{r}_i = \bar{y}_{i.} - \bar{y}, \quad \hat{c}_j = \bar{y}_{.j} - \bar{y}, \quad \text{and} \quad \hat{e}_{ij} = y_{ij} - [\hat{a} + \hat{r}_i + \hat{c}_j] \quad \text{or}$$

$$\hat{e}_{ij} = y_{ij} - \bar{y}_{i.} - \bar{y}_{.j} + \bar{y}.$$

Example

For example, a 2 by 3 table of data that conform perfectly to the additive model ($e_{ij} = 0$) is

	B_1	B_2	B_3	Mean
A_1	10	20	30	20
A_2	0	10	20	10
mean	5	15	25	15

Then

$$\hat{a} = \bar{y} = 15 \quad \hat{r}_1 = \bar{y}_{1.} - \bar{y} = 20 - 15 = 5 \quad \hat{c}_1 = \bar{y}_{.1} - \bar{y} = 5 - 15 = -10$$

$$\hat{r}_2 = \bar{y}_{2.} - \bar{y} = 10 - 15 = -5 \quad \hat{c}_2 = \bar{y}_{.2} - \bar{y} = 15 - 15 = 0$$

$$\hat{c}_3 = \bar{y}_{.3} - \bar{y} = 25 - 15 = 10.$$

For example, $\hat{y}_{22} = \hat{a} + \hat{r}_2 + \hat{c}_2 = 15 + (-5) + 0 = 10 = y_{22}$ (since $e_{22} = 0$). The defining characteristic of the additive model is

$$y_{ki} - y_{kj} = (a + r_k + c_i) - (a + r_k + c_j) = c_i - c_j$$

and then

$$\bar{y}_{.i} - \bar{y}_{.j} = (a + c_i) - (a + c_j) = c_i - c_j.$$

That is, differences between the column values and column mean values are not influenced by the row variable. An analogous relationship exists among the row mean values.

An additive relationship between categorical variables A and B is a kind of independence. That is, the influences of the level of variable A on the observed values are the same regardless of the level of variable B; conversely, the influences of the level of variable B are the same regardless of the level of variable A. The influences of one categorical variable are totally unaffected by the other.

When influences are additive (no interaction), the marginal mean values directly reflect the separate influences of the row and column variables. That is, the row and column mean values are useful summaries of the row and column influences. For the exactly additive data, the difference between the values in columns B_3 and B_1 is 20 for both levels A_1 and A_2, and the difference between the corresponding mean values $\bar{y}_{.3}$ and $\bar{y}_{.1}$ is also 20.

Geometrically, perfect additivity of the observations translates into parallel lines. If the y_{ij}-values are plotted for each row, additivity requires that the distances associated with each column be equal (parallel lines). Plotting the column values for each row also forms parallel lines.

When the structure underlying an r by c table fails to be additive (interaction), the influences of levels of A depend on the level of B; conversely, the influences of the levels of B depend on the level of A. An extreme case is illustrated by the following data:

	B_1	B_2	B_3	Mean
A_1	5	15	25	15
A_2	25	15	5	15
mean	15	15	15	15

Clearly, the differences between the rows depends on the columns, and vice versa. For example, the difference between B_3 and B_1 is 20 for A_1, and the difference between B_3 and B_1 is -20 for A_2. The influences from B_3 and B_1 have exactly opposite effects, depending on the level of A. Therefore, the row and column mean values do not summarize the relationships among the row and column observations. All row and column mean values are equal to 15, giving no indication that the cell frequencies vary substantially (in opposite directions) within the table. When data in a two-way table do not conform to an additive structure, summarizing the influences of the categorical variables A and B becomes more complex than simply comparing column or row mean values.

14. TWO BY c TABLE

A 2 by c table is frequently constructed to explore a trend or a dose–response relationship between a binary variable (denoted Y) and a measured response variable (denoted X) sorted into c categories. The resulting table contains $2c$ counts of observations (denoted f_{ij}). The notation is

	x_1	x_2	x_3	. . .	x_c	Total
$Y = 1$	f_{11}	f_{12}	f_{13}	. . .	f_{1c}	n_1
$Y = 0$	f_{21}	f_{22}	f_{23}	. . .	f_{2c}	n_2
total	f_1	f_2	f_3	. . .	f_c	n
proportion	$\hat{p}_1$	$\hat{p}_2$	$\hat{p}_3$	. . .	$\hat{p}_c$	1.0

and $\hat{p}_j = f_{1j}/f_j$ is the proportion of observations recorded in the first row ($Y = 1$) for each of the c levels of the column variable X.

As with all two-way tables containing counts, the data can be viewed as n pairs of x-values and y-values. The cell frequencies f_{ij} are the number of identical pairs. In symbols, for the 2 by c table,

row 1 $(Y = 1)$	row 2 $(Y = 0)$
f_{11} sets of pairs $(x_1, 1)$	f_{21} sets of pairs $(x_1, 0)$
f_{12} sets of pairs $(x_2, 1)$	f_{22} sets of pairs $(x_2, 0)$
f_{13} sets of pairs $(x_3, 1)$	f_{23} sets of pairs $(x_3, 0)$
. . . .	. . . .
. . . .	. . . .
. . . .	. . . .
f_{1c} sets of pairs $(x_c, 1)$	f_{2c} sets of pairs $(x_c, 0)$.

Consider the linear regression model applied to data from a 2 by c table

$$p_j = a + bx_j$$

where p_j represents the probability estimated by $\hat{p}_j$ or $p_j = P(Y = 1 \mid x_j)$. An ordinary least squares estimate applied to the n pairs (not tabulated) yields an estimate of the regression coefficient or slope b where

$$\hat{b} = \frac{S_{xy}}{S_{xx}}$$

when $S_{xy} = \Sigma(x_i - \bar{x})(y_i - \bar{y})$ and $S_{xx} = \Sigma(x_i - \bar{x})^2$ for $i = 1, 2, 3, \ldots, n$. An estimated variance of the estimated slope is

$$\text{variance}(\hat{b}) = \frac{S_{yy}}{nS_{xx}}$$

when $S_{yy} = \Sigma(y_i - \bar{y})^2 = n_1 n_2 / n$.

Three test statistics measuring the strength of the relationship between X and Y are

$$z = \frac{\hat{b}}{\sqrt{\text{variance}(\hat{b})}}$$

or

$$z = \frac{\bar{x}_1 - \bar{x}_2}{\sqrt{\dfrac{S_{xx}}{n}\left(\dfrac{1}{n_1} + \dfrac{1}{n_2}\right)}} \qquad (\bar{x}_i = \text{mean of the } i\text{th row})$$

and

$$z = \sqrt{n}\, r_{xy} \quad (r_{xy} = \text{product–moment correlation coefficient}).$$

The resulting values of z reflect the degree of linear association across the c-levels of x and are identical regardless of the form. Additionally, the value z has an approximately normal distribution (mean $= 0$ and variance $= 1$) when no linear relationship exists between the proportions p_j and the independent variable x_j, that is, when $b = 0$. The equivalence of these three assessments of the association between x and y confirms that the slope, the difference between two means, and the correlation coefficient ($\hat{b}$, $\bar{x}_1 - \bar{x}_2$ and r_{xy}) are different ways of expressing the same thing: the degree to which a simple linear relationship summarizing a trend or a dose–response relationship differs from a horizontal line (no association). The assessment of z is sometimes called the *test for linear trend*.

Partition

A bit of algebra produces the relationship

$$\sum f_j\,(\hat{p}_j - \bar{p})^2 = \sum f_j\,(\tilde{p}_j - \bar{p})^2 + \sum f_j\,(\hat{p}_j - \tilde{p}_j)^2 \quad j = 1,\, 2,\, 3,\, \ldots,\, c$$

where

$\hat{p}_j = f_{1j}/f_j$, as before,
$\tilde{p}_j = \hat{a} + \hat{b}x_j = \bar{y} + \hat{b}\,(x_j - \bar{x})$ is estimated from the linear regression model, and
$\bar{p} = n_1/n$.

Dividing each component of this expression by $\bar{p}(1 - \bar{p})$ partitions the overall Pearson chi-square statistic (X^2) into the sum of two chi-square distributed statistics or

$$X^2 = \frac{1}{\bar{p}(1 - \bar{p})}\sum f_j\,(\hat{p}_j - \bar{p})^2$$

$$X_L^2 = \frac{1}{\bar{p}(1 - \bar{p})}\sum f_j\,(\tilde{p}_j - \bar{p})^2$$

$$X^2_{NL} = \frac{1}{\bar{p}(1 - \bar{p})} \sum f_j \, (\hat{p}_j - \tilde{p}_j)^2$$

and
$$X^2 = X^2_L + X^2_{NL}$$

where

$X^2 =$ the overall Pearson chi-square statistic (degrees of freedom $= c - 1$),
$X^2_L =$ a chi-square statistic reflecting linearity (degrees of freedom $= 1$), and
$X^2_{NL} =$ a chi-square statistic reflecting nonlinearity (degrees of freedom $= c - 2$).

This partition allows the overall chi-square statistic (X^2) to be divided into two meaningful pieces, a linear piece (X^2_L) and a nonlinear piece (X^2_{NL}). The relative magnitudes of the respective pieces yield yet another measure of the linear association in a 2 by c table. In fact, $X^2_L = z^2$ when z represents any of the previous three measures of the linear trend.

The quantity of $\hat{c} = X^2_L/X^2$ is the proportion of the variability in $\hat{p}_j$ explained by a linear regression model based on x_j. That is, $\hat{c} = 0$ means that the line describing the data is perfectly horizontal ($b = 0$ or no linear relationship exists between x and the proportion p_j), and $\hat{c} = 1$ means that all estimated values of $\hat{p}_j$ lie perfectly on a line. Other values of $\hat{c}$ simply indicate the degree of association, summarized by a number between 0 and 1.

15. KAPLAN-MEIER ESTIMATED SURVIVAL PROBABILITIES

The Kaplan-Meier procedure produces estimates of survival probabilities, denoted P_m. A survival probability is the probability that an individual survives beyond a specified time or

$$P_m = P \, (\text{survival time} \geq t_m) = P \, (\text{survive from time 0 to time } t_m)$$

where t_m represents the endpoint of a specific time interval (denoted m) 0 to t_m. The estimation of these probabilities is straightforward if all survival times are complete (all failure times are known). Then the survival probability P_m is directly estimated by the total number of individuals who failed before or at time t_m divided by the number of individuals who could have failed. However, survival data frequently contain censored observations. The failure time of a censored observation is not known. A censored observation is simply an observation that did not fail during the time the data were observed.

The Kaplan-Meier estimation process includes censored observations when they are relevant to the survival probability calculation and excludes them otherwise. A survival time, censored or not, contributes to the calculation of interval specific survival probabilities when the observation either fails at time t_m or survives beyond the interval. Consequently, censored observations that are not observed over an entire interval are not used in calculations pertaining to that interval or any subsequent interval.

The estimation of the survival probabilities begins with the following table of survival data:

Notation

Interval	From − to	Failure times	Failures	Censored	At risk
0	0	$t_0 = 0$	$d_0 = 0$	c_0	n
1	$0 - t_1$	t_1	d_1	c_1	n_1
2	$t_1 - t_2$	t_2	d_2	c_2	n_2
3	$t_2 - t_3$	t_3	d_3	c_3	n_3
. . .	. . .	. . .	. . .	. . .	. . .
. . .	. . .	. . .	. . .	. . .	. . .
m	$t_{m-1} - t_m$	t_m	d_m	c_m	n_m
. . .	. . .	. . .	. . .	. . .	. . .
. . .	. . .	. . .	. . .	. . .	. . .
k	$t_{k-1} - t_k$	t_k	d_k	c_k	n_k

where

n = total number of participating individuals
t_i = the ith unique observed failure time
d_i = number of individuals who failed at the time t_i, usually one,
c_i = count of individuals censored between times t_{i-1} and t_i
n_i = number of individuals at risk t_{i-1} to t_i

The interval endpoints are equal to complete survival times and are chosen so that the interval contains as few failures as possible. In most cases the number of failures is one.

Important elements in the estimation of a survival probability $\hat{P}_m$ are estimates of the conditional failure and survival probabilities calculated for each time interval, t_0 to t_1, t_1 to t_2, t_2 to t_3, . . . , t_{k-1} to t_k, where k is the total number of intervals. These estimates are

$$\hat{q}_i = \frac{d_i}{n_i} = P \text{ (failing in the } i\text{th interval } | \text{ survived up to the } i\text{th interval)}$$

$$\hat{p}_i = 1 - \hat{q}_i = P \text{ (surviving the } i\text{th interval } | \text{ survived up to the } i\text{th interval).}$$

That is, the symbol $\hat{p}_m$ represents the conditional probability of surviving from time t_{m-1} to time t_m for all individuals who survived to time t_{m-1}. These

interval specific probabilities are combined to give an estimate of the uncon-
ditional survival probability $\hat{P}_m$ where

$$\hat{P}_m = \hat{p}_1 \hat{p}_2 \hat{p}_3 \ldots \hat{p}_m = \hat{P}\,(\text{survival beyond the } m\text{th interval})$$
$$= \hat{P}\,(\text{survival time} \geq t_m).$$

Estimates

The time to develop AIDS for HIV-positive individuals with CD4 counts above
900 ($n = 16$) provides the data to illustrate a Kaplan-Meier estimated survival
curve. The survival times are 97^+, 59, 37^+, 6^+, 84^+, 54, 100^+, 21, 102, 98^+,
102^+, 98^+, 98^+, 57, 42, and 12. The "+" denotes a censored survival time.
These data in tabular form are:

Interval	t_i	d_i	c_i	n_i	$\hat{q}_i$	$\hat{p}_i$	$\hat{P}_i$
0	0	0	1	16	0	1.0	1.0
0–12	12	1	0	15	0.067	0.933	0.933
12–21	21	1	0	14	0.071	0.929	0.867
21–42	42	1	1	12	0.083	0.917	0.794
42–54	54	1	0	11	0.091	0.909	0.722
54–57	57	1	0	10	0.100	0.900	0.650
57–59	59	1	0	9	0.111	0.889	0.578
59–102	102	1	6	2	0.500	0.500	0.289

For example, $P_4 = P\,(\text{surviving beyond 54 weeks}) = ?$ Then

$$m = 4, \quad t_4 = 54, \quad \text{and } \hat{P}_4 = \hat{p}_1 \hat{p}_2 \hat{p}_3 \hat{p}_4 = (0.933)(0.929)(0.917)(0.909) = 0.722.$$

Variance of the Estimated Survival Probability $\hat{P}_m$

Question: variance $(\hat{P}_m) = $ variance $(\hat{p}_1 \hat{p}_2 \ldots \hat{p}_m) = ?$

To start (a.2),

$$\text{variance } [\log (\hat{P}_m)] = \text{variance } [\log (\hat{p}_1 \hat{p}_2 \ldots \hat{p}_m)] = \text{variance } [\Sigma \log (\hat{p}_i)]$$
$$= \Sigma \text{variance } [\log (\hat{p}_i)] \quad i = 1, 2, 3, \ldots, m.$$

Note again (a.9) that

$$\text{variance } [\log (x)] \approx \frac{1}{(EX)^2} \text{variance } (x).$$

Then

$$\text{variance} [\log (\hat{p}_i)] \approx \frac{1}{p_i^2} \left[\frac{p_i q_i}{n_i} \right] = \frac{q_i}{n_i p_i} \approx \frac{d_i}{n_i (n_i - d_i)}$$

making

$$\text{variance} [\log (\hat{P}_m)] \approx \sum \frac{d_i}{n_i (n_i - d_i)} \quad i = 1, 2, 3, \ldots, m$$

when, for each interval t_{i-1} to t_i, the estimated probability $\hat{p}_i$ results from an associated binomial distribution (parameters n_i and p_i (a.3)—making $E(\hat{p}_i) = p_i$ and variance $(\hat{p}_i) = p_i q_i / n_i$). In addition, the failures must be unrelated events; that is, p_i-values must be uncorrelated.

Since

$$\text{variance} [\log (\hat{P}_m)] \approx \frac{1}{P_m^2} \text{variance} (\hat{P}_m)$$

an estimated variance of the estimated survival probability $\hat{P}_m$ is

$$S_{\hat{P}_m}^2 = [\hat{P}_m]^2 S_{\log (\hat{P}_m)}^2 = [\hat{P}_m]^2 \sum \frac{d_i}{n_i (n_i - d_i)} \quad i = 1, 2, 3, \ldots, m$$

sometimes called *Greenwood's formula*.

Continuing the HIV/AIDS data example, the estimated variance associated with the estimate $\hat{P}_4 = 0.722$ is

$$S_{\hat{P}_4}^2 = (0.722)^2 \left[\frac{1}{15(14)} + \frac{1}{14(13)} + \frac{1}{12(11)} + \frac{1}{11(10)} \right] = (0.722)^2 (0.027) = 0.014$$

and the estimated standard error is

$$S_{\hat{P}_4} = \sqrt{0.014} = 0.119.$$

16. MEAN AND MEDIAN SURVIVAL TIME

If all n observed survival times (denoted t_i) are complete, then the mean survival time is estimated by the usual sample mean value $\bar{t} = (1/n) \sum t_i$. However, when censored observations are present, the total survival time $\sum t_i$ is likely too small (biased downward) and needs to be adjusted to produce an unbiased estimate of the mean survival time, denoted μ.

When n survival times t_i are sampled,

1. d values t_i will be complete $(d \leq n)$ and
2. $n - d$ values of t_i will be incomplete (too small).

For a censored value t_i, an estimated *complete* survival time is an estimate of the total survival time that would have been observed if the censored observation was followed until failure. When the hazard function underlying the sampled data is constant or at least approximately constant, every censored observation has the same expected time to failure, regardless of the observed value t_i. That is, an individual who has survived up to t_i has the same expected time to failure as an individual who has survived up to another time t_j. Therefore, adding the expected remaining survival time (μ) to each censored observation regardless of the previous survival time t_i produces an estimate of the complete survival time for censored observations with the same constant hazard function. In symbols, a complete survival time estimate becomes $t_i + \mu$ when the observed survival time t_i is a censored observation.

An unbiased estimate of the mean based on all n observations, complete and all estimated complete survival times, is then

$$\hat{\mu} = \frac{\sum_{\text{complete}} t_i + \sum_{\text{censored}} (t_i + \hat{\mu})}{n} = \frac{\Sigma t_i + (n - d)\,\hat{\mu}}{n}$$

and

$$n\hat{\mu} = \Sigma t_i + (n - d)\hat{\mu} \quad \text{or} \quad \hat{\mu} = \frac{1}{d}\Sigma t_i \quad i = 1, 2, 3, \ldots, n.$$

That is, each censored observation is "missing" a time equal, on average, to μ, making the observed total survival time too small by an expected amount $(n - d)\,\mu$. This missing time is estimated and added to the total observed complete time, making the estimate of the mean time unbiased with respect to the influence of censoring. As a result, the sum of all n observed survival times, both complete and incomplete, is divided by d and not by n, compensating for the amount of unobserved survival time associated with the censored observations.

Also, note that the estimated constant hazard rate (denoted $\hat{\lambda}$) is the total number of failures divided by the total time at risk or

$$\hat{\lambda} = \frac{d}{\Sigma t_i} = \frac{1}{\bar{t}}.$$

The estimated constant hazard rate is the reciprocal of the estimated survival time ($\hat{\lambda} = 1/\bar{t}$) when the hazard rate is constant.

Median Survival Time

When a hazard rate is constant, the survival function is estimated[35-37] by

$$\hat{S}(t) = e^{-\hat{\lambda}t}.$$

The median survival time is directly estimated from $\hat{S}(t)$ since t_{median} is the survival time such that $\hat{S}(t_{median}) = 0.5$. Then

$$\hat{S}(t_{median}) = 0.5 = e^{-\hat{\lambda}t_{median}}$$

and

$$t_{median} = -\frac{1}{\hat{\lambda}} \log(0.5) = \bar{t}\log(2).$$

Also, an estimate of the median can be interpolated from the survival probabilities generated by the Kaplan-Meier process free of any assumptions about the hazard function.

17. TWO PROPERTIES OF THE MULTIVARIABLE LOGISTIC MODEL

Property 1

For a sample of n binary outcomes each associated with k measurements (denoted x_{ij}—the jth measurement of the ith observation), the log-odds for the ith observation can be represented by a linear function or

$$\text{log-odds}_i = b_0 + \Sigma b_j x_{ij}.$$

More specifically, if p_i denotes the probability of the ith binary event occurring, then

$$\log\left[\frac{p_i}{1 - p_i}\right] = b_0 + \Sigma b_j x_{ij} \qquad i = 1, 2, 3, \ldots, n \quad j = 1, 2, 3, \ldots, k$$

giving

$$\frac{p_i}{1 - p_i} = e^{b_0 + \Sigma b_j x_{ij}}$$

$$p_i = (1 - p_i)e^{b_0 + \Sigma b_j x_{ij}}$$

and

$$p_i = \frac{e^{b_0 + \Sigma b_j x_{ij}}}{e^{b_0 + \Sigma b_j x_{ij}} + 1} = \frac{1}{1 + e^{-(b_0 + \Sigma b_j x_{ij})}} = \frac{1}{1 + e^{-(\text{log-odds}_i)}}.$$

In words, if the log-odds is a linear function of the x-values, then the probabilities p_i have a linear logistic form; conversely, a linear logistic representation of p_i makes the log-odds a linear function of a series of x-values.

Property 2

If $x_{u1}, x_{u2}, x_{u3}, \ldots, x_{uk}$ and $x_{v1}, x_{v2}, x_{v3}, \ldots, x_{vk}$ are two independent observations (denoted u and v) made up of k measurements, then the additive logistic model yields an odds ratio of

$$or_{uv} = \frac{p_u/(1 - p_u)}{p_v/(1 - p_v)} = \frac{e^{b_0 + \Sigma b_j x_{uj}}}{e^{b_0 + \Sigma b_j x_{vj}}} = e^{\Sigma b_j(x_{uj} - x_{vj})}.$$

Therefore, the additive logistic model–derived odds ratio (a.11) reflecting the differences in risk between observations u and v factors into k pieces. Each piece is associated with an independent variable, where

$$or_{uv} = e^{b_1(x_{u1} - x_{v1})} \times e^{b_2(x_{u2} - x_{v2})} \times e^{b_3(x_{u3} - x_{v3})} \times \cdots \times e^{b_k(x_{uk} - x_{vk})}$$

or

$$or_{uv} = or_1^{(x_{u1} - x_{v1})} \times or_2^{(x_{u2} - x_{v2})} \times or_3^{(x_{u3} - x_{v3})} \times \cdots \times or_k^{(x_{uk} - x_{vk})}$$

and $e^{b_i} = or_i$ is called the *adjusted odds ratio* measuring the risk associated with the ith independent variable accounting for the other $k - 1$ variables in the model. For an additive logistic model, adjusted odds ratios multiply to equal the overall risk.

Corollary

If $x_{ul} = x_{vl} + 1$ $(x_{ul} - x_{vl} = 1)$ for variable l and for the other $k - 1$ variables $x_{uj} = x_{vj}$ $(x_{uj} - x_{vj} = 0)$, then the adjusted odds ratio is

$$or_{uv} = e^{b_l} = or_l \quad \text{or} \quad \log(or_{uv}) = b_l = \log(or_l).$$

For this special case, or_{uv} is the adjusted odds ratio associated with a one unit increase in the risk variable x_l when the other $k - 1$ variables are held constant. More generally, for an m-unit difference in the risk variable x_l when the other $k - 1$ variables are held constant, the change in risk measured by the adjusted odds ratio is $or_{uv} = (e^{b_l})^m$ or $(or_l)^m$. This property provides a compact interpretation of the k logistic model regression coefficients b_j and adjusted odds ratios or_j from an additive model.

Index

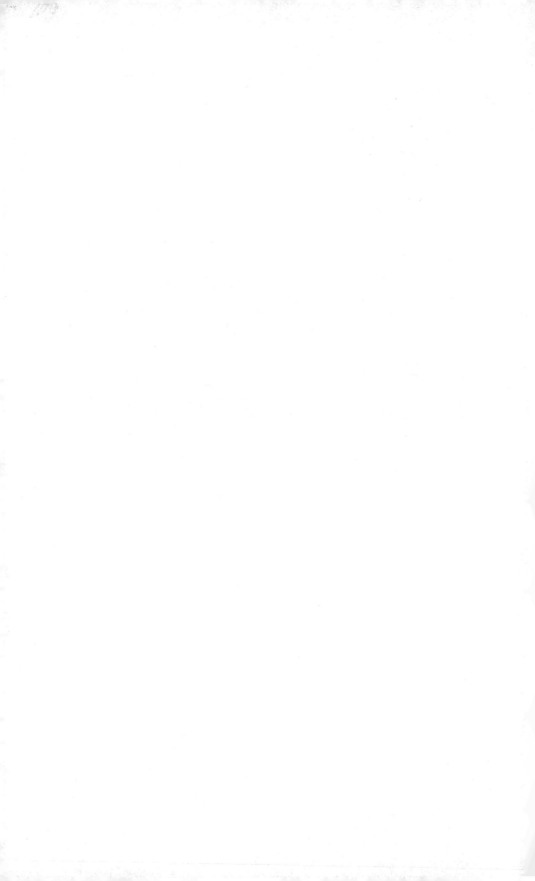